# Advances in Sports Medicine and Fitness
## Volume 3

# Advances in Sports Medicine and Fitness

## Volume 1

## Volume 2

# Advances in Sports Medicine and Fitness

## Editor-in-Chief

### William A. Grana, M.D.

Clinical Professor of Orthopedic Surgery and Rehabilitation
University of Oklahoma College of Medicine
Director, Oklahoma Center for Athletes
Oklahoma City, Oklahoma

## Associate Editors

### John A. Lombardo, M.D.

Associate Clinical Professor of Family Practice
Case Western Reserve University School of Medicine
Medical Director, Section of Sports Medicine
Cleveland Clinic Foundation
Cleveland, Ohio

### Brian J. Sharkey, Ph.D.

Dean, College of Human Performance and Leisure Studies
University of Northern Colorado
Greeley, Colorado

### Jennifer A. Stone, M.S., A.T.C.

Head Athletic Trainer
Colorado Springs Olympic Training Center
United States Olympic Committee
Colorado Springs, Colorado

## Volume 3 · 1990

Year Book Medical Publishers, Inc.
Chicago · London · Boca Raton · Littleton, Mass.

International Standard Serial Number: 0889-3977
International Standard Book Number: 0-8151-3580-7

*Sponsoring Editor:* Christopher W. Freiler
*Associate Managing Editor:* Denise M. Dungey
*Assistant Director, Manuscript Services:* Frances M. Perveiler
*Production Coordinator:* Max Perez
*Proofroom Supervisor:* Barbara M. Kelly

# Contributors

**Keith Blase**

Assistant Executive Director, Amateur Hockey Association of the United States, Colorado Springs, Colorado

**Kenneth E. DeHaven, M.D.**

University of Rochester School of Medicine and Dentistry, Department of Orthopaedics, Section of Athletic Medicine, Rochester, New York

**Jesse C. DeLee, M.D.**

Associate Clinical Professor, Department of Orthopaedics, University of Texas Health Science Center at San Antonio, San Antonio, Texas

**E. Randy Eichner, M.D.**

Professor of Medicine, University of Oklahoma Health Sciences Center, Oklahoma City, Oklahoma

**Kathleen A. Ellickson, Ph.D.**

Department of Psychiatry, Ohio State University College of Medicine, University Hospitals Clinic, Columbus, Ohio

**Patty S. Freedson, Ph.D.**

Associate Professor, University of Massachusetts, Department of Exercise Science, Amherst, Massachusetts

**Jack Harvey, M.D.**

Director of Sports Medicine, Orthopaedic Center of the Rockies, Fort Collins, Colorado

**Teresa A. Hazucha, M.A., A.T.C.**

Director, St. Ann's HEALTHletics, St. Ann's Hospital, Westerville, Ohio

**William A. Herndon, M.D.**

Associate Professor, Department of Orthopedic Surgery, University of Oklahoma College of Medicine, Oklahoma City, Oklahoma

**Donna L. Hull, M.S., A.T.C.**

Head Athletic Trainer, Dublin City Schools, Dublin, Ohio

**Ben R. Londeree, Ed.D.**

Associate Professor of Physical Education, Director, Human Performance Lab, University of Missouri—Columbia, Columbia, Missouri

**Julie Ann Moyer, Ed.D.**
Adjunct Professor, University of Delaware, Newark, Delaware; Adjunct Professor and Athletic Trainer, Delaware Technical and Community College, Wilmington, Delaware; Clinical Assistant Professor, Thomas Jefferson University, Philadelphia, Pennsylvania; Director, Pike Creek Sports Medicine, Physical Therapy, Wilmington, Delaware

**Daniel O'Neill, M.D.**
Director, Plymouth Sports and Orthopaedic Clinic, Plymouth, New Hampshire

**Russell R. Pate, Ph.D.**
Department of Exercise Science, School of Public Health, University of South Carolina, Columbia, South Carolina

**John C. Pearce, M.D.**
Venable-Stuck Fellow in Lower Extremity Reconstruction, Department of Orthopaedics, University of Texas Health Science Center at San Antonio, San Antonio, Texas

**James M. Rippe, M.D.**
Associate Professor, Director, Exercise Physiology and Nutrition Laboratory, University of Massachusetts Medical Center, Division of Cardiovascular Medicine, Worcester, Massachusetts

**Kenneth M. Singer, M.D.**
Clinical Instructor in Orthopaedic Surgery, University of Oregon Health Sciences Center, Eugene, Oregon

**Keith Stanley, M.D.**
Eastern Oklahoma Orthopaedic and Sports Medicine Center, Tulsa, Oklahoma

**Richard Sterba, M.D.**
Pediatric Cardiologist, The Cleveland Clinic Foundation, Cleveland, Ohio

**Ann Ward, Ph.D.**
Assistant Professor, Co-director, Exercise Physiology and Nutrition Laboratory, University of Massachusetts Medical Center, Division of Cardiovascular Medicine, Worcester, Massachusetts

**Dianne S. Ward, Ed.D.**
Department of Exercise Science, School of Public Health, University of South Carolina, Columbia, South Carolina

**Daniel C. Wascher, M.D.**
University of Rochester School of Medicine and Dentistry, Department of Orthopaedics, Section of Athletic Medicine, Rochester, New York

# Preface

While there has been an explosion in the participation of young people in organized, competitive sports, there also has been a significant decline in the overall fitness of the school-age and adolescent child. There are far-reaching implications for this decreased fitness in the adult. More and more concerns are expressed about the results of early competition and the potential detrimental effects of this on our young athletes. At the same time, competitive sports often exclude young children from the opportunity to take part in activities that promote fitness and health because of inadequate skills. Volume 3 of *Advances in Sports Medicine and Fitness* addresses many of the concerns and problems related to participation of the young person in sports.

In the section on Sports Science, concerns about the effects of endurance and weight training on the young athlete are addressed, as well as testing methods that are available to predict performance outcomes in the young person. These three chapters, along with the chapters on acute and chronic injury in the young athlete and the psychological effects of competition, form the essence of most parents' concern about their child's participation in sports. This information should prove useful to anyone who sees a young athletic population and desires information for counselling.

It is in the young athlete that preparticipation evaluation is first accomplished. Therefore, the chapter on this topic is particularly timely. A major part of that preparticipation evaluation is directed towards the cardiovascular system, and the chapter on this area provides an update on this clinical assessment.

In the Sports Traumatology section, the chapters on meniscal repair and ligamentous injury in the young athlete provide a slightly different perspective and insight than we see in the adult, but emphasize the importance of meniscal preservation and ligamentous function in this age group. Much of the interest in sports medicine, especially the physical well-being of the young, began with a concern about the occurrence of elbow pain in the Little League baseball pitcher. Therefore, I asked Dr. Ken Singer, an author of one of the classic studies on elbow problems in the Little League pitcher, to update that information to provide a fresh perspective.

Finally, in the section on Rehabilitation, we look at special concerns about rehabilitation in the young athlete along with providing an overview of the organization of youth sports and the health care that is provided to the young athlete. These topics are crucial for anyone in providing adequate care to a young population. This volume closes with a discussion of how the various disciplines and expertise work together to become an elite athletic team.

In this third year of the *Advances,* we are sorry to bid farewell to our sponsoring editor, Jim Shanahan, but happy to welcome our new editor,

Chris Freiler. The organizational job that Jim has done and which Chris now takes over facilitates the composition, editing, and publication of each volume. It certainly makes the job of the editors significantly easier. Again, I would like to thank the other members of the editorial board for their diligence in selecting experts in each area and for their continued individual interest and participation in this series.

*William A. Grana, M.D.*
*Editor-in-Chief*

# Contents

# An Overview of the Pediatric Athlete

## Jack Harvey, M.D.

Director of Sports Medicine, Orthopaedic Center of the Rockies,
Fort Collins, Colorado

As has been stated often, children are not merely small adults and their bodies do not respond to training stimuli in the same manner as do adult bodies. Research is just beginning to accrue regarding the trainability of enzymes, muscles, nerves, and organ systems of children. From a molecular level, the cell anatomy and enzyme systems for aerobic trainability are in place. To what degree and how best to train them is the question. Recent research has shown that prepubescent males and females can improve their aerobic capacity by endurance training, and that this capacity increases with age. In adolescent athletes, aerobic power correlates with lean body mass and maturity. In males, maximal $O_2$ power increases with age to 18 years, while in females maximal $O_2$ power does not increase much beyond the age of 14 years.[1, 2]

Practical experience and research indicate that anaerobic potential can be developed in the adolescent athlete. However, recent data also indicate that prepubescent children have limited potential for development of the anaerobic system.[3] Therefore, the advisability of using this type of training in the prepubescent athlete and in the younger, more inexperienced, adolescent athlete is questionable. In general, the longer-duration, higher-frequency, and higher-intensity training programs should be utilized for the more advanced teenage athlete. Intense training programs run the risk of physical and psychological injury to the younger, less experienced athlete.

Strength training is often of interest to many youth sport coaches, parents, and athletes. It certainly has its place for the more experienced adolescent athlete, but again it must be questioned in the prepubescent athlete. It is well known that the presence of testosterone greatly enhances the effect of a strength program. The two groups of young athletes that lack this hormone are prepubescent males and all females. This does not mean that these groups of athletes cannot develop strength with a properly designed exercise program that enhances recruitment patterns of muscles. However, hypertrophy of muscle mass will not occur, as this aspect of weight training does require the presence of testosterone.

In younger athletes, strength training should be a very minor part of the overall training regimen. It should probably be pursued only in the few prepubescent children who enthusiastically want to participate in a weight program. Fun, proper technique, and perhaps some strength gains should be the focus of the closely supervised program for younger athletes.[4] Calisthenics, light free-weights, or machines that can accommodate pediatric-size anatomy should be the tools which are used. A higher number of repetitions (15 to 25), a low number of sets (1 to 2), and proper technique should be emphasized. However, the adolescent athlete will perform better and perhaps be less injury-prone if a good pre-season strength program is combined with an in-season strength maintenance program. Recent trends indicate that this is important to the female athlete as well. This properly designed program will require increased frequency and number of sets (3 to 5) but fewer repetitions (6 to 10). Again, proper supervision with free-weights and/or machines, and emphasis on good technique and intensity will give the best results.[5]

As has been mentioned previously, hypertrophy of muscle mass requires the presence of testosterone. Augmentation of this process by the use of anabolic steroids is condemned. These substances are not only unethical and illegal in competition and training, but they present several hazards to the performance and health of the athlete. Although steroids do produce profound strength increases, they do not necessarily enhance in any manner the endurance performance of the athlete. Psychological changes induced by steroids, including aggressiveness and impatience, jeopardize athlete-coach and athlete-athlete relationships. The positive aspects of teamwork are often destroyed by these drugs. Health consequences are many, with shortness of stature being one result that is unique to the growing athlete. Female athletes develop permanent masculine changes of voice, hirsutism, and other secondary male sexual characteristics. The alteration of several body enzyme systems and reproductive function present health concerns for the future. Of particular concern is an increase in atherosclerotic deposits in the coronary arteries. This may well accelerate the

## TABLE 1.
## Bill of Rights For Young Athletes

Right to participate in sports.
Right to participate at a level commensurate with each child's maturity and ability.
Right to have a qualified adult leadership.
Right to play as a child and not as an adult.
Right to share in the leadership and decision-making of their sport participation.
Right to participate in safe and healthy environments.
Right to proper preparation for participation in sports.
Right to an equal opportunity to strive for success.
Right to be treated with dignity.
Right to have fun in sports.

development of coronary artery disease in steroid abusers.[6] In no way do the benefits justify the risks of steroid use.

More important than a strength program for the younger or inexperienced athlete is learning the basic skills of the sport and perfecting these skills. The athlete's performance and enjoyment of the sport will be influenced more profoundly by learning these skills than by participating in a strict conditioning program. Only after mastery of the skills has been acquired should strength training or other aspects of conditioning be emphasized.

The psychological status of the young athlete needs to be monitored carefully. Young athletes need to have reached a maturational level that coincides with the demands of the sport in which they participate. Readiness to compete in a sport also requires parental tolerance and a willing coach to prepare the child for the sport.[7] Young athletes can grasp the idea of competition at around 6 to 8 years of age. However, undue emphasis on competition and winning likely will result in early burnout. Therefore, rigorous training and competition need to be delayed for later years. As long as the competitive concept is used constructively in goal setting, motivation, and striving to do one's best, the psychological effect of sports participation will be positive. Coaches, parents, and team physicians need to understand and fulfill the psychological needs of the young athlete. The athletes' Bill of Rights needs to be practiced by those who care for the pediatric athlete (Table 1). The positive attributes of fun, worthiness, teamwork, goal setting, and accomplishment should not be overshadowed by anxiety, fear of failure, and undue emphasis on the outcome of the competition.

# References

1. Rowland TW: Aerobic response to endurance training in prepubescent children: A critical analysis. Med Sci Sports Exerc 1985; 17:493–497.
2. Bar-Or O: Metabolic response to acute exercise, in Bar-Or O (ed): Pediatric Sports Medicine. New York, Springer-Verlag, 1983, pp. 1–18.
3. Inbar O, Bar-Or O: Anaerobic characteristics in male children and adolescents. Med Sci Sports Exerc 1986; 18:264–269.
4. Micheli L: Physiological and orthopedic considerations for strengthening the prepubescent athlete. Natl Strength Conditioning Assoc J 1986; 8:38–40.
5. Tottem L: Practical considerations in strengthening the prepubescent athlete. Natl Strength Conditioning Assoc J 1986; 8:38–40.
6. Cohen HC, Faber WM, Spinnler Benade AJ, et al: Altered serum lipoprotein profiles in male and female power lifters ingesting anabolic steroids. The Physician and Sportsmedicine, 1986; 14:131–136.
7. Malina R: Readiness for youth sport, in Weiss M, Gould D (eds): Sport for Children and Youth. Champaign, Ill, Human Kinetics Press, 1986, pp

**Part I**

# *Sports Science*

Edited by
BRIAN J. SHARKEY, Ph.D.

# Prediction of Athletic Potential: Implications for Children

## Ben R. Londeree, Ed.D.

Associate Professor of Physical Education, Director, Human Performance Lab, University of Missouri-Columbia, Columbia, Missouri

**Editor's Introduction**

There is a general belief in the world of sport that children can be carefully selected for participation and success in a specific sport, and that the selection process is more effective than chance in identifying athletic potential. In this chapter on the prediction of athletic potential, Dr. Londeree addresses two main questions: Can we predict performance in adults? And, if so, is it possible to predict the future performance potential of young athletes? The answers to these questions may surprise many readers.

*Brian J. Sharkey, Ph.D.*

Can exercise scientists predict athletic performance from laboratory tests? If so, how accurate are the predictions? The answer to the former question probably is a qualified yes, with the degree of success dependent upon the activity. Can laboratory measurements accurately predict potential athletic performance? That is, if developed through appropriate training, can performance be predicted several years into the future? This question is more difficult, but elite athletic profiles suggest that some predictions might be possible. However, it is more difficult to predict the athletic potential of children 5 to 15 years into the future, because of individual differences in maturation. As a result of these differences, some children with promising profiles will continue to develop while others will not; conversely, some children who do not score very well on tests when they are young may mature later.

The relative importance of heredity and environment is central to the problem of predicting athletic potential in children. As a result, the heritability of basal performance characteristics has received considerable research attention in the past 18 years. During the last 6 years, the interaction of heredity and environment, or the inheritance of trainability, has been an especially important focus of research. However, if exercise scientists are able to predict the athletic potential of children from laboratory

**7**

and/or field tests, the question arises whether they should. The potential negative side effects of steering children into a strenuous and narrow training regimen at an early age need to be examined.

The purpose of this chapter is to review the research relating to the prediction of athletic potential with the goal of answering the questions posed above. In some cases, answers can be provided; in others, more questions will be raised than answered. Overall, this review should provide researchers with many important problems to study in the next few years.

## Predicting Current Athletic Performance

This review of sports profiling and prediction will be limited to individual activities and to those activities in which all participants perform the same tasks (e.g., rowing). In addition, it will be limited to those activities which are vigorous and about which enough research data were available to permit conclusions. The order of the review is as follows: (1) running (long-distance, middle-distance, and sprinting); (2) cycling (road cycling); (3) water activities (swimming and rowing); (4) winter activities (cross-country skiing, alpine skiing, and speed skating); (5) strength/skill activities (wrestling, gymnastics, and judo); and (6) weight-lifting activities (body building, weight lifting, and power lifting).

## Long Distance Running

The most thoroughly studied elite athlete (based on published research) has been the long-distance runner. Elite male runners were studied at the Aerobics Center (Dallas, Tex.) in 1977[1] and in Japan in 1989,[2] and an entire issue of *The International Journal of Sports Medicine* was devoted to studies of elite women distance runners in 1987.[3] Many other studies were found also.

Success in long-distance running is dependent upon the ability to run at a fast pace while accumulating very little lactic acid. The best predictor of long-distance running performance is the speed of running at some measure of aerobic-anaerobic threshold (i.e., lactate threshold, ventilatory threshold, onset of plasma lactate accumulation, onset of blood lactate accumulation, or maximal steady state) with correlations of .76 to .99 reported for events ranging from 2 miles to the marathon.[4-12] Factors which contribute to this ability include a relatively high maximal oxygen consumption, a low percentage of body fat, a low body weight per unit of height, an economical running style, and a highly oxidative musculature. Marathoners whose times are less than 2 hours and 15 minutes have had maximal oxygen consumption values ranging from 62 to 83 $ml \cdot kg^{-1} \cdot min^{-1}$ (most values were in the 70s).[1, 2] The importance of a high maximal oxygen consumption becomes apparent when considering the oxygen consumption for running at a 5 minute per mile pace (55 to 68 $ml \cdot kg^{-1} \cdot min^{-1}$ in elite marathoners).[13] These elite marathoners work near their maximal oxygen consumption throughout the race. Since excess body weight reduces maximal oxygen consumption when expressed relative to weight, it is not surprising to find that elite marathoners have body fat values below 10% and body mass index (BMI=$W \cdot H^{-2}$) values averaging 19.66,[1, 2] the lowest of all athletic groups. Marathoners who finished in less than 2 hours and 15 minutes averaged less oxygen consumption at a 5 minute per mile pace than did those who finished 1 to 5 minutes later.[1] One factor contributing to the ability to work close to maximal oxygen consumption with little lactate accumulation is the oxidative capacity of muscle fibers. In a study performed in Dallas, Texas, all of the long-distance runners had 80% or more slow-twitch (ST) muscle fibers except Don Kardong, who had a very high succinate dehydrogenase activity level.[14]

Other factors which appear to contribute to successful long-distance running include knee flexion and extension strength,[2] age and/or years of training,[15] and a personality profile that is high on mood states.[16, 17] Elite, male marathoners averaged 175.6 cm and 60.6 kg for height and weight, respectively.[1, 2] Carter[18] reported somatotypes of athletes involved in three Olympic Games with the averages for male marathoners being 1.4 for endomorphy, 4.4 for mesomorphy, and 3.4 for ectomorphy. Other long-distance runners had average somatotype values of 1.4, 4.2, and 3.7, respectively. Mean aerobic threshold values as high as 88% of maximal oxygen consumption[19] and mean anaerobic threshold values as high as 90% of maximal oxygen consumption[12] have been reported. Crielaard and Pirnay[20] reported that anaerobic power in runners is inversely related to maximal oxygen consumption, with marathoners showing the lowest values (8.93 $W \cdot kg^{-1}$), which were less than those of normal students (10.1 $W \cdot kg^{-1}$).

Elite, female long-distance runners had a mean height of 161.3 cm and a mean weight of 47.0 kg. The calculated BMI was 18.06; mean body fat was 14.3%; mean maximal oxygen consumption was 66.4 $ml \cdot kg^{-1} \cdot min^{-1}$; and mean slow-twitch muscle fibers was 82%.[3]

In summary, long-distance runners are of average height and very low body weight and percent fat, and have a somatotype classified as ectomesomorphy. They have a high maximal oxygen consumption and a very high aerobic-anaerobic threshold, factors which are useful in predicting performance. Long-distance runners have a very high proportion of slow-twitch muscle fibers with very high oxidative enzyme levels.

## Middle Distance Running

Elite middle-distance runners have been studied nearly as often as long-distance runners.[3, 13, 21] Elite, male middle-distance runners had higher values for maximal oxygen consumption than did elite, male long-distance runners (78.7 vs. 74.1 $ml \cdot kg^{-1} \cdot min^{-1}$), slightly higher oxygen consumption when running at 12 mph (66.7 vs. 63.8 $ml \cdot kg^{-1} \cdot min^{-1}$), higher lactic acid values when running at 12 mph (when other factors were statistically controlled,[13] a lower percentage of slow-twitch muscle fibers (<80% ST vs. ≥80% ST), and enlargement of slow-twitch (ST) and fast-twitch (FT) muscle fibers (vs. only ST fibers in long-distance runners).[14] Otherwise, elite, male middle- and long-distance runners were similar. Elite, female middle- and long-distance runners have not demonstrated the differences reported in their male counterparts[3] except that the percentage of slow-twitch muscle fibers was lower in female middle-distance runners than in long-distance runners (71%).[22]

Since oxygen consumption is tied significantly to running speed, maximal oxygen consumption would be expected to be an important predictor of endurance running performance. However, Baumgartner and Jackson[23] prepared a table from the results of a literature review of maximal oxygen consumption vs. running time for distances ranging from .75 mile to 3 miles. The correlations ranged from −.22 to −.91. In elite athletes, the correlations have ranged from .25 to −.54 (reported or calculated from their data).[1, 21, 24] These data indicate that an elite performance in a middle-distance event requires a large maximal oxygen consumption. However, in homogeneous groups, other variables such as running economy[25] become important. Noakes[26] reported that running speed at maximal oxygen consumption (horizontal treadmill test) and running velocity at the lactate turnpoint were correlated with running performance with values of −.90 and −.88, respectively. No studies were found which correlated a lactate threshold variable with middle-distance performance. However, LaFontaine et al.[7] reported correlations of .99 at 2 miles and .84 at .25 mile, while Farrel et al[4] found a correlation of .91 at 2 miles. Crielaard and Pirnay[20] found that elite middle-distance runners had fairly normal anaerobic powers, while marathoners had below normal values. Perhaps the best approach to predicting middle-distance running performance would involve multiple regression, utilizing some combination of maximal oxygen consumption, anaerobic power, running economy, and velocity at lactate threshold.

In summary, middle-distance runners are similar to long-distance runners, except for a slightly higher maximal oxygen consumption; a slightly lower aerobic-anaerobic threshold; slightly less running economy; and a higher, more normal anaerobic power.

## Sprint Running

Surprisingly, not much published research exists regarding elite sprinters. Their most obvious characteristic is the ability to run fast, and this is very easy to determine in a field setting. Their laboratory-determined characteristics include a somatotype of 1.7, 5.2, and 2.8; a height of 174.5 to 179.0 cm; a weight of 68.4 to 72.8 kg; a BMI of 22.46 to 23.31; a low percentage of fat (<9%); a slightly above-average maximal oxygen consumption (52 to 60+ ml·kg$^{-1}$·min$^{-1}$); a high anaerobic power (14.2 W·kg$^{-1}$ on a modified Margaria Anaerobic Bicycle Test); and high isokinetic strength values for knee flexion, knee extension, and leg press.[18, 20, 27, 28] In addition, Gollnick et al[29] and Costill et al[30] reported high proportions of fast-twitch muscle fibers (73% to 79%) in elite sprint athletes. The mean heights Olympic female sprinters reported in these studies ranged from 164.5 to 166.3 cm and the mean weights ranged from 55.8 to 57.8 kg.[28] Calculated BMI values were 20.25 to 20.90. The somatotypes reported for the Mexico Olympics were 2.6, 3.8, and 3.0 compared to 0.9, 0.7, and 0.8 for the Montreal Olympics.[18]

## Road Cycling

Maximal oxygen consumption has been shown to differentiate elite road cyclists from those in lesser categories.[31–36] However, this variable has not been significantly different between the very best cyclists in some studies.[31, 34] On the other hand, one study developed a regression equation using maximal oxygen consumption for selecting the best cyclists (based on 16.1-km performance time) with a correlation of .945.[33] Another study used maximal oxygen consumption and excess carbon dioxide production (an anaerobic measure) to predict 84-km performance times accurately ($r=.96$).[35] However, Hagberg et al[34] reported that an anaerobic power test did not differentiate between team members and non-team members on an American national team.

Mean maximal oxygen consumption values for elite male road cyclists have been reported to be from 4.89 to 5.53 $L \cdot min^{-1}$ (67 to 76 $ml \cdot kg^{-1} \cdot min^{-1}$).[31–39] Lower values have been reported for females (3.27 $L \cdot min^{-1}$, 53.2 $ml \cdot kg^{-1} \cdot min^{-1}$).[40] Miller and Manfredi[41] reported that ventilation threshold was correlated with 15-km performance time ($r=.935$).

Generally, road cyclists have been reported to have percent fat values under 10%,[31, 33, 34, 42] although Malhotra et al[35] reported a mean of 12.27% fat for Indian cyclists. The mean heights of elite road cyclists in these studies have been reported to be between 175.8 and 181.3 cm, while mean weights have ranged between 69.5 and 72.0 kg.[31–36, 43] These size values calculate out to BMI values between 21.90 and 22.49, which suggest that road cyclists have more muscular development than do long-distance runners. The percentage of slow-twitch fibers in elite road cyclists has been reported to range from 31% to 73%, with mean values of 56.8% and 61.4%.[29, 32] Elite road cyclists have elevated muscle oxidative enzymes.[29, 32, 36] Ventilatory and lactate threshold values have been reported to be 71.1% of maximal oxygen consumption.[41, 44] Hagberg et al[34] reported that elite cyclists were able to work at a power output above 3,780 kpm·min− for an average of 52.8 seconds. Malhotra et al[35] reported mean oxygen debt values of 8.72 L.

In summary, it appears that success in road cycling requires a high maximal oxygen consumption (although perhaps not as high as long-distance running), probably a high anaerobic power and/or capacity, a low percentage of body fat, and highly oxidative muscle tissue. It appears that aerobic threshold is an excellent predictor of performance time.

## Swimming

Swimming rivals running when it comes to research interest. There have been several national and international symposia which have resulted in books about research on swimming. In contrast to running, swimming competitions typically do not include pure sprints (50 meters of swimming might be equivalent to 250 meters of running in terms of time) or very long distances (1,500 meters of swimming might be equivalent to 7 to 8 km of running). Another important difference between swimming and running is the higher density of water vs. air which makes drag, or resistance to motion, much higher in water.

Maximal oxygen consumption has been shown to be a poor to moderate predictor of 100-yard or 100-meter swim times.[45, 46] However, maximal oxygen consumption is a good estimator of 400-yard or 400-meter swim times ($r=.80$ to .90) and of 1,500 meter swim times ($r=.91$).[45, 47] Even at 400 yards, though, maximal oxygen consumption is a poor to moderate predictor of performance in non-elite swimmers.[46, 47]

Several factors mitigate against high correlations between maximal oxygen consumption and performance times. For shorter events, anaerobic factors contribute significantly to performance.[46, 48] For all swimming events, drag plays an important part. All swimming events also are affected by the swimmer's technique, which involves reducing drag and optimizing the application of forces.[48] Holmer[48] calculated that there is a threefold difference in the energy cost of swimming between elite and poor swimmers.

Researchers have proposed a variety of other methods for predicting swim performance. Via multiple correlation, Costill et al.[47] found that maximal oxygen consumption plus distance per stroke correlated at 0.97 with 400-yard swim times in competitive swimmers. Craig et al[49] developed elaborate charts for each swimmer, relating velocity to stroke rate and stroke distance. Treffene[50] developed an extrapolation method for determining the lowest speed (Vcr) that elicits maximal heart rate. Percent of Vcr for each competitive distance was graphed as follows: 100 m=112%, 200 m=106%, 400 m=102%, 800 m=99%, and 1,500 m=98%, with correlations between actual and predicted performance times of 0.98 to 0.99. Klissouras and Sinning[51] proposed a complicated process of developing pairs of regression lines utilizing the percentage of maximal oxygen consumption that could be used for various time periods, the maximal oxygen consumption, the amount of oxygen available from oxygen consumption plus oxygen debt and time. The predicted time for a particular distance was determined by noting the point at which the pairs of regression lines crossed. Elliot and Haber[52] proposed determining lactic acid concentration of blood at two or three submaximal speeds, graphing the results using a semilog plot of lactate change from rest versus time, and extrapolating to maximal lactate to determine maximal speed for that distance. The correlation between actual and predicted speed for the 100-meter breast stroke was 0.86. Troup[53] described a series of submaximal and maximal tests to determine oxygen consumption and lactic acid profiles for a swimmer; from these results, current performance could be predicted and suggestions for appropriate training to enhance performance could be provided.

Male elite swimmers have been reported to have mean maximal oxygen consumptions of 4.68 to 6.26 L·min$^{-1}$ and 67.0 to 79.9 ml·kg$^{-1}$· min$^{-1}$.[38, 54, 55] Female elite swimmers had average values of 3.10 to 3.37 L·min$^{-1}$ and 52.1 to 57.0 ml·kg$^{-1}$·min$^{-1}$.[38, 54, 55]

The elite male swimmers in these studies averaged 178 to 191 cm in height with a tendency toward increasing height in recent years.[29, 43, 54, 56, 57] Female heights averaged 166.9 to 172.8 cm.[43, 54, 56] Weights have averaged 70.8 to 78.3 kg for males,[29, 43, 54, 56, 57] and 57.8 to 64.7 kg for females.[43, 54, 56] Calculated BMI figures are 21.46 to 22.35 for males and 20.75 to 21.67 for females. The values for males suggest that male swimmers have greater muscular development than male middle- and long-distance runners. The percentage of fat values for males have averaged between 5% and 10%.[42, 57] The percentage of fat values for females have been reported to average from 14% to 19%.[42, 57]

The proportion of slow-twitch muscle fibers in the deltoid muscle of swimmers tended to be above normal.[29, 58] However, Gerard et al[56] found that male sprint swimmers had fairly normal fiber type proportions. Costill[59] found that sprint swimmers had elevated glycolytic and oxidative muscle enzymes, while endurance swimmers had only elevated oxidative enzymes. Sharp et al[60] found that sprint performance was increased following an isokinetic strength training program. The research of Miyashita and Kanehisa[61] and Manning et al[62] did not support these results. In fact, Miyashita and Kanehisa found that the increases in isokinetic muscular endurance were related to improved sprint times. Gerard et al[56] found that long-distance swimmers had lower isokinetic strength than other swimmers.

Elite swimmers have been reported to have very high anaerobic threshold values (85% of maximal speed for 100 meters,[63] or 90% of maximal oxygen consumption[64]). Smith et al[64] reported that endurance swimmers had a higher anaerobic threshold than sprint swimmers (90.4% vs. 65.9% of maximal oxygen consumption). Elite swimmers have been reported to have a high oxygen debt capacity[65] and high peak lactate values.[66]

In summary, elite swimmers have a high maximal oxygen consumption, a low percentage of body fat, a well-developed musculature (especially in the upper body), a high oxidative muscle metabolism, an above-average proportion of slow-twitch muscle, a high anaerobic threshold (endurance swimmers), a high oxygen debt capacity, a high tolerance for lactic acid, and an above-average height.

## Rowing

No studies were found that attempted to predict rowing performance with physiological and other variables. Perhaps the lack of such equations is due to the fact that rowing, for the most part, is a team sport. However, several studies were found which provided characteristics of elite rowers.

Elite rowers on average are quite tall (191 to 193 cm), and are built heavily (88 to 93 kg).[43, 67-69] BMI ratios calculated from these values are 24.14 to 24.97, which are among the highest found among elite endurance athletes. Percent fat values for heavyweights (those in the heavier of two weight classes) recently have been reported to be below 10%,[42, 69] while older data reported a figure of 11%.[67] Clarkson et al[70] reported oarswomen with a mean height of 173 cm, a mean weight of 70 kg, and a fat percentage of 12% to 14%, while Hagerman et al[67] reported values of 173 cm, 68 kg, and 14%, respectively. Calculated BMI ratios were 22.72 to 23.39. Maximal oxygen consumption values reported in the earlier literature were presented in table form by Secher, et al;[69] mean values were 3.40 to 6.10 L·min$^{-1}$ and 43 to 72 ml·kg$^{-1}$·min$^{-1}$. Higher values clustered in recent years. Female maximal oxygen consumption mean values have been reported to be about 4.10 L·min$^{-1}$ and 60.2 ml·kg$^{-1}$·min$^{-1}$.[67] Hagerman[71] stated that to be successful at the international level maximal oxygen consumption values must exceed 6.0 L·min$^{-1}$ for men and 4.0 L·min$^{-1}$ for women. Anaerobic threshold values for elite rowers have been reported to be 83% to 90% of maximal oxygen consumption[68, 72, 73] and 71% of peak power.[68] Oxygen consumption during simulated and actual rowing has been reported to be 98% to 99% of maximal oxygen consumption for almost the entire test period.[67] The same investigators reported maximal lactate values of 168 mg·100ml$^{-1}$, oxygen debts of 13.4 L, and oxygen deficits of 7.7 L. After reviewing the literature, Hagerman[71] concluded that rowing is 20% to 30% anaerobic. Maximum power has been reported to be 374 to 392.5 watts for men and 284 watts for women.[67, 68] Hagerman[71] reported data for three oarsmen over a period of 8 years. Average maximal oxygen consumption increased only slightly, while maximal power increased an average of 23%. The percentage of slow-twitch muscle fibers has been reported to be 70% or higher in men[74-76] and 55% to 68% in women.[70, 71]

In summary, elite oarsmen are very tall, heavily muscled, and have a low percentage of body fat. They have high maximal oxygen consumption values when expressed in liters per minute, high anaerobic thresholds, high anaerobic capacity and power, and a high proportion of slow-twitch muscle fibers.

## Cross-Country Skiing

No reports were found which predicted the performance of elite cross-country skiers from laboratory data. Two studies conducted multiple regression analyses with sub-elite skiers. Niinimaa et al[77] studied Canadian intercollegiate skiers and calculated a correlation value of .95 using racing experience, maximal oxygen consumption, and percentage of body fat to predict success. Ng et al[78] predicted 10-km times for recreational skiers based on upper body strength, maximal oxygen consumption, isokinetic knee extension strength, and weight with a correlation value of .78.

Bergh[74] found that successful, male, world-class skiers weighed more and had higher values for maximal oxygen consumption than less successful skiers; these differences were not found among females.

Elite cross-country skiers were reported to have mean heights ranging from 174 to 185 cm and mean weights ranging from 60.6 to 78.6 kg.[79-84] Calculated BMI ratios range from 20.02 to 22.97. Values for the percentage of body fat ranged between 4.0% and 10.2%.[80, 81, 83-85] Haymes and Dickinson[81] reported a mean height of 163.4 cm, a mean weight of 55.9 kg, and a mean percentage of body fat of 15.7% for U.S. female cross-country skiers. Their BMI ratio averaged 20.94. Sinning et al[85] reported mean somatotype scores of 1.95, 4.45, and 3.00 for males and 3.50, 4.30, and 2.30 for females.

Mean maximal oxygen consumption values for elite, male, cross-country skiers have been reported from 5.34 to 6.54 $L \cdot min^{-1}$ and from 67.3 to 83.8 $ml \cdot kg^{-1} \cdot min^{-1}$.[38, 79-84, 86] Values for females have ranged from 3.44 to 3.90 $L \cdot min^{-1}$ and from 61.5 to 68 $ml \cdot kg^{-1} \cdot min^{-1}$.[38, 81, 86] Haymes and Dickinson[81] found that elite cross-country skiers had higher maximal oxygen consumption values than alpine and nordic combined skiers (73.0, 66.6, and 67.5 $ml \cdot kg^{-1} \cdot min^{-1}$, respectively, for males) while elite female cross-country skiers had higher values than alpine skiers (61.5 and 52.7 $ml \cdot kg^{-1} \cdot min^{-1}$, respectively).

Haymes and Dickinson[81] also found that cross-country skiers had less leg strength than alpine and nordic combined skiers, and less leg power than alpine skiers. Similarly, the cross-country skiers had slower response times and were less agile than alpine skiers.

Bergh[87] stated that all elite cross-country skiers tested had at least 63% slow-twitch muscle fibers. He also reported that their oxidative enzyme levels were double normal values. Mackova et al[83] reported more modest enzyme levels than those claimed by Bergh. Sharkey[86] reported anaerobic threshold (OBLA-4mM lactate) values between 80% and 92% of maximal oxygen consumption for cross-country skiers on the U.S. team. Rusko[88] found similar values in young Finnish female skiers.

In summary, elite cross-country skiers have very high maximal oxygen consumption values, a high percentage of slow-twitch muscle fibers, a high level of muscle oxidative enzymes, and a high anaerobic threshold. A lower percentage of body fat and higher BMI ratios than long-distance runners suggests more muscle development in cross-country skiers.

## Alpine Skiing

No multiple regression studies involving elite alpine skiers were found. However, three studies reported correlations between laboratory tests and performance. Haymes and Dickinson[81] reported significant correlations between FIS (Federation de International de Ski) points and isokinetic muscular leg endurance in males (−.80) and females (−.78); and between percentage of body fat (.78), weight (.76), lean body weight (.64), and power (.64) in males. In males, giant slalom performance was related to leg endurance (−.75), power (.80), and vertical jump (.64). Downhill performance was correlated with the percentage of body fat in males (−.67) and females (−.74), and with maximal oxygen consumption in females (−.66). Song[89] reported moderate correlations between downhill performance and lower leg length, grip strength, maximal oxygen consumption, and anaerobic power. He also found that slalom performance was related to grip strength and strength of elbow flexion, hip flexion, and trunk flexion. Andersen et al.[90] reported good correlations (.80 to .86) between slalom performance and the following three field tests: hexagonal obstacle course (a jumping agility test), high box test (sideways jumping on and off a 40-cm box for 90 seconds), and the 5 double leg jump test. This group also found that skilled alpine skiers had higher values than club skiers on the following variables: peak anaerobic power, maximal blood lactate values, hexagonal obstacle course, and 20-meter shuttle run. Brown and Wilkinson[91] reported that Canadian national level alpine skiers had better values than club skiers on the 2-mile run, the number of situps they can do in 60 seconds, the vertical jump, the big box jump, the anaerobic treadmill test, the isokinetic knee extension, and isokinetic leg endurance. Differences between national and divisional level skiers were not significant.

Elite male alpine skiers have mean heights reported to be between 173.1 and 178.5 cm, mean weights between 65.5 and 77.6 kg, and mean percentages of body fat between 10% and 11%.[81, 84, 91, 92] The corresponding values for females were 165.1 cm, 58.8 kg, and 20.6%.[81] Calculated BMI ratios were 21.86 to 24.35 for males and 21.57 for females.

Maximal oxygen consumption mean values for elite males have been reported to be between 4.20 and 5.03 $L \cdot min^{-1}$ and between 63.1 and 68.0 $ml \cdot kg^{-1} \cdot min^{-1}$.[38, 81, 84, 91] Female values have been reported as 3.10 $L \cdot min^{-1}$ and 51 to 52.7 $ml \cdot kg^{-1} \cdot min^{-1}$.[38, 81]

The mean percentage of slow-twitch muscle fibers has ranged between 53% and 63%.[84, 92] Rusko et al[84] reported a relatively normal muscle oxidative enzyme activity level in alpine skiers.

In summary, elite alpine skiers have moderately high values for maximal oxygen consumption, normal height, a low percentage of body fat, more muscularity than long-distance runners, a relatively normal percentage of slow-twitch muscle fibers and oxidative capacity, high anaerobic power and capacity, and high leg strength and endurance. Alpine skiers scored well on field tests of agility and leg power/endurance.

## Speed Skating

Any prediction of speed skating performance is complicated by the fact that wind resistance is a major factor.[93, 94] Consequently, the ability to assume a low-profile position and still apply stroking power effectively are very important to success.[95, 96] In the latter study, the velocity of elite skaters was correlated highly with the following variables: the knee angle of the new supporting leg at the moment of weight transfer ($\theta_b$) (−.70), $\theta_b$ minus pre-extension knee angle (.80), and the angle of the push-off leg to the ice surface (.70). Geijsel et al[97] found that anaerobic capacity on a bicycle ergometer for 30 seconds was correlated highly with the skating power developed during 500 meters (.78) and 1,500 meters (.85); correlations between skating power and maximal oxygen consumption were lower (.62 and .63, respectively). Multiple correlations using the 30-second anaerobic power test and stroke frequencies during skating were .85 for the 500-meter power and .90 for the 1,500-meter power. Compared to trained skaters, Ingen Schenau et al[95] found that elite skaters had a shorter upper leg relative to total leg length, a higher aerobic power during cycling, a higher stroke frequency, a smaller pre-extension knee angle coupled with higher work per stroke, a higher efficiency during skating, and a higher external power during skating and cycling. Pollock et al[98] found that successful and unsuccessful Olympic speed skating candidates did not differ on body composition or aerobic power variables. The only exception was Eric Heiden, whose maximal oxygen consumption and body weight were considerably higher than the other Olympic candidates. Nemoto et al.[99] reported that elite skaters had a higher maximal oxygen consumption than did trained skaters. Nemoto also found that all rounders (longer lap events) had higher aerobic threshold values than sprinters. For marathon speed skating (35 to 40 km), Geijsel[100] found that the only variable which discriminated between winners and losers was endurance time on an anaerobic capacity test on a bicycle ergometer (5 $W \cdot kg^{-1}$); nonsignificant variables included training variables and submaximal and maximal physiological variables.

Elite speed skaters have mean heights reported to be between 174.4 and 183.1 cm and mean weights between 71.1 and 82.4 kg.[84, 93, 95, 98, 99, 101–105] Calculated BMI ratios are 23.38 to 24.58. Elite female speed skaters' mean reported heights range from 164.5 to 168.1 cm while mean weights range from 60.8 to 65.4 kg.[98, 101, 102] BMI ratios are 22.47 to 23.14. The mean percentage of body fat among elite speed skaters ranges from 6.8% to 10.6%.[98, 99, 105] Pollock et al[98] reported a mean percentage of body fat value of 16.5% for female Olympic speed skating candidates.

Reported maximal oxygen consumption mean values for elite speed skaters range between 3.47 and 5.80 $L \cdot min^{-1}$ (4.39 to 5.80 $L \cdot min^{-1}$, excluding Terry McDermott) and 41.4 to 79 $ml \cdot kg^{-1} \cdot min^{-1}$ (59.3 to 79.3 $ml \cdot kg^{-1} \cdot min^{-1}$, excluding Terry McDermott).[38, 93, 95, 97–103] Corresponding values for females are 2.71 to 3.40 $L \cdot min^{-1}$ and 46.1 to 52.2 $ml \cdot kg^{-1} \cdot min^{-1}$.[98, 101, 102]

Nemoto et al[99] reported aerobic and anaerobic threshold values for Japanese elite male sprinters and all rounders vs. trained skaters. Aerobic and anaerobic thresholds were not significantly higher in the elite vs. the trained skaters (60.1% vs. 61.7% and 71.0% vs. 75.0% of maximal oxygen consumption). However, all rounders had significantly higher anaerobic thresholds than sprinters (75.6% vs. 71.1%).

In summary, elite speed skaters are normal in height, but their weight-to-height ratio is higher than average, suggesting an above average musculature. Their percentage of body fat values are normal for athletes, while their maximal oxygen consumption values are moderate to high. Aerobic anaerobic threshold values are slightly above average and anaerobic capacity is very high. Important variables for success are related mostly to technique, although maximal oxygen uptake and anaerobic capacity also play a role.

## Wrestling

Three studies were found which compared small numbers of elite and sub-elite wrestlers.[106–108] Stine et al[108] found nonsignificant differences in favor of All-American wrestlers vs. moderately successful wrestlers on the following variables: height, weight, sum of six skinfolds, percentage of body fat, maximal oxygen consumption, submaximal heart rate response, grip strength, upper body strength, lower body strength, reaction time, situps in 30 seconds, and sit and reach. Nagle et al.[107] reported nonsignificant differences in favor of successful over nonsuccessful Olympic trials candidates for height, weight, grip strength, maximal lactate, and submaximal ratings of perceived exertion. The percentage of body fat was equal, and maximal heart rate was nonsignificantly lower. Successful candidates exhibited slightly higher maximal ventilation and oxygen consumption, but were significantly better on bench- press endurance and submaximal exercise heart rate. Psychological differences in favor of the successful candidates existed for tension, confusion, vigor, and fatigue. Gale and Flynn[106] found no significant differences between successful and nonsuccessful Olympic candidates for height, weight, fat-free weight, calculated percentage of body fat, and maximal oxygen consumption. No studies were found which compared skill levels between elite and sub-elite wrestlers. BMI ratios for the successful vs. the unsuccessful wrestlers in the above studies appeared to be slightly higher in the successful groups; this would suggest that they have slightly more muscle mass.

Mean heights for elite wrestlers in the studies reviewed ranged from 175.6 to 179.8 cm, and mean weights ranged from 71.9 to 81.8 kg.[106–109] Calculated BMI ratios were 23.32 to 25.30. Values for the percentage of body fat ranged from 3.7% to 9.8%,[106–110] except for a 13% fat value reported for the 1968 Olympics.[111]

Mean maximal oxygen consumption values for elite wrestlers have ranged from 53 to 64 ml·kg$^{-1}$·min$^{-1}$.[38, 106–111] DiPrampero et al[111] reported relatively high anaerobic power on a stair climb test (equivalent to 225 ml·kg$^{-1}$·min$^{-1}$ of oxygen consumption). Sharatt et al[110] reported that elite wrestlers ran for 55.6 seconds on a treadmill set at 8 mph and a 20% grade. Sharatt et al[110] also reported 48% slow-twitch muscle fibers, a slow-twitch area of 4,452 μm, a fast-twitch area of 7,211 μm, and normal levels of phosphofructokinase activity (34.5 μM·g$^{-1}$·min$^{-1}$ of wet weight). Although several studies reported measures of strength, the measurements generally were not comparable. Grip strength was reported by Nagle et al[107] (59.5 kg) and Stine et al[108] (61 kg). Stine et al[108] concluded that elite wrestlers have superior strength and muscle endurance. Sharatt et al[110] stated that strength and power are important contributors to wrestling success.

In summary, elite wrestlers have a well-developed musculature; a low percentage of body fat; slightly above-average maximal oxygen consumption; high strength, power, and muscular endurance; high anaerobic power; normal proportions of slow-twitch muscle fibers; and large fast-twitch muscle fibers. Psychologically, successful wrestlers may exhibit less tension, confusion, and fatigue, and more vigor.

## Gymnastics

Surprisingly little published research was found on gymnasts. No studies attempted to predict performance in elite gymnasts; perhaps this is due to the importance of skill in this activity. However, Nelson et al[112] developed a discriminant analysis equation for young (7, 10, and 13 years), female competitive gymnasts vs. recreational gymnasts and physical education students. The equation correctly classified 85.2% of the competitive gymnasts, 68.4% of the recreational gymnasts, and 85% of the physical education students. The competitors had a higher ponderal index, greater strength, and more hip flexibility, and they weighed less and were more slender.

Elite male gymnasts are reported to be short (164.3, 169.3, and 178.5 cm),[43, 113, 114] while female gymnasts are more normal in height (159.7 and 163.0 cm).[101, 115] The weights of the male athletes are low (61.4 to 69.2 kg),[43, 113, 114] while the weights of the female athletes varied (57.9 and 48.8 kg).[101, 115] Calculated BMI ratios ranged from 21.72 to 22.75 for males and from 18.37 to 22.70 for females. Fat content of both males and females was very low (6% and 11.2% fat, respectively).[42, 116]

LeVeau et al[113] compared elite male American and Japanese gymnasts on numerous anthropometric values. Primary differences were found in segmental lengths and upper body development. The Japanese had shorter body segments, although total height was not significantly different (169.6 vs. 164.3 cm). The chest circumference relative to total height was greater in the Japanese. Both groups had a large biacromial breadth relative to biiliac breadth, giving an inverted trapezoid or triangle shape. Both groups also had a high sitting height relative to total height. Conversely, femoral and humeral bicondrial breadth was less than that found in other athletes. LeVeau et al concluded that gymnasts are short, stout, have low weights, and are trapezoidal in form, with a heavy upper body and relatively short legs.

In contrast to these findings, Caldarone et al[117, 118] found that elite European junior gymnasts had a long arm span and a short trunk. These gymnasts also were short and lightweight (except the older males). The percentage of body fat was low (7.1% and 16.3% for males and females, respectively).

Only one study reported maximal oxygen consumption for male gymnasts and the mean value was 55.5 ml·kg$^{-1}$·min$^{-1}$.[114] Two studies reported very different maximal oxygen consumption values for females: 36.3 ml·kg$^{-1}$·min$^{-1}$ [115] and 49.8 ml·kg$^{-1}$·min$^{-1}$.[101]

In summary, gymnasts tend to be short, with lower than normal weights and very low percentages of body fat. They are very flexible and have excellent muscular development, particularly in the upper body. Their maximal oxygen consumption values are average.

## Judo

No studies were found which attempted to predict the performance of judoists. Taylor and Brassard[119] stated that success in international judo competition was not correlated to any laboratory measures or field tests (i.e., maximal oxygen consumption, anaerobic capacity, anthropomorphic values, strength, flexibility, or muscular endurance). However, Claessens et al[120] found numerous differences between elite judo athletes and a reference group. Some of the anthropomorphic differences were correlated with weight classes, although all weight classes except the top class had low skinfold fat values. Strength and sit-and-reach also were high in the heavier weight classes. Judoists performed considerably better than the reference group in measures of muscular endurance (leg lifts and flexed arm hang) and on a 50-meter shuttle run. Tests in which judoists scored similar to the reference group included limb speed, sit and reach (lower weight group), vertical jump, and strength (lower weight group).

The mean reported heights of male judo athletes ranged from 167.8 to 170.7 cm for the light classes, and from 177.8 to 178.9 cm for the heavier classes.[43, 119-122] BMI ratios ranged from 22.62 to 23.69 in the low weight classes, and from 25.60 to 28.29 in the heavy weight classes. The mean percentage of body fat ranged from 7.2% to 14.0%, with the latter figure coming from a heavy weight group.[42, 119, 122] One way to circumvent the effect of weight classes in analyzing the structure of these athletes is via somatotyping. The lower weight classes had the following values reported: 2.3 to 3.0 for endomorphy, 4.8 to 6.57 for mesomorphy, and 1.79 to 2.40 for ectomorphy. The somatotypes reported for the heavier weight classes were: 3.10 to 4.32 for endomorphy, 5.6 to 7.23 for mesomorphy, and 1.41 to 1.7 for ectomorphy. In other words, judoists are endomesomorphs.[120-123]

Only one study reported a maximal oxygen consumption value (57.7 ml·kg$^{-1}$·min$^{-1}$),[119] and anaerobic capacity appeared to be low in the same study. As stated previously, the judo athletes in the heavier weight classes tended to have greater strength, and all judoists had high muscular endurance scores.

In summary, judo athletes are robustly built with relatively large breadths and circumferences. They tend to have a low percentage of body fat, especially in the lower weight classes. Generally, judoists are average to high on motor performance tests.

## Body Builders and Weight Lifters

No studies were found correlating laboratory data or field test results with performance in body building or power lifting. However, two studies of elite Olympic weight lifters (one involving sub-elite weight lifters and one involving novice lifters) reported correlations between various test data and performance. Hakkinen et al[124] found significant correlations between the squat jump and counter movement jump vs. performance in the snatch and the clean and jerk (r=.73 to .79) in elite lifters. In another study involving elite lifters,[125] the same researchers found modest correlations between the snatch and the clean and jerk performance, and between the standing long jump and the standing triple jump (r=.41 to .55). In sub-elite lifters, Ward et al[126] found that, of all the anthropometric measures, only weight correlated significantly with snatch (r=.97) and clean and jerk (r=.95) performances. In other words, lifters in heavier weight classes lifted more. Ward et al also found that the master lifters were heavier and stouter than first-class lifters. Using novice lifters who had trained about 6 months, Stone et al[127] found that weight correlated with performance (r=.62 to .63), and that vertical jump power correlated with performance somewhat better (r=.74 to .77).

Elite lifters and body builders tended to be shorter than most athletes (164.6 to 179.3 cm with one group of heavy body builders at 183.2 cm). Mean weights ranged from 68.7 to 99 kg,[43, 109, 124, 125, 128–137] and calculated BMI ratios were 25.36 to 29.50. The mean percentage of body fat values ranged from 8.3% to 19.9%, although the body builders were leaner than the lifters.[42, 109, 124, 125, 129–131, 133–135] Mean heights and weights for females were reported to range from 160.8 to 162.3 cm and from 53.8 to 63.9 kg, respectively.[138–140] Calculated BMI ratios were 20.81 to 24.26, compared to 21.58 for a reference group.[140] Freedson et al[140] reported a percentage of body fat value of 13.2% in female body builders, compared to 23.6% in a reference group. In other words, the body builders and probably the lifters had less fat but more muscle than nonathletes, producing similar BMI ratios. Two other anthropometric measures commonly reported on the weight athletes are thigh and upper arm circumferences; these are 55.1 to 64.8 cm and 36.7 to 43.6 cm, respectively. Corresponding values for females are 53.0 to 57.9 cm and 28.9 to 30.9 cm, respectively. Male somatogram values are as follows: 1.42 to 3.9 for endomorphy, 6.8 to 9.0 for mesomorphy, and 0.8 to 1.5 for ectomorphy.[123, 128, 133]

Mean maximal oxygen consumption values for males ranged from 2.55 to 4.50 $L \cdot min^{-1}$ and from 35.3 to 56.0 $ml \cdot kg^{-1} \cdot min^{-1}$.[38, 109, 125, 129, 133–135, 137] Anaerobic power was reported as 6.4 to 6.6 $W \cdot kg^{-1}$.[129] The percentage of fast-twitch muscle fibers in elite body builders and weight lifters fell within a fairly narrow range (58.6% to 66%), while the proportion of fast-twitch area to slow-twitch area ranged from 1.29 to 1.68.[129, 132, 136] Comparisons of these fiber characteristics to those of normal individuals produced mixed results, although the differences that occurred favored the athletes. Bell et al[141] reported 58.0% fast-twitch muscle fibers in female body builders. They also found enlarged fibers, but not as much as in their male counterparts.

In summary, elite body builders, Olympic weight lifters, and power lifters tend to be short and heavily muscled. The body builders, in particular, had relatively low percentages of body fat. Maximal oxygen consumption values were low to modest, especially when expressed relative to weight.

## Effect of Inheritance on Variables Related to Elite Performances

Numerous characteristics which deviate from average have been identified in elite athletes. Heritability studies have shown that some of these traits have a high genetic component, while others do not. In addition, many studies in the last few years have shown that the trainability of some traits is significantly genetically influenced. Identification of potential elite athletes would depend on locating individuals who rate high on important variables that have a high genetic component. Then other important variables can be developed through appropriate training.

Several excellent reviews have been written about the heritability of numerous traits. For the sake of efficiency, only the conclusions of these reviews will be presented. Most of the studies conducted on heritability have examined only the main effect of genetics; summaries of these will be in tabular form (Table 1). The interaction of genetics and trainability will be covered later in this chapter.

Height and body lengths have high heritability (80% to 90%). Breadth and physique values are moderate (40% to 60%).

Although a wide range of maximal oxygen consumption heritability estimates have been reported, the actual value probably is 30%,[143] or less than 40% to 60%.[144] However, the trainability of maximal oxygen consumption varies considerably, and Bouchard[143] estimated that the genetic × trainability interaction heritability was about 40%. Combining the genetic and genetic × trainability estimates suggests that about 70% of the variance in maximal oxygen consumption after training is determined genetically.

The ability to work at submaximal intensities has a relatively low pure genetic component. In addition, the genetic × trainability heritability has been estimated to be 25% for aerobic capacity (the highest amount of work that can be done in 90 minutes).[143] Prud Homme et al[151] estimated that the genetic × trainability heritability was about 50% for the first ventilatory threshold and about 30% for the second ventilatory threshold.

Although some investigators have reported very high genetic components for anaerobic power,[145, 146] others have found more moderate values.[147] Bouchard et al[152] reported that training improved anaerobic power by 22% and anaerobic capacity by 35% with genetic × trainability heritability estimates of 31% and 69%, respectively. Combining the genetic and

## TABLE 1.
## Heritability Estimates of Selected Variables

| Variable | | % Genetic | Reference |
|---|---|---|---|
| **Physique Variables** | | | |
| Height | | 85±7 | Bouchard and Lortie, 1984[142] |
| Leg length | | 80±10 | Bouchard and Lortie, 1984[142] |
| Arm length | | 84±4 | Bouchard and Lortie, 1984[142] |
| Biacromial diameter | | 64±22 | Bouchard and Lortie, 1984[142] |
| Biiliac diameter | | 60±13 | Bouchard and Lortie, 1984[142] |
| Ponderal index | | 53±19 | Bouchard and Lortie, 1984[142] |
| Ectomorphy | | 35–50 | Bouchard and Lortie, 1984[142] |
| Mesomorphy | | 42 | Bouchard and Lortie, 1984[142] |
| Endomorphy | | 50 | Bouchard and Lortie, 1984[142] |
| Sitting height | | 71±29 | Bouchard and Lortie, 1984[142] |
| Skinfold fat | | 55±26 | Bouchard and Lortie, 1984[142] |
| **Physiological Variables** | | | |
| $VO_2$ max | | 30 | Bouchard, 1986[143] |
| | | 0–93 | Bouchard and Lortie, 1984[142] |
| | | <40–60 | Bouchard and Malina, 1983[144] |
| Aerobic capacity | (90 min) | 20 | Bouchard, 1986[143] |
| $PWC_{150}$ | | 30–48 | Bouchard and Lortie, 1984[142] |
| Anaerobic power | (Margaria) | 97.8 | Komi and Karlsson, 1979[145] |
| Anaerobic power | (Arm crank) | 97.0 | Jones and Klissouras, 1986[146] |
| Anaerobic power | 10″ bike | 44–66 | Simoneau et al, 1986[147] |
| Ventilatory threshold (1) | | 30 | Bouchard, 1986[143] |
| Ventilatory threshold (2) | | 24 | Bouchard, 1986[143] |
| % slow-twitch fibers | | 92–100 | Komi et al, 1977[148] |
| | | 55 | Lortie et al, 1986[149] |
| Fiber areas | | low | Lortie et al, 1986[149] |
| Metabolic enzymes | | low | Bouchard and Lortie, 1984[142] |
| | | | Komi et al, 1977[148] |
| Strength | | 11–81 | Bouchard and Malina, 1983[144] |
| | | | Malina, 1986[150] |
| Muscle endurance | | 22–83 | Bouchard and Malina 1983[144] |
| | | | Malina, 1986[150] |
| **Field Test Variables** | | | |
| Dashes | | 45–91 | Bouchard and Malina, 1983[144] |
| | | | Malina, 1986[150] |
| Jumping | | 33–86 | Malina, 1986[150] |
| | | 45–86 | Bouchard and Malina, 1983[144] |
| Throwing | | 14–71 | Bouchard and Malina, 1983[144] |
| | | | Malina, 1986[150] |
| Flexibility | | 69–91 | Bouchard and Malina, 1983[144] |
| Balance | | 24–85 | Bouchard and Malina, 1983[144] |
| | | 27–86 | Malina, 1986[150] |

genetic trainability components in the latter studies suggests that the post-training heritability would approach the values reported by the first two groups of investigators.

Different labs have reported moderate to very high heritability estimates for muscle fiber type proportions. Since recent work has shown that conversion of type II to type I muscle fibers is possible, with appropriate training,[153–156] the heritability estimates of Komi et al[148] probably are too high. Conversely, the different laboratories agreed that muscle enzyme levels and fiber areas have a low genetic component. Strength, muscle endurance, running speed, jumping, and balance heritability estimates range from low to moderate, to moderate to high. Flexibility estimates have been higher.

Bouchard and associates have reviewed a series of studies regarding the inheritance of trainability which they performed.[143, 152] These investigators have studied the genetic × trainability interaction for maximal oxygen consumption, maximal aerobic capacity, anaerobic power (10 seconds all-out bicycle ride), and anaerobic capacity (90 seconds all-out bicycle ride), and have reported heritability estimates of 40%, 25%, 69%, and 31%, respectively. The mean improvements and range of improvements demonstrated were as follows: maximal oxygen consumption = 33% (5% to 88%); maximal aerobic capacity = 51% (16% to 97%); maximal anaerobic power = 22% (3% to 66%); and maximal anaerobic capacity = 35% (11% to 77%). Although there was no sex difference in the trainability of maximal oxygen consumption, males appeared to be more trainable for maximal oxygen capacity. Since only sedentary subjects were used in these studies, the effect of previous training was unknown. Bouchard[143] cited a review of 50 training studies and concluded that the trainability of maximal oxygen consumption is moderately and negatively related to initial values. Although no efforts to determine the inheritance of trainability for other variables have been reported, it seems reasonable to expect similar results. Unfortunately, no markers have been found which will identify individuals who are low, high, early, or late responders to appropriate training.[152]

## Effect of Training in Children

Several recent reviews of research on the effects of training in children have been conducted.[157–160] Therefore, only a brief summary of some of their conclusions will be presented here.

Numerous studies have been conducted which monitored changes in maximal oxygen consumption during a longitudinal training program. At least one half of the studies found no improvement in maximal oxygen consumption ($ml \cdot kg^{-1} \cdot min^{-1}$), but many of these included training programs that either were not very vigorous or were very short. Rowland[159] and Vaccaro and Mahon[160] concluded that 75% of the studies that provided an adequate training stimulus (by adult standards) produced a significant improvement. In some of the studies which found no change, the subjects were active prior to the study and/or had high initial values for maximal oxygen consumption. Bar-Or[157] analyzed performance on running tests for those studied where little or no change occurred in maximal oxygen consumption; in two-thirds of the cases running times improved. Several studies analyzed longitudinal data before, during, and after peak growth velocity with conflicting results. Most of the training studies which looked at pre- to post-training responses to the same absolute or relative intensity found that the post-training heart rate was lower. One study found that running economy improved.

Almost all of the studies that have used strength training with prepubescent children found improvements; most studies showed improvements greater than those which would have been expected from growth alone. Several studies compared strength training responses between different maturational periods; these showed generally similar results in three of four studies.[157] No studies have determined whether increases in muscle mass occurred with the strength gains.

Bar-Or[157] summarized three training studies that assessed pre- to post-training measures of peak power and mean power on the Wingate anaerobic test. Training consisted of (1) cycling or sprinting (boys only), (2) interval running (boys only), or (3) participation in a sports class (boys and girls). Peak power and mean power improved in all cases. Another study conducted at the end of a competitive sports season found no improvement in anaerobic power during a 4-week program of interval isokinetic and all-out cycling training.

Hardly any well-controlled studies were located which investigated the effect of appropriate training on other performance variables in children. There were studies which compared athletes to normals, studies which followed athletes longitudinally, and studies which failed to use an equivalent control group. Since the first 20 years of life are so dynamic, it is imperative that self-selection and maturation be controlled in training studies.

## Summary and Implications for Children

Elite athletes in various sports have been profiled. Some characteristics were generalized among most athletic categories, e.g., low body fat. However, most characteristics were generalized within clusters of related activities. High maximal oxygen consumption, the ability to perform close to maximum without accumulating significant amounts of lactate, efficiency, a high proportion of slow-twitch muscle fibers, and high levels of muscle oxidative enzymes were found in elite endurance athletes, while very high scores on mesomorphy and strength were found in elite strength athletes. Other characteristics were unique to specific events. Long distance runners tended to be short and very lightly built; swimmers tended to be tall, well-muscled in the upper body, and able to develop a large oxygen debt; and rowers tended to be very tall, heavily muscled, and to have a high absolute maximal oxygen consumption, anaerobic power, and oxygen capacity. Finally, some events were found to require very high levels of specific skills (gymnastics, wrestling, alpine skiing, and judo). Even though specific profiles were found for these sports, it was obvious in reviewing the scatter of data that some elite athletes deviate considerably from their sport-specific profile. Attempts to predict current or near-term performance have produced mixed results; in some areas prediction has been excellent (long distance running), and in other areas little research has been done (gymnastics, judo, and body building).

The review of the heritability of sports characteristics showed that most mean heritability estimates were moderate at best. The major exceptions to this generalization were height and body length. Other lesser exceptions probably include running dash speed, flexibility, and perhaps percentage of slow-twitch muscle fibers. At the other end of the spectrum, muscle fiber areas and enzyme patterns have very low heritability estimates. A relatively unknown factor in the heritability equation is the heritability of trainability. The additive effect of the main effect of heritability and its interaction with trainability is relatively unknown and may be substantial. Unfortunately, no methods for predicting the interaction effect have been discovered. Therefore, some individuals may show the potential for success in a particular sport at a young age but never develop, while others may develop rapidly. On the other hand, some individuals who appear to be only slightly above average at a young age eventually may attain or exceed the abilities of those who mature earlier. However, it is probably safe to conclude that young individuals who are below average for a particular characteristic probably will never become very high on that characteristic.

What are the implications of the research findings on sports profiling and heritability? Is it possible to identify young individuals who are likely to become elite athletes? The available evidence suggests that many errors are likely to be made in attempting to classify young individuals in this manner. The younger the individual is, the less likely that the predictions would come true. The success rate probably would be better in those sports which rely heavily on a relatively pure physiological parameter i.e., maximal oxygen consumption probably places an upper limit on development in endurance activities). Conversely, in those activities where sports profiling and prediction are in their infancy, it is not possible to predict even current performance from laboratory tests, much less future performance. Even in those sports where profiling and prediction are more advanced, it is impossible at this time to predict trainability. Probably the best profiling advice would be to encourage children who are likely to be tall to participate in those activities where height is an advantage and to encourage children who are likely to be short to participate in those activities where the lack of height is an advantage.

The best policy for identifying sports potential is for parents and appropriate public and private organizations to sponsor and encourage participation in a broad-based sports program that is available to all children. Such programs should remain broadly based at least through the late teens to allow late-maturers a chance to recognize their potential. Workshops, clinics, and/or camps should be available so that interested athletes can benefit from expert teaching and coaching. At some point (which would vary with the sport), individuals with promising potential could be organized into "select" teams that could receive more advanced coaching, training, and competition. Depending on the sport, there will be a time when laboratory testing of individuals with apparent national and international potential would be justified. With such a broadly based program the "cream will rise to the top" and many children will have the opportunity to have fun and develop their potential. On a cautionary note, however: safeguards should be built into such a system to maximize positive experiences and minimize negative ones.

## References

1. Pollock ML: Characteristics of elite class distance runners. *Ann N Y Acad Sci* 1977; 301:278–410.
2. Ebashi H, Goto Y, Nishijima Y, et al: Maximal aerobic power and maximal isokinetic strength of male Japanese elite marathon runners. *Bulletin of the Physical Fitness Research Institute* 1989; 71:10–24.
3. Sparling PB: A comprehensive profile of elite women distance runners. *Int J Sports Med* 1987; 8(suppl 2):71–136.
4. Farrel PA, Wilmore JH, Coyel EF, et al: Plasma lactate accumulation and distance running performance. *Med Sci Sports Exerc* 1979; 11:338–344.
5. Fohrenbach R, Moader A, Hollman W: Determination of endurance capacity and prediction of exercise intensities for training and competition in marathon runners. *Int J Sports Med* 1987; 8:11–18.
6. Kumagai S, Tanaka K, Matsuura Y, et al: Relationships of the anaerobic threshold with the 5 km, 10 km, and 10 mile races. *Eur J Appl Physiol* 1982; 49:13–23.
7. LaFontaine TP, Londeree BR, Spath WK: The maximal steady state versus selected running events. *Med Sci Sports Exerc* 1981; 13:190–192.
8. Powers SK, Dodd S, Deason R, et al: Ventilatory threshold, running economy and distance running performance of trained athletes. *Res Quart Exerc Sport* 1983; 54:179–182.
9. Reybrouck T, Ghesquiere J, Weymans M, et al: Ventilatory threshold measurement to evaluate maximal endurance performance. *Int J Sports Med* 1986; 7:26–29.
10. Rhodes EC, McKenzie DC: Predicting marathon time from anaerobic threshold measurements. *Physician Sportsmed* 1984; 12:95–98.
11. Sjodin B, Jacobs I: Onset of blood lactate accumulation and marathon running performance. *Int J Sports Med* 1981; 2:23–26.
12. Tanaka K, Matsuura Y: Marathon performance, anaerobic threshold, and onset of blood lactate accumulation. *J Apply Physiol* 1984; 57:640–643.
13. Pollock ML, Jackson AS, Pate RR: Discriminant analysis of physiological differences between good and elite distance runners. *Res Quart Exerc Sport* 1980; 51:521–532.
14. Fink WJ, Costill DL, Pollock ML: Submaximal and maximal working capacity of elite distance runners. Part II. Muscle fiber composition and enzyme activities. *Ann N Y Acad Sci* 1977; 301:323–327.

15. Sjodin B, Svendenhag J: Applied physiology of marathon running. *Sports Med* 1985; 2:83–99.
16. Morgan WP, Pollock ML: Psychological characterization of the elite distance runner. *Ann N Y Acad Sci* 1977; 301:382–403.
17. Morgan WP, O'Connor PJ, Sparling PB, et al: Psychological characterization of the elite female distance runner. *Int J Sports Med* 1987; 8(suppl 2):103–106.
18. Carter JEL: Somatotypes of Olympic athletes from 1948 to 1976, in Carter JEL (ed): *Physical Structure of Olympic Athletes, Part II.* Basel, S Karger, 1982, pp 80–109.
19. Martin DE, Vroon DH, May DF, et al: Physiological changes in elite male distance runners training for the Olympics. *Physician Sportsmed* 1986; 14:152–171.
20. Crielaard JM, Pirnay F: Anaerobic and aerobic power of top athletes. *Eur J Appl Physiol* 1981; 47:295–300.
21. Ready AE: Physiological characteristics of male and female middle distance runners. *Can J Appl Sport Sci* 1984; 9:70–77.
22. Costill DL, Fink WJ, Flynn M, et al: Muscle fiber composition and enzyme activities in elite female distance runners. *Int J Sports Med* 1987; 8(suppl 2):103–106.
23. Baumgartner TA, Jackson AS: *Measurement for Evaluation in Physical Education,* ed 2. Dubuque, Iowa, Wm C Brown, 1982.
24. Boileau RA, Mayhew JL, Riner WF, et al: Physiological characteristics of elite middle and long distance runners. *Can J Apply Sport Sci* 1982; 7:167–172.
25. Conley DL, Krahenbuhl GS: Running economy and distance running performance. *Med Sci Sports Exerc* 1980; 12:357–360.
26. Noakes TD: Implications of exercise testing for prediction of athletic performance: A contemporary perspective. *Med Sci Sports Exerc* 1988; 20: 319–330.
27. Barnes WS: Selected physiological characteristics of elite male sprint athletes. *J Sports Med Phys Fitness* 1981; 21:49–54.
28. Carter JEL: Age and body size of Olympic athletes, in Carter JEL (ed): *Physical Structure of Olympic Athletes, Part II.* Basel, S Karger, 1982, pp 53–79.
29. Gollnick PD, Armstrong RB, Saubert CW IV, et al: Enzyme activity and fiber compositions in skeletal muscle of untrained and trained men. *J Appl Physiol* 1972; 33:312–319.
30. Costill DL, Daniels J, Evans W, et al: Skeletal muscle enzymes and fiber composition in male and female track athletes. *J Appl Physiol* 1976; 40: 149–154.
31. Burke ER: Physiological characteristics of competitive cyclists. *Physician Sportsmed* 1980; 8:79–84.
32. Burke ER, Cerny F, Costill D, et al: Characteristics of skeletal muscle in competitive cyclists. *Med Sci Sports Exerc* 1977; 9:109–112.
33. Foster C, Daniels JT: Aerobic power of competitive cyclists. *Aust J Sports Med* 1974; 7:111–112.
34. Hagberg JM, Mullin JP, Bahrke M, et al: Physiological profiles and selected psychological characteristics of national class American cyclists. *J Sports Med Phys Fitness* 1979; 19:341–346.
35. Malhotra MS, Verma SK, Gupta RK, et al: Physiological basis for selection of competitive road cyclists. *J Sports Med* 1984; 24:49–57.

36. Sjogaard G: Muscle morphology and metabolic potential in elite road cyclists during a season. *Int J Sports Med* 1984; 5:250–254.
37. Folinsbee LJ, Wallace ES, Bedi JF, et al: Exercise respiratory pattern in elite cyclists and sedentary subjects. *Med Sci Sports Exerc* 1983; 15:503–509.
38. Saltin B, Astrand PO: Maximal oxygen uptake in athletes. *J Appl Physiol* 1967; 23:353–358.
39. Stromme SB, Ingjer F, Meen HD: Assessment of maximal aerobic power in specifically trained athletes. *J Appl Physiol* 1977; 42:833–837.
40. Holloway EC, Rogers CA, Dressendorfer RH: Maximal aerobic power of elite female cyclists: Treadmill running vs bicycle ergometry. *Med Sci Sports Exerc* 1981; 13:110.
41. Miller FR, Manfredi TG: Physiological and anthropometrical predictors of 15-kilometer time trial cycling performance time. *Res Quart Exerc Sport* 1987; 58:250–254.
42. Carter JEL: Body composition of Montreal Olympic athletes, in Carter JEL (ed): *Physical Structure of Olympic Athletes.* New York, Karger, 1982, pp 107–116.
43. Carter JEL, Ross WD, Aubury SP, et al: Anthropometry of Montreal Olympic athletes, in Carter JEL (ed): *Physical Structure of Olympic Athletes.* New York, Karger, 1982, pp 25–52.
44. Lopategui E, Perez HR, Smith TK, et al: The anaerobic threshold of elite and novice cyclists. *J Sports Med Phys Fitness* 1986; 26:123–127.
45. Charbonnier JP, Lacour JR, Riffat J, et al: Experimental study of the performance of competition swimmers. *Eur J Appl Physiol* 1975; 34:157–167.
46. Van Huss WD, Cureton TK: Relationship of selected tests with energy metabolism and swimming performance. *Res Quart* 1955; 26:205–221.
47. Costill DL, Kovaleski J, Porter D, et al: Energy expenditure during front crawl swimming: Predicting success in middle-distance events. *Int J Sports Med* 1985; 6:266–270.
48. Holmer I: Physiology of swimming man, in Hutton RS, Miller DI (eds): *Exercise and Sport Sciences Reviews.* Salt Lake City, Utah, Franklin Institute Press, 1979, pp 87–123.
49. Craig AB Jr, Boomer WL, Gibbons JF: Use of stroke rate, distance per stroke, and velocity relationships during training for competitive swimming, in Terauds J, Bedingfield EW (eds): *Swimming Medicine III.* Baltimore, University Park Press, 1979, pp 265–274.
50. Treffene RJ: Heart rate measurement technique in swimming performance prediction, in Hollander AP, Huijing PA, de Groot G (eds): *Biomechanics and Medicine in Swimming.* Champaign, Ill, Human Kinetics, 1983, pp 339–344.
51. Klissouras V, Sinning WS: Metabolic prediction of swimming performance, in Eriksson B, Furberg B (eds): *Swimming Medicine IV.* Baltimore, University Park Press, 1978, pp 262–273.
52. Elliot M, Haber P: Estimation of peak performance in the 100-meter breast stroke on the basis of serum lactate measurement during two submaximal test heats at different velocities, in Hollander AP, Huijing PA, de Groot G (eds): *Biomechanics and Medicine in Swimming.* Champaign, Ill, Human Kinetics, 1983, pp 335–338.
53. Troup J: Setting up a season using scientific training. *Swimming Technique* 1986; 23:8–16.

54. Eriksson BO, Holmer I, Lundin A: Physiological effects of training in elite swimmers, in Eriksson B, Furberg B (eds): *Swimming Medicine IV*. Baltimore, University Park Press, 1978, pp 177–187.
55. Gullstrand L, Holmer I: Physiological characteristics of champion swimmers during a five-year follow-up period, in Hollander AP, Huijing PA, de Groot G (eds): *Biomechanics and Medicine in Swimming*. Champaign, Ill, Human Kinetics, 1983, pp 258–262.
56. Gerard ES, Caiozzo VJ, Rubin BD, et al: Skeletal muscle profiles among elite long, middle, and short distance swimmers. *Am J Sports Med* 1986; 14:77–82.
57. Lavoie JM, Montpetit RR: Applied physiology of swimming. *Sports Med* 1986; 3:165–189.
58. Nygaard E, Nielsen E: Skeletal muscle fiber capillarization with extreme endurance training in man, in Eriksson B, Furberg B (eds): *Swimming Medicine IV*. Baltimore, University Park Press, 1978, pp 282–293.
59. Costill DL: Adaptation in skeletal muscle during training for sprint and endurance swimming, in Eriksson B, Furberg B (eds): *Swimming Medicine IV*. Baltimore, University Park Press, 1978, pp 233–248.
60. Sharp RL, Troup JP, Costill DL: Relationship between power and sprint freestyle swimming. *Med Sci Sports Exerc* 1982; 14:53–56.
61. Miyashita M, Kanehisa H: Effects of isokinetic, isotonic and swim training on swimming performance, in Hollander AP, Huijing PA, de Groot G (eds): *Biomechanics and Medicine in Swimming*. Champaign, Ill, Human Kinetics, 1983, pp 329–334.
62. Manning JM, Dooley-Manning CR, Terrell DT, et al: Effects of a power circuit weight training program on power production and performance. *J Swimming Research* 1986; 2:24–29.
63. Cazorla G, Dufort C, Cervetti JP, et al: The influence of active recovery on blood lactate disappearance after supramaximal swimming, in Hollander AP, Huijing PA, de Groot G (eds): *Biomechanics and Medicine in Swimming*. Champaign, Ill, Human Kinetics, 1983, pp 244–250.
64. Smith BW, McMurray RG, Symanski JD: A comparison of the anaerobic threshold of sprint and endurance trained swimmers. *J Sports Med* 1984; 24:94–99.
65. Hermansen L: Anaerobic energy release. *Med Sci Sports Exerc* 1969; 1:32–38.
66. Holmer I, Lundin A, Eriksson BO: Maximal oxygen uptake during swimming and running by elite swimmers. *J Appl Physiol* 1974; 36:711–714.
67. Hagerman FC, Hagerman GR, Mikelson TC: Physiological profiles of elite rowers. *Physician Sportsmed* 1979; 7:74–83.
68. Mickelson TC, Hagerman FC: Anaerobic threshold measurements of elite oarsmen. *Med Sci Sports Exerc* 1982; 14:440–444.
69. Secher NH, Vaage O, Jensen K, et al: Maximal aerobic power in oarsmen. *Eur J Appl Physiol* 1983; 51:155–162.
70. Clarkson PM, Johnson J, Melchionda A, et al: Isokinetic strength, fatigue, and fiber type in elite oarswomen. *Med Sci Sports Exerc* 1983; 15:178.
71. Hagerman FC: Applied physiology of rowing. *Sports Med* 1984; 1:303–326.
72. Mahler DA: Comparison of six-minute "all-out" and incremental exercise tests in elite oarsmen. *Med Sci Sports Exerc* 1984; 16:567–571.
73. Mahler DA, Andersen DC, Parker HW, et al: Physiologic comparison of row-

ing performance between national and collegiate women rowers. *Med Sci Sports Exerc* 1983; 15:157.

74. Bonde-Petersen F, Gollnick PD, Hansen TI, et al: Glycogen depletion pattern in human muscle fiber during work under curarization, in Howald H, Poortmans JR (eds): *Metabolic Adaptation To Prolonged Physical Exercise.* Basel, Birkhauser, Verlag, 1975, pp 422–430.

75. Hagerman FC, Staron RS: Seasonal variations among physiological variables in elite oarsmen. *Can J Appl Sports Sci* 1983; 8:143–148.

76. Larsson L, Forsberg A: Morphological muscle characteristics in rowers. *Can J Appl Sports Sci* 1980; 5:239–244.

77. Niinimaa V, Dyon M, Shephard RJ: Performance and efficiency of intercollegiate cross-country skiers. *Med Sci Sports Exerc* 1978; 10:91–93.

78. Ng AV, Demment RB, Bassett DR, et al: Characteristics and performance of male citizen cross-country skill racers. *Int J Sports Med* 1988; 9:205–209.

79. Bergh U: The influence of body mass in cross-country skiing. *Med Sci Sports Exerc* 1987; 19:324–331.

80. Hanson JS: Maximal exercise performance in members of the US nordic team. *J Appl Physiol* 1973; 35:592–595.

81. Haymes EM, Dickinson AL: Characteristics of elite male and female ski racers. Med Sci Sports Exerc 1980; 12:153–158.

82. Jette M, Thoden JS, Spence J: The energy expenditure of a 5 km cross-country ski run. *J Sports Med Phys Fitness* 1976; 16:134–137.

83. Mackova EV, Bass A, Sprynarova S, et al: Enzyme activity patterns of energy metabolism in skiers of different performance levels. *Eur J Appl Physiol* 1982; 48:315–322.

84. Rusko H, Havu M, Karvinen E: Aerobic performance capacity in athletes. *Eur J Appl Physiol* 1978; 38:151–159.

85. Sinning WE, Cunningham LE, Racaniello AP, et al: Body composition and somatotype of male and female nordic skiers. *Res Quart* 1977; 48:741–749.

86. Sharkey BJ: *Training for Cross-Country Ski Racing.* Champaign, Ill, Human Kinetics, 1982.

87. Bergh U: *Physiology of Cross-Country Ski Racing.* Champaing, Ill, Human Kinetics, 1982.

88. Rusko H, Rahkila P, Karvinen E: Anaerobic threshold, skeletal muscle enzymes, and fiber composition in young female cross-country skiers. *Acta Physiol Scand* 1980; 108:263–268.

89. Song TMK: Relationship of physiological characteristics to skiing performance. *Physician Sportsmed* 1982; 10:97–102.

90. Andersen RE, Montgomery DL, Turcotte RA: An on-site test battery to evaluate a giant slalom skiing performance. *Can Appl J Sports Sci* 1988; 13:40P.

91. Brown SL, Wilkinson JG: Characteristics of national, divisional, and club male alpine ski racers. *Med Sci Sports Exerc* 1983; 15:491–495.

92. Thorstenssen A, Larsson L, Tesch P, et al: Muscle strength and fiber composition in athletes and sedentary men. *Med Sci Sports Exerc* 1977; 9: 26–30.

93. diPrampero PE, Cortili G, Mognoni P, et al: Energy cost of speed skating and efficiency of work against air resistance. *J Appl Physiol* 1976; 40:585–591.

94. Ingen Schenau GJ van: The influence of air friction in speed skating. *J Biomech* 1982; 15:449–458.

95. Ingen Schenau GJ van, de Groot G, Hollander AP: Some technical, physio-

logical and anthropometrical aspects of speed skating. *Eur J Appl Physiol* 1983; 50:343–354.

96. Ingen Schenau GJ van, de Groot G, deBoer RW: The control of speed elite female speed skaters. *J Biomech* 1985; 18:91–96.

97. Geijsel J, Bomhoff G, van Velzen J, et al: Bicycle ergometry and speed skating performance. *Int J Sports Med* 1984; 5:241–245.

98. Pollock ML, Pels AE III, Foster C, et al: Comparison of male and female Olympic candidates, in Landers DM (ed): *Sport and Elite Performers*. Champaing, Ill, Human Kinetics, 1986, pp 143–152.

99. Nemoto I, Iwaoka K, Funato K, et al: Aerobic threshold, anaerobic threshold, and maximal oxygen uptake of Japanese speed-skaters. *Int J Sports Med* 1988; 9:433–437.

100. Geijsel JSM: The endurance time on a bicycle ergometer as a test for marathon speed skaters. *J Sports Med Phys Fitness* 1980; 20:333–340.

101. Hermansen L: Oxygen transport during exercise in human subjects. *Acta Physiol Scand* 1973; 399(suppl):1–104.

102. Maksud MG, Wiley RL, Hamilton LH, et al: Maximal $Vo_2$, ventilation, and heart rate of Olympic speed skating candidates. *J Appl Physiol* 1970; 29:186–190.

103. Maksud MG, Hamilton LH, Balke B: Physiological responses of a male Olympic speed skater—Terry McDermott. *Med Sci Sports Exerc* 1971; 3:107–109.

104. Maksud MG, Hamilton LH, Coutts KD, et al: Pulmonary function measurements of Olympic speed skaters from the US. *Med Sci Sports Exerc* 1971; 3:66–71.

105. Pollock ML, Foster C, Anholm J, et al: Body composition of Olympic speed skating candidates. *Res Quart Exerc Sports* 1982; 53:150–155.

106. Gale JB, Flynn KW: Maximal oxygen consumption and relative body fat of high ability wrestlers. *Med Sci Sports Exerc* 1974; 6:232–234.

107. Nagle FJ, Morgan WP, Hellickson RO, et al: Spotting success traits in Olympic contenders. *Physician Sportsmed* 1975; 3:31–34.

108. Stine G, Ratliff R, Shierman G, et al: Physical profile of the wrestlers at the 1977 NCAA Championships. *Physician Sportsmed* 1979; 7:98–105.

109. Fahey TD, Akka L, Rolph R: Body composition and $Vo_2$ max of exceptional weight-trained athletes. *J Appl Physiol* 1975; 39:559–561.

110. Sharatt MT, Taylor AW, Song TMK: A physiological profile of elite Canadian freestyle wrestlers. *Can J Appl Sports Sci* 1986; 11:100–105.

111. diPrampero PE, Limas FP, Sassi G: Maximal muscular power, aerobic and anaerobic, in 116 athletes performing at the XIXth Olympic Games in Mexico. *Ergonomics* 1970; 13:665–674.

112. Nelson JK, Johnson BL, Smith GC: Physical characteristics, hip flexibility, and arm strength of female gymnasts classified by intensity of training across age. *J Sports Med Phys Fitness* 1983; 23:95–101.

113. LeVeau B, Ward T, Nelson RC: Body dimensions of Japanese and American gymnasts. *Med Sci Sports Exerc* 1974; 6:146–150.

114. Novak LP, Hyatt RE, Alexander JF: Body composition and physiologic function of athletes. *JAMA* 1968; 205:764–770.

115. Conger PR, MacNab RBJ: Strength, body composition, and work capacity of participants and nonparticipants in women's intercollegiate sports. *Res Quart* 1967; 38:184–192.

116. Malina RM, Mueller WH, Bouchard C, et al: Fatness and fat patterning

among athletes at the Montreal Olympic Games, 1976. *Med Sci Sports Exerc* 1982; 14:445–452.

117. Caldarone G, Leglise M, Giampietro M, et al: Anthropometric measurements, body composition, biological maturation and growth predictions in young female gymnasts of high agonistic level. *J Sports Med Phys Fitness* 1986; 26:263–273.

118. Caldarone G, Leglise M, Giampietro M, et al: Anthropometric measurements, body composition, biological maturation and growth predictions in young male gymnasts of high agonistic level. *J Sports Med Phys Fitness* 1986; 26:406–415.

119. Taylor AW, Brassard L: A physiological profile of the Canadian judo team. *J Sports Med Phys Fitness* 1981; 21:160–164.

120. Claessens ALM, Beunen GP, Simons JM, et al: Body structure, somatotype, and motor fitness of top-class Belgian judoists, in Day JAP (ed): *Perspectives in Kinathropometry*. Champain, Ill, Human Kinetics, 1986, pp 155–163.

121. Claessens A, Beunen G, Wellens R, et al: Somatotype and body structure of world top judoists. *J Sports Med Phys Fitness* 1987; 27:105–113.

122. Farmosi I: Body composition, somatotype and some motor performance of judoists. *J Sports Med Phys Fitness* 1980; 20:431–434.

123. Carter JEL, Aubry SP, Sleet DA: Somatotypes of Montreal Olympic athletes, in Carter JEL (ed): *Physical Structure of Olympic Athletes*. Basel, S Karger, 1982, pp 53–80.

124. Hakkinen K, Komi PV, Kauhanen H: Electromyographic and force production characteristics of leg extensor muscles of elite weight lifters during isometric, concentric, and various stretch-shortening cycle exercises. *Int J Sports Med* 1986; 7:144–151.

125. Hakkinen K, Kauhenen H, Komi PV: Aerobic, anaerobic, assistant exercise and weight lifting performance capacities in elite weight lifters. *J Sports Med Phys Fitness* 1987; 27:240–246.

126. Ward T, Groppel JL, Stone M: Arthropometry and performance in master and first class Olympic weight lifters. *J Sports Med Phys Fitness* 1979; 19:205–212.

127. Stone MH, Byrd R, Tew J, et al: Relationship between anaerobic power and Olympic weightlifting performance. *J Sports Med Phys Fitness* 1980; 20:99–102.

128. Borms J, Ross WD, Duquet W, et al: Somatotypes of world class body builders, in Day JAP (ed): *Perspectives in Kinanthropometry*. Champaign, Ill, Human Kinetics, 1986, pp 81–90.

129. Hakkinen K, Alen M, Komi PV: Neuromuscular, anaerobic, and aerobic performance characteristics of elite power lifters. *Eur J Appl Physiol* 1984; 53:97–105.

130. Katch FI, Katch VL: The body composition profile. *Clin Sports Med* 1984; 3:31–63.

131. Katch VL, Katch FI, Moffatt R, et al: Muscular development and lean body weight in body builders and weight lifters. *Med Sci Sports Exerc* 1980; 12:340–344.

132. MacDougall JD, Sale DG, Elder GCB, et al: Muscle ultrastructural characteristics of elite powerlifters and bodybuilders. *Eur J Appl Physiol* 1982; 48:117–126.

133. Pipes TV: Physiological characteristics of elite body builders. *Physician Sportsmed* 1979; 7:116–120.
134. Spitler DL, Diaz FJ, Horvath SM, et al: Body composition and maximal aerobic capacity of bodybuilders. *J Sports Med Phys Fitness* 1980; 20:181–188.
135. Sprynarova S, Parizkova J: Functional capacity and body composition in top weightlifters, swimmers, runners and skiers. *Int Z Angew Physiol* 1971; 29:184–194.
136. Tesch PA, Thorsson A, Kaiser P: Muscle capillary supply and fiber type characteristics in weight and power lifters. *J Appl Physiol* 1984; 56:35–38.
137. Veicsteinas A, Feroldi P, Dotti A: Ventilatory response during incremental exercise tests in weight lifters and endurance cyclists. *Eur J Appl Physiol* 1985; 53:322–329.
138. Bale P, Williams H: An anthropometric prototype of female power lifters. *J Sports Med Phys Fitness* 1987; 27:191–196.
139. Bond V Jr, Gresham KE, Tuckson LE, et al: Strength comparisons in untrained men and trained women body builders. *J Sports Med Phys Fitness* 1985; 25:131–134.
140. Freedson PS, Mihevic PM, Loucks AB, et al: Physique, body composition, and psychological characteristics of competitive female body builders. *Physician Sportsmed* 1983; 11:85–93.
141. Bell DG, Jacobs I, Laufer J: Muscle fiber area, fiber type distribution and capillary supply in male and female body builders. *Can J Sports Science* 1988; 13:42P.
142. Bouchard C, Lortie G: Heredity and endurance performance. *Sports Med* 1984; 1:38–64.
143. Bouchard C: Genetics of aerobic power and capacity, in Malina RM, Bouchard C (eds): *Sports and Human Genetics.* Champaign, Ill, Human Kinetics, 1986, pp 59–88.
144. Bouchard C, Malina RM: Genetics of physiological fitness and motor performance, in Terjung RL (ed): *Exercise and Sport Sciences Reviews.* Salt Lake City, Utah, Franklin Institute, 1983, pp 306–339.
145. Komi PV, Karlsson J: Physical performance skeletal muscle, enzyme activities, and fiber types in monozygous and dizygous twins of both sexes. *Acta Physiol Scand* 1979; (suppl 462) pp 1–43.
146. Jones B, Klissouras V: Genetic variation in the force-velocity relation of human muscle, in Malina RM, Bouchard C (eds): *Sport and Human Genetics.* Champaign, Ill, Human Kinetics, 1986, pp 155–163.
147. Simoneau JA, Lortie G, Boulay MR, et al: Inheritance of human skeletal muscle and anaerobic capacity adaptation in high-intensity intermittent training. *Int J Sports Med* 1986; 7:167–171.
148. Komi PV, Viitasalo JHT, Havu M, et al: Skeletal muscle fibers and muscle enzyme activities in monozygous and dizygous twins of both sexes. *Acta Physiol Scand* 1977; 100:385–392.
149. Lortie G, Simoneau JA, Boulay MR, et al: Muscle fiber type composition and enzyme activities in brothers and monozygotic twins, in Malina RM, Bouchard C (eds): *Sport and Human Genetics.* Champaign, Ill, Human Kinetics, 1986, pp 147–153.
150. Malina RM: Genetics of motor development and performance, in Malina RM, Bouchard C (eds): *Sport and Human Genetics.* Champaign, Ill, Human Kinetics, 1986, pp 23–57.

151. Prud Homme D, Bouchard C, Leblanc C, et al: Sensitivity of maximal aerobic power to training is genotype-dependent. *Med Sci Sports Exerc* 1984; 16:489–493.
152. Bouchard C, Boulay MR, Simoneau JA, et al: Heredity and trainability of aerobic and anaerobic performances. *Sports Med* 1988; 5:69–73.
153. Andonian MH, Fahim MA: Endurance exercise alters the morphology of fast- and slow-twitch rate neuromuscular junction. *Int J Sports Med* 1988; 9:218–223.
154. Jansson E, Sjodin B, Tesch P: Changes in muscle fiber distribution in man after physical training. A sign of fiber type transformation. *Acta Physiol Scand* 1977; 104:235–237.
155. Schantz P, Billeter R, Henriksson, et al: Training-induced increase in myofibrillar ATPase intermediate fibers in human skeletal muscle. *Muscle Nerve* 1982; 5:628–636.
156. Schantz PG: Plasticity of human skeletal muscle. *Acta Physiol Scand* 1986; (suppl 558) pp 1–62.
157. Bar-Or O: Trainability of the prepubescent child. *Physician Sportsmed* 1989; 17:65–82.
158. Krahenbuhl GS, Skinner JS, Kohrt WM: Developmental aspects of maximal aerobic power in children, in Terjung RL (ed): *Exercise and Sport Sciences Reviews*. New York, MacMillan, 1985, 13:503–538.
159. Rowland TW: Aerobic response to endurance training in prepubescent children: A critical analysis. *Med Sci Sports Exerc* 1985; 17:493–497.
160. Vaccaro P, Mahon A: Cardiorespiratory responses to endurance training in children. *Sports Med* 1987; 4:352–363.

# Endurance Exercise Trainability in Children and Youth

## Russell R. Pate, Ph.D.

Department of Exercise Science, School of Public Health, University of South
Carolina, Columbia, South Carolina

## Dianne S. Ward, Ed.D.

Department of Exercise Science, School of Public Health, University of South
Carolina, Columbia, South Carolina

---

**Editor's Introduction**

There is disagreement concerning the endurance trainability of children and youth.
Some studies show improvement with training while others do not. Moreover,
some medical organizations caution against serious distance training for children.
Drs. Pate and Ward review the studies on endurance trainability and comment on
the design and methods of the studies. They then address the issue of development as a factor in trainability, and identify factors that may influence trainability in
children and youth. They conclude with a discussion of future research needs and
the implications of their observations in real-world settings.

*Brian J. Sharkey, Ph.D.*

---

By 1990, the proportion of children and adolescents ages 10 to 17 participating
in appropriate physical activities, particularly cardiorespiratory fitness programs
which can be carried into adulthood, should be greater than 90% (U.S. Department of Health and Human Services).

The physiologic adaptations of adults to endurance exercise training
have been studied extensively. It is now well documented that groups of
initially sedentary young and middle-aged adults can be expected to manifest mean increases in maximal aerobic power of 15% or more.[22, 23] Such
increases can be explained by adaptive increases in maximal stroke volume and cardiac output,[28] total blood volume,[7] and skeletal muscle oxidative capacity.[17] On the basis of these observations, guidelines for the prescription of exercise in healthy adults have been adopted and widely dis-
seminated.[2, 3, 6]

The importance of high levels of habitual physical activity during childhood have been acknowledged by educational authorities for many dec-

ades.[33] Recently, the U.S. Department of Health and Human Services[31] and several medical organizations[1, 4] have recommended that children and youths participate regularly in endurance exercise. Often, recommendations for increased exercise in children have emerged from discussions about the status of physical fitness in American youngsters. Typically, it has been stated that U.S. children and youths do not perform as well as is recommended on tests of physical fitness and should participate more regularly in endurance exercise training activities. The obvious, but usually unstated, assumption is that such training would enhance performance on such tests. That is, it usually is blithely assumed that children and youths are physiologically trainable (i.e., physiologically adaptive to endurance exercise) in a manner similar to that documented in adults. Some authorities have even gone so far as to recommend application of the "adult exercise prescription" to youngsters.[3, 25]

This chapter is dedicated to the proposition that exercise programming with children and youths should not be based on either unexamined assumptions or observations of adults. Rather, such programming should be based on the critically evaluated results of properly designed, scientific studies of children like those who populate our school physical education classes, youth sport programs, and pediatric clinics. Accordingly, the overall purpose of this chapter is to conduct a critical review of the current scientific literature on endurance exercise training in children and youths. The major focus will be the identification and analysis of those studies which meet pre-established, stringent criteria with regard to research design, methodology, and statistical analysis. Specific purposes of this chapter are as follows:

1. To review the existing scientific literature on exercise training in children and youths and to identify those studies that meet designated criteria in design and methodology.
2. To compare children of various developmental stages in terms of physiologic adaptations to endurance exercise training.
3. To identify factors that might be associated with the magnitude of the training effect in children and youths.
4. To recommend future directions for research on endurance exercise training in youngsters.
5. To discuss the practical significance of the observations mentioned above.

## Review of Training Studies in Children and Youth

### Review Procedure

The existing literature includes several well-researched reviews of the adaptations that children and youths exhibit to exercise training.[9, 25, 26, 32] These reviews have employed various strategies in organizing, evaluating, and interpreting the research studies published thus far on exercise training in youngsters. Typically, these reviews have organized the available studies according to the age of the subjects, the nature of the training program, and/or the types of measures administered. To our knowledge, no previously published review of this topic has been structured so as to identify and critique only those studies which employed designs and methodologies that meet stringent, pre-established criteria. This chapter is an effort to fill this void.

In selecting research papers for inclusion in this review, the following criteria were employed:

1. **Control group.**— Only studies which included a control group that was well-matched to the training group(s) were included. This criterion was considered essential because, in our view, the changes associated with growth and development greatly complicate the interpretation of uncontrolled training studies in children. Key factors in matching experimental and control groups were age, sex, developmental status, and initial fitness and activity levels.

2. **Training protocol.**— A study was included in this review as long as the training protocol was readily interpretable in terms of mode, frequency, intensity, and duration of exercise sessions, and overall length of the intervention. Some ambiguity was acceptable in one of these factors if most were described with adequate clarity and specificity.

3. **Physiologic measures.**— A study was not included if it did not employ physiologic measures, preferably taken during maximal exercise, which could be used to document training adaptations. Thus, studies that presented only performance measures were not included.

4. **Design and statistical analysis.**— Only controlled training studies employing statistical analysis of data were included. Longitudinal observations of physically active children were included only if there was a clear exercise intervention (i.e., experiment) and an appropriate control group. Random assignment to treatment and control groups, though considered desirable, was not required for inclusion in the review, as long as an apparently well-matched control group was used. Only studies that used statistical procedures deemed appropriate were incorporated into this review.

5. **Study published in peer-reviewed scientific journal.**— To enhance the likelihood that all studies included in the review met acceptable scientific standards, only those that had been published in recognized, peer-reviewed scientific journals were considered.

## Evidence of Trainability

### Prepubescent Children

Table 1 provides summaries of 12 training studies in which the age of the subjects did not exceed 13 years. Although developmental status was evaluated systematically in only a few of these studies, it is likely that most of the subjects were prepubescent, because the vast majority were males un-

## TABLE 1.
## Exercise Training Studies With Children Aged 13 Years and Younger*

| Author | Experimental Group | Control Group | Design | Statistical Analysis | Physiologic Variables | Performance Variables |
|---|---|---|---|---|---|---|
| Becker & Vaccaro[5] | N=11<br>X̄ age 9.5<br>Boys | N=11<br>X̄ age 9.95 | Randomized, pre-, post- | ANCOVA | V̇o₂max anaerobic threshold | None |
| Docherty et al[10] | 2 groups<br>N=11   N=12<br>Boys   Boys<br>Age 12   Age 12 | N=11<br>Boys<br>Age 12 | 3 groups, random assignment | 2-way ANOVA | Max (cycle)<br>V̇o₂<br>HR<br>RER<br>Modified Wingate | None |
| Ekblom[11] | N=6<br>Boys<br>Age 11 | N=7<br>Boys<br>Age 11 | 2 groups, self-selection | Change plotted versus L³ | Max (treadmill)<br>V̇o₂<br>HR<br>VE<br>HLa cycle<br>Submax (KPM 300)<br>450<br>HR<br>VE<br>HLa<br>Vital capacity<br>Heart volume | None |
| Gatch & Byrd[14] | N=16<br>Age 9–10<br>Boys | N=16<br>Age 9–10<br>Boys | Randomized, pre-, post- | ANOVA | Submax<br>Cardiac output<br>HR<br>SV<br>O₂ pulse<br>A-V̇o₂<br>O₂ uptake | |
| Gilliam & Freedson[15] | N=11<br>X̄ age 8.5<br>Boys & Girls | N=12<br>X̄ age 8.5<br>Boys & Girls | Randomized, pre-, post-, 2 groups | ANOVA | V̇o₂max | |
| Lussier & Buskirk[19] | N=16<br>X̄ age 10.3<br>11 Boys,<br>5 Girls | N=10<br>X̄ age 10.5<br>9 Boys,<br>1 Girl | 2 groups, non-random assignment | Paired t-test | V̇o₂max<br>Submax HR<br>SV | |
| Massicotte & MacNab[20] | 3 groups<br>N=9 in each<br>Boys<br>Age 11–13 | N=9<br>Boys<br>Age 11–13 | 4 groups, stratified, random assignment | ANOVA | Max (Cycle)<br>V̇o₂<br>HR<br>VE<br>RER<br>HLa<br>Submax (cycle, 450 KPM)<br>V̇o₂<br>HR<br>VE<br>RER<br>HLa | |
| Rotstein et al[24] | N=16<br>X̄ age 10.78<br>Boys | N=12<br>X̄ age 10.78<br>Boys | Non-random, age/activity matched control, 2 groups | paired t test, | Max V̇o₂<br>anaerobic threshold (4 measures)<br>WAnT | 1,200-meter run |

| | Training Protocol | | | | Observation | | |
|---|---|---|---|---|---|---|---|
| **Mode** | **Frequency** | **Intensity** | **Duration** | **Length** | **$\dot{V}O_2$Max (ml·kg$^{-1}$·min$^{-1}$)** | **HR Submax** | **Other** |
| Cycle | 3/week | 80% VO$_2$max | 40 minutes | 8 weeks | T$_1$ T$_2$ %Δ<br>E 39.0 46.99 20.55<br>C 41.7 44.0 5.51 | AT<br>E %Δ<br>C +28<br>+13 | |
| Mixed circuit (mostly resistance) | 3/week | E$_1$ High resistance/low velocity; E$_2$ Low resistance/high velocity | Unknown | 4 weeks | T$_1$ T$_2$ %Δ<br>E$_1$ 47.0 55.1 17.2<br>E$_2$ 46.2 54.7 18.3<br>C 47.0 49.0 4.3 | | No change in Wingate |
| Mixed | 2/week | Variable | 45 to 60 minutes | 6 months | T$_1$ T$_2$ %Δ<br>E 53.9 59.4 10.2<br>C 49.9 50.2 0.6 | T$_1$ T$_2$ %Δ<br>E 147 139 −5.4<br>C 156 153 −1.9 | No change in VC, HV |
| Interval cycling | 5/week | 80% to 90% max HR | 30 minutes | 8 weeks | | E −8.9%<br>C −0.6<br>SV<br>E +6.5%<br>C +2.0%<br>O$_2$ Pulse<br>E +9.3%<br>C +1.4% | |
| Mixed "Feeling Good" control—regular physical education 2/week | 4/week | 165 beats/minute (78% max) | 25 minutes | 12 weeks | T$_1$ T$_2$ %Δ<br>E 43.4 42.9 −1.0<br>C 40.5 40.9 1.0 | | |
| Running | 4/week | 92% HR | 45 minutes | 12 weeks | T$_1$ T$_2$ %Δ<br>E 55.6 59.4 6.8<br>C 53.1 53.9 1.5 | 40% %Δ<br>E −7.3<br>C +0.4<br>80%<br>E −7.2<br>C +0.3 | SV (at 68% max)<br>E +11%<br>C +12% |
| Cycle | 3/week | E$_1$ HR 170–80<br>E$_2$ HR 150–60<br>E$_3$ HR 130–40 | 12 minutes | 6/weeks | T$_1$ T$_2$ %Δ<br>E$_1$ 46.7 51.8 10.9<br>E$_2$ 47.4 48.0 1.3<br>E$_3$ 46.6 48.2 3.4<br>C 45.7 44.2 −3.3 | T$_1$ T$_2$ %Δ<br>E$_1$ 150 134 −10.7<br>E$_2$ 163 151 −7.4<br>E$_3$ 169 153 −9.5<br>C 155 155 | |
| Running (interval) | 3/week | Unknown | 45 minutes | 9/weeks | T$_1$ T$_2$ %Δ<br>E 54.2 58.6 8.0<br>C 57.1 58.3 2.0 | | AT<br>E improved in 3 of 4 measures by 5%<br>C < 2%<br>WAnT<br>Mean power<br>E +10%<br>C 2%<br>Peak<br>E +14%<br>C 0.1%<br>1,200 meter run time<br>E −10%<br>C −1% |

*Continued.*

## TABLE 1. (continued)

| Author | Experimental Group | | Control Group | Design | Statistical Analysis | Physiologic Variables | Performance Variables |
|---|---|---|---|---|---|---|---|
| Savage et al[27] | 2 groups | | N=10 | 3 groups, random | ANCOVA | Max (treadmill) | None |
| | N=14 | N=11 | Boys | assignment | One analysis | $\dot{V}O_2$ | |
| | Boys | Boys | Age 9.0 | | including data | HR | |
| | Age 8.0 | Age 8–9 | | | of boys and 3 | RER | |
| | | | | | groups of men | | |
| Stewart & Gutin[29] | N=13 | | N=11 | 2 groups, random | 2-way ANOVA | Max (treadmill) | None |
| | Boys | | Boys | assignment | | $\dot{V}O_2$ | |
| | Age 10–12 | | Age 10–12 | | | HR | |
| | | | | | | Submax (cycle, 300 KPM) | |
| | | | | | | $\dot{V}O_2$ | |
| | | | | | | HR | |
| Weber et al[34] | N=4 | N=4 | Identical twins | 2 groups, | Wilcoxon test, | Max (cycle) | None |
| | Boys | Boys | | twin pairs, | Mason-Whitney | $\dot{V}O_2$ | |
| | Age 10 | Age 13 | | self-selection to | University | HR | |
| | | | | E or C | | RER | |
| | | | | | | VE | |
| | | | | | | HLa | |
| | | | | | | Near max (cycle) | |
| | | | | | | Q | |
| | | | | | | HR | |
| Yoshida et al[35] | Two groups | | Boys & Girls | Non-random, | T-tests | $\dot{V}O_2$max | Running speed |
| | N=21 | | N=11 | 3 groups, | | Submax HR | max |
| | Boys & Girls | | X̄ age 4.95 | pre-, post- | | | Running speed |
| | X̄ age 5.03 | | | | | | submax |
| | Boys & Girls | | | | | | |
| | X̄ age 5.04 | | | | | | |

der 13 years of age. Each of the studies met the research design criteria discussed above.

The information presented in Table 1 provides, we believe, convincing evidence that prepubescent boys are physiologically adaptive to endurance exercise training. This conclusion is based primarily on an examination of the changes in weight-relative maximal aerobic power ($\dot{V}O_2$max) that were reported in the 12 studies. In 8 of the 12 studies, $\dot{V}O_2$max (ml·kg$^{-1}$) clearly was increased in at least one experimental group (several of the studies included more than one exercise training group). Among these 8 studies, the range of increases in $\dot{V}O_2$max in 13 experimental groups was 1.3% to 20.5% (average increase 10.4%). In the 9 control groups in these studies,

| | Training Protocol | | | | Observation | | |
|---|---|---|---|---|---|---|---|
| | | | | | $\dot{V}O_2$Max | | |
| Mode | Frequency | Intensity | Duration | Length | (ml·kg$^{-1}$·min$^{-1}$) | HR Submax | Other |
| Walk/jog/run | 3/week | $E_1$ 75% $\dot{V}O_2$max $E_2$ 40% $\dot{V}O_2$max | 2.4–4.8 km | 10 weeks | $T_1$ $T_2$ %$\Delta$<br>$E_1$ 55.9 58.5 4.7<br>$E_2$ 52.2 54.6 4.6<br>C 57.0 55.7 −2.3 | | No change in blood lipid profiles |
| Interval running | 4/week | HR 185 | 5–12 minutes | 8 weeks | $T_1$ $T_2$ %$\Delta$<br>E 49.8 49.5 −0.6<br>C 48.4 49.2 1.6 | $T_1$ $T_2$ %$\Delta$<br>E 162 149 8.0<br>C 174 170 2.3 | |
| Mixed | 7/week | HR 160+ | 8–10 minutes | 10 weeks | Age 10<br>$T_1$ $T_2$ %$\Delta$<br>E 55.6 66.0 18.7<br>C 55.6 58.8 6.5<br>Age 13<br>E 43.9 48.6 10.7<br>C 44.6 49.0 9.9 | | HLa max in 10 year–olds |
| Running | $E_1$ 5/week $E_2$ 1/week | 190 beats/ minute† | 5–10 minutes | 14 months‡ | $T_1$ $T_2$ %$\Delta$ %$\Delta$<br>$E_1$ 42.1 38.9 −7.6 $E_1$ −6.4<br>$E_2$ 43.5 41.6 −4.4 $E_2$ −3.2<br>C 41.6 42.8 2.9 C −3.99 | | Max running (m/sec) speed %$\Delta$<br>$E_1$ +36.4<br>$E_2$ +27.3<br>C +27.1<br>Submax %$\Delta$<br>$E_1$ +6.6<br>$E_2$ +3.1<br>C +3.95 |

*Max = maximum; C = control; E = experimental; HR = heart rate; N = number; Submax = submaximum; T = training group; AT = anaerobic threshold; HLa = lactate; HV = heart volume; Q = cardiac output; RER = respiratory exchange ratio; SV = stroke volume; VC = vital capacity; VE = minute ventilation; WAnT = Wingate Anaerobic Test.
†No indication of how determined.
‡Training did not occur every week but averaged 19.6 weeks for $E_1$ and 27 weeks for $E_2$.

change in $\dot{V}O_2$max ranged from −3.3 to +9.9%, with the average being a +2.7% increase. The approximate 10% average increase seen in the experimental groups is within the range of increases typically reported in studies of adults, albeit at the low end of this range.[4, 23] $\dot{V}O_2$max was not measured in a ninth study,[14] but clear evidence of a training effect was reported. In 3 studies,[15, 29, 35] no appreciable change in $\dot{V}O_2$max was observed in the trained groups. However, as will be discussed later, this observation may be explained readily by the nature of either the training protocol or the measurement procedures used in each of these cases.

The conclusion that prepubescent children are physiologically adaptive to endurance training must be qualified in several ways. First, the presently available data only document the trainability of prepubescent boys. Only three of the studies summarized in Table 1 included female subjects, and two of those were among the studies in which no change in $\dot{V}O_2$max was observed. Second, few of the studies reviewed included extensive batteries of physiologic measures; consequently, conclusions must be based almost exclusively on $\dot{V}O_2$max data. In general, variables such as cardiac output and skeletal muscle oxidative enzymes have not been included in well-controlled training studies of prepubescent children. Third, the available studies have used a rather heterogeneous array of training protocols, and few have examined more than one. Thus, our ability to relate a given magnitude of change in $\dot{V}O_2$max to a particular level of training is limited.

**TABLE 2.**
**Exercise Training Studies With Youngsters Aged 14 Years and Older***

| Author | Experimental Group | Control Group | Design | Statistical Analysis | Physiologic Variables | Performance Variables |
|---|---|---|---|---|---|---|
| Hagberg et al.[16] | N=25 Boys & Girls Age 15–17 Hypertensive | N=17 Boys & Girls Age 15–17 Hypertensive | 2 groups, self-selection to E or C | ANOVA | Max (treadmill) $\dot{V}O_2$ Rest HR SV Cardiac index BP | None |
| Stransky et al.[30] | N=16 Girls Age 15.8 | N=14 Girls Age 15.9 | 2 groups, self-selection | T-tests | Max (cycle) $\dot{V}O_2$ VE $Q_2$ pulse HR VC Hematological variables Skinfolds | None |
| Weber et al.[34] | N=4 Boys Age 16 | Identical twins | Twin pairs, self-selection to E or C | Wilcoxon test Mason-Whitney University | Max (cycle) $\dot{V}O_2$ HR RER VE HLa Near max (cycle) Q HR | None |

*BP = blood pressure; C = control; E = experimental; HR = heart rate; Max = maximum; N = number; Submax = submaximum; T = training group; HLa = lactate; LBW = lean body weight; MBC = maximal breathing capacity; Q = cardiac output; RER = respiratory exchange ratio; SV = stroke volume; VC = vital capacity; VE = minute ventilation.

## Adolescent Youth

As indicated by the material in Table 2, a surprisingly small number of controlled training studies have been conducted with adolescent youngsters. However, the three studies reviewed were consistent in that all observed appreciable increases in weight-relative $\dot{V}O_2$max in the trained groups. The range of increases was 9.7% to 17.3%, with the average increase being 14.4%. Negligible changes were reported for each of the control groups.

Although $\dot{V}O_2$max clearly was increased in all three of these studies, the small number of studies greatly limits our ability to draw general conclusions. One of these studies included only female subjects,[30] one only

| Training Protocol | | | | | Observation | | | | |
|---|---|---|---|---|---|---|---|---|---|
| **Mode** | **Frequency** | **Intensity** | **Duration** | **Length** | **$\dot{V}O_2$max (ml · kg$^{-1}$ · min$^{-1}$)** | | | **HR Submax** | **Other** |
| Walk/jog | 3/week | 60% to 65% $\dot{V}O_2$max | 30 minutes | 6 months | E | T$_1$ 43.4 | T$_2$ 47. 6 | %Δ 9.7 | Resting BP in |
| | | | | | C | ? | ? | NC | E |
| Swim | 4/week | Unknown | 12,800 yards/ week | 7 weeks | E | T$_1$ 41.6 | T$_2$ 48.3 | %Δ 16.1 | LBW, MBC, Max O$_2$ pulse in E |
| | | | | | C | 42.9 | 42.9 | 0 | |
| Mixed (run, cycle, step) | 7/week | HR 160+ | 8–10 minutes | 10 weeks | E | T$_1$ 48.1 | T$_2$ 56.4 | %Δ 17.3 | Max HLa |
| | | | | | C | 48.3 | 49.2 | 1.9 | |

males,[34] and another both males and females.[16] One study used mixed training modes,[34] one used walking/jogging,[16] and another used swimming.[30] In the swimming study, physiologic responses to maximal exercise were observed only during leg cycling.[30] The procedures applied in these studies are quite different and the research literature on training in adolescent youngsters is sorely lacking in replication.

## Potential Determinants of Trainability in Children and Youth

The cumulative findings of the studies reviewed in this paper provide substantial evidence of the trainability of youths. It is important, however, to identify key factors that determine the magnitude of the training effect. Thus, in this section we attempt to identify the determinants of trainability in youths.

Although the studies just reviewed were organized into two age categories, this section will consider all the studies as a single group. Among the factors to be examined across these studies are subject age, gender, and initial fitness level, and several characteristics of the training protocol (e.g., mode, length, intensity, frequency, and duration).

### Subject Age

That differences in trainability exist across developmental levels (prepubescent, pubescent, and postpubescent) has been suspected for a long time. However, few experimental data exist to document such differences.[32] Much of what is available in the literature is derived from cross-sectional comparisons of the maximal aerobic power of children at different stages of development.[18, 21] The "critical stage" hypothesis suggests that a certain level of maturity must be reached before improvement in maximal aerobic power can be made.[32]

Of the studies reviewed, few assessed developmental status. Consequently, the role of maturity cannot be examined directly and age must be used as a surrogate. In the 14 studies reviewed, subject ages ranged from 5 to 17 years. No change in $\dot{V}O_2max$ was observed in 2 of the 4 studies conducted with the youngest subjects (ages 5 to 9 years),[15, 35] but positive changes were seen in all but one of the studies using 10 to 13 year–old children. In the oldest category, all of the training groups experienced an increase in $\dot{V}O_2max$, while the control groups demonstrated no change. This examination suggests that older children are more likely than their younger counterparts to show increased $\dot{V}O_2max$ with endurance training. However, it should be noted that measurement of $\dot{V}O_2max$ in young children is difficult, and this technical limitation may explain some of the observations summarized in Table 1. For example, Yoshida et al,[35] working with 4-year-old subjects, developed an over-ground assessment of $\dot{V}O_2max$, the validity of which is suspect.

There does seem to be evidence that younger children (<9 years) are not as trainable as are older youths. Increases in $\dot{V}O_2max$ for young children were in the range of 5% to 10%, rather than the 16% to 17% observed in older youths. One of the studies attempted to address directly the role of developmental stage as a determinant of endurance trainability. Weber[34] examined training in three different groups of twin boys, age 10, 13, and 16 years. Improvement in $\dot{V}O_2$max occurred in all three age groups, but the change was less than half as great in the middle age group. These results seem to support the notion that trainability is reduced during the transition period of pubescence.

## Gender

Since none of the studies reviewed attempted to compare trainability across the sexes, it is difficult to draw a conclusion regarding the role of gender differences. Only male subjects were used in nine studies and, among these, subjects from six showed trainability. Significant pre- to post-training changes were observed in three of the four studies using girls and boys. Only female subjects were used in one study,[30] and a significant 16% change in $\dot{V}O_2$max was reported. Based on this very limited analysis, gender does not appear to be an important determinant of trainability.

## Initial Fitness Level

Several authors have hypothesized that children might be less trainable than adults because of their relatively high initial fitness levels.[19, 26] In the present review, initial $\dot{V}O_2$max values ranged from 36.5 to 55.9 ml/kg/min. Interestingly, in the studies in which aerobic power was initially high (>53.0 ml/kg/hr), significant increases in $\dot{V}O_2$max were observed in every case. This was not true in studies in which the children had lower initial fitness levels ($\dot{V}O_2$max < 44.0 $ml \cdot kg^{-1} \cdot min^{-1}$). No firm conclusion can be drawn from this preliminary analysis except that children apparently can increase their maximal aerobic power with systemic training regardless of their initial $\dot{V}O_2$max level. It may be that the initial fitness level per se does not affect trainability; the initial level of habitual physical activity may be a more important factor. This theory has been discussed in a number of review papers,[26, 32] but no systematic study has been undertaken to evaluate its validity.

## Training Protocol

Another area which is questioned often in training studies is the appropriateness of the training stimulus. Was it of sufficient length (i.e., weeks or months)? Did it occur frequently enough (days/week)? Was the duration adequate (minutes/session)? Was it intense enough (% $\dot{V}O_2$max)? At present, there are no widely accepted standards for training protocols used with young people.[26, 32] When an attempt is made to establish minimal criteria for training, usually an adult standard has been applied.[3, 25] The potential importance of several key components of an endurance training regimen are examined as follows:

**Mode.**—In the studies reviewed, the mode of exercise did not seem to be a major determinant of the magnitude of the training adaptation. Three studies used cycling, with significant improvements in maximal aerobic power observed in each. Six studies used running (walk/jog); of these, five found significant improvements. Two studies demonstrated trainability using a combination of running, cycling, and stepping. One study used a swimming protocol and produced successful results even though measures were performed on the leg cycle. Docherty et al[10] used circuit weight training which included a cycling station, and the increase in $\dot{V}O_2$max was substantial (17% to 18%). The remaining study[15] was conducted during physical education classes and used a packaged aerobic training program ("Feeling Good"). Changes with that program were non-significant. It may be that a physical education curricular package, such as "Feeling Good," does not provide adequate stimulus to be classified as a training study. Of note, the average training heart rate was 165 beats/min in the "Feeling Good" group, while the control group (typical physical education class) had an average heart rate of 150 beats/min).

**Continuous vs. Interval Training.**—Type of training, described as either continuous or interval, has been targeted as a controversial aspect of endurance training in children.[26] The efficacy of interval training in children has been questioned because of its similarity to the spontaneous play (short bouts of high-intensity activity, followed by periods of rest) that is characteristic of youngsters. Four of the studies reviewed used an interval training approach—two with running,[24, 29] one with cycling,[14] and one with circuit weight training[10] which included a cycling station. Only one of these studies (running) failed to demonstrate trainability.[29] Seven of the nine studies using continuous aerobic training were able to produce a significant change in a measure of aerobic endurance. These observations suggest that both continuous and interval training can produce increased $\dot{V}O_2$max in youngsters.

**Length.**—The lengths of the training programs reviewed ranged from 4 weeks to 14 months. Four weeks was a period sufficient to produce an increased $\dot{V}O_2$max using the circuit weight training protocol of Docherty et al.[10] Using a more standard continuous cycling protocol, Massicotte and MacNab[20] observed an 11% increase in maximal aerobic power over a 6-week period. A similar finding was reported by both Gatch and Byrd,[14] and Becker and Vaccaro,[5] during 8-week training periods. However, one study, also 8 weeks in length, failed to demonstrate significant changes in $\dot{V}O_2$max.[29]

The study with the longest training period (14 months) did not demonstrate any significant alteration in aerobic power.[35] However, training did not occur weekly throughout this time period. The 5-day training group actually had 98 sessions, or an average of 20 weeks for the 5 sessions per week group. It is interesting to note that the training protocol of Ekblom[11] lasted 6 months, but did not produce a percent change in $\dot{V}O_2$max (+10%) greater than that observed in comparable studies of 6 or 8 weeks in length.

**Frequency and Duration.**—An examination of training outcomes as related to the frequency and duration of the training programs yields an equivocal finding. A 2-day per week protocol produced a significant training effect,[11] as did a 7-times per week protocol.[34] Of the 12 studies that used 3-, 4- or 5-days per week protocols, 9 demonstrated trainability and 3 did not.

The duration of training ranged from 5 to 10 minutes to 60 minutes per session. An analysis of the role of session length indicates that there was a greater chance of increasing aerobic fitness with programs that were 25 minutes or more in length (8 out of 9 demonstrated trainability) than with those that were less than 25 minutes (3 out of 5 demonstrated trainability).

**Intensity.**—In 4 of the studies reviewed, the intensity of training was not specified. Of the 10 studies that did quantify training intensity, levels ranged from 50% to 92% of maximal heart rate (HRmax). In the lower intensity ranges (85% HRmax and less), 5 of 7 studies demonstrated a significant increase in $\dot{V}O_2max$. At the higher range (> 85% HRmax), 2 of 4 training studies reported a significant increase in $\dot{V}O_2max$. Attempting to draw a firm conclusion based on this superficial examination of intensity is hazardous and probably is not appropriate at this time. It should be noted that most of the studies reviewed used percentages of HRmax that would be considered high by adult standards.

Only three of the studies reviewed for this paper failed to demonstrate trainability in their subjects. Gilliam and Freedson[15] used the "Feeling Good" program as the basis for their training protocol. As indicated earlier, the nature and amount of training stimulus provided by this physical education program probably was insufficient to induce changes in $\dot{V}O_2max$. However, the estimated intensity for this program was 79% HRmax.

In one of the remaining studies, Yoshida et al[35] estimated training heart rate to be approximately 88% of maximal for the 5-year-old children. The study employed continuous running for very short periods of time (initially 5 minutes, increasing to 10 minutes by the end of the training period) as the mode of training. Young children have higher maximum heart rates, making it necessary that the training heart rate be higher in order to elicit a training response. The short time period (almost interval in nature), the intensity level, and a questionable test protocol contribute to suspicion regarding this study's validity (see previous section).

The remaining study which failed to demonstrate trainability in youth was that of Stewart and Gutin.[29] Although intensity was estimated at 90% HRmax, the time spent exercising at this level was very short (34 minutes per week). The authors also used interval training, which is designed for short bursts of high intensity activity. It may be that the low number of minutes per week interacted with the nature of the training (work/rest intervals) and the selected intensity level to result in non-significant findings.

Two studies did compare different intensity levels. Using a walk/jog protocol, Savage[27] had subjects work at 50% and 85% HRmax. Both groups improved about 6% in $\dot{V}O_2max$. Massicotte and MacNab[20] compared three intensity levels and found that only in the highest intensity group (approximately 84% $\dot{V}O_2max$) were changes detectable in 12-year-old boys. It may be that intensity alone is an inadequate clue to differences in trainability, and age, type of training (interval/continuous), or other factors must be included also.

**Dosage Interactions.**—In an effort to clarify the sources of variance in training adaptations observed with various training protocols, it seems appropriate to examine the interaction between frequency and duration. It is likely, of course, that training outcomes in children are best related to total work done (i.e., energy expended) in the training program. Total work should be reasonably well related to the product of duration and frequency of training (minutes/week). This product was computed for the studies included in this review and, while somewhat helpful, the analysis was not conclusive. Of the training programs that provided 10 to 70 "session-minutes" per week, 50% induced significant increases in $\dot{V}O_2$max. Sixty percent of the protocols providing a training stimulus between 70 and 120 minutes per week induced an increase in $\dot{V}O_2$max. All of the training programs involving between 120 and 180 minutes per week were successful in increasing maximal power. Thus, there is an apparent association between the amount of training each week and changes in $\dot{V}O_2$max. It would be desirable to factor intensity into this analysis, but this was not attempted because intensity was not quantified precisely in many of the studies reviewed.

## Future Directions for Research on Trainability of Children

The preceding review indicates clearly that the current body of knowledge concerning the endurance exercise trainability of children is quite limited. The small number of well-controlled training studies leaves many gaps in our knowledge of the trainability of certain sub-groups of children, and in our understanding of the physiologic basis of the training adaptation in children. In this section we will identify important directions for future research on endurance training in children.

A clear deficiency in the current literature is the lack of studies on certain sub-groups of youngsters. Particularly notable is the small number of studies involving female subjects. It is often assumed that sex differences are of minimal significance before puberty, but are large and important after puberty. The endurance training literature, as it currently exists, does not allow these assumptions to be examined. A similar problem is apparent with adolescent youth. Despite the fact that massive numbers of adolescents engage in endurance exercise training in athletic programs, the current literature includes very few studies with adolescent subjects. The suspicion that postpubescent youths are more adaptive to training than are their prepubescent counterparts presently is just that—a suspicion. Future studies should focus directly on gender and developmental status as potential determinants of trainability. This could be approached by exposing, in the same studies, groups of prepubescent and postpubescent males and females to comparable training regimens. Such an approach has been employed very rarely in the past.

Over the past 3 decades a major focus of training studies in adults has been a description of the "dose-response" relationship. The goal has been to understand the nature and degree of adaptation that might be expected with various types of training protocols. This goal, which has been attained to a limited extent with adults,[22, 23] is a worthy one for children and youths as well. However, with youngsters it is presently a distant goal. Very few published studies have compared directly different modes, frequencies, durations, and intensities of training in children. Future studies should attempt to fill this void. In these studies it will be important that training programs be quantified carefully.

As is evident from a review of Tables 1 and 2, precise quantification of training procedures has not always been incorporated into studies of youngsters. A particularly important issue seems to be the extent to which training adaptations are related to intensity of exercise. A key question is whether there is an intensity threshold and, if so, whether this threshold is different from that seen in sedentary adults. Direct comparisons of training protocols using different and carefully quantified intensities with young subjects have been performed in only a few studies thus far.[20, 27] Over the years, a relatively large number of controlled training studies has been undertaken with adult subjects.[23] The accumulated findings and collective data generated by these studies greatly facilitate the generation of conclusions regarding the trainability of adults. Unfortunately, the pediatric exercise literature does not provide the luxury of replication at the present time. Consequently, conclusions cannot be drawn confidently about the levels of physiologic adaptation that are expected with various levels of training. The solution is to increase markedly the number of training studies which are undertaken with children and youths. Even small-scale studies will contribute importantly to the body of knowledge as long as they use appropriate research designs, carefully quantify training programs, and measure key variables (such as $\dot{V}O_2max$).

A somewhat surprising deficiency in the current pediatric exercise literature is a lack of knowledge of the expected changes in field performance measures that occur with endurance training. As demonstrated in Tables 1 and 2, few of the studies reviewed included performance measures such as the 1-mile run/walk.[24] This is regrettable, because such tests are used very commonly in assessing physical fitness in children. Often these tests are used in physical education programs to determine changes in physical fitness and are associated frequently with elaborate reward systems.[8] Because performance measures like the 1-mile run generally have not been measured in well-controlled training studies in children, little is known about the degree of change in gross endurance performance that accompanies an increase in physiologic measures such as $\dot{V}O_2max$. To remedy this deficiency, we recommend that future studies include measures like the 1-mile run in their procedures.

In contrast to the exercise literature on adults, training studies involving children and youths are notable for the infrequency with which underlying physiologic and biochemical mechanisms have been studied. It is understandable that investigators might be reluctant to apply invasive procedures such as muscle biopsies and vascular catheterizations on youthful subjects. Because of ethical considerations and concerns about subject recruitment, it seems likely that invasive procedures will continue to be used less frequently with children than adults. However, it should be noted that invasive procedures have been used in some studies of children.[12, 13] Unfortunately, these previously published studies have tended not to employ control groups. Thus, it is recommended that future studies employing invasive data collection procedures with youngsters also employ controlled research designs.

## Practical Application

The major, global conclusion of this review is that children and youths are physiologically adaptive to endurance exercise training. While there are currently many limitations and gaps in the relevant body of knowledge, there is compelling evidence to indicate that maximal aerobic power can be increased in youngsters via endurance training programs. In this section we reflect on the potential practical applications of this conclusion for practitioners who design and implement exercise regimens for children and youths.

Perhaps the most common setting for the delivery of structured exercise programs for youngsters is school physical education classes. The findings of this review indicate that the potential exists for children to improve endurance fitness in physical education. However, the feasibility of this actually occurring on a large scale is suspect. In the typical school physical education program, time is rather limited and objectives such as the promotion of motor skill acquisition tend to be given primary attention. As noted previously, the dose of exercise needed to increase $\dot{V}O_2$max in youngsters is substantial; in order to achieve such an increase, most of the available time in the physical education program would have to be committed to vigorous endurance exercise. This probably is not practical and may not be desirable from the standpoint of the effect on the child's attitude toward exercise. A reasonable compromise would be to dedicate substantial time to endurance training 4 to 5 week periods in physical education, perhaps once or twice per year. During these periods, much of the available physical education time would be dedicated to vigorous exercise. At other times such activity would be used less frequently and for shorter periods. With this approach, all youngsters would gain familiarity with appropriate exercise procedures and most would experience an increase in fitness (maximal aerobic power). Our review suggests that a few weeks of exposure to an adequate training stimulus is sufficient to produce a measurable training effect. At the present time, little is known about the long-term behavioral effects of participation in heavy endurance training programs during childhood. Therefore, we recommend that the results of this review be applied cautiously in school physical education programs.

Youth sport programs constitute the other major setting in which youngsters are exposed to endurance training programs. Available evidence indicates that young athletes can increase $\dot{V}O_2$max as long as the dose of training is adequate. While the precise dose needed has not been identified, it probably approximates three or more sessions per week in which high intensity activity is sustained for 30 or more minutes. Research has not yet provided a description of the relationship between change in $\dot{V}O_2$max and change in endurance performance. Likewise, we currently do not know whether or not youngsters are more or less trainable at certain phases of development, or what risks exist with overtraining. Therefore, youth sport coaches are advised to establish modest performance goals and to avoid extreme training programs for their young athletes.

## Summary

Our review of 14 well-designed training studies indicates that children and youths are physiologically adaptive to chronic endurance exercise. This is demonstrated principally by statistically significant increases in weight-relative maximal aerobic power in the training groups. Other conclusions, all of which must be considered tentative because of the small number of relevant studies, are as follows:

1. Percentage increases in $\dot{V}O_2$max elicited by endurance training appear to be smaller in youths than in adults, and may be somewhat smaller in younger children than in adolescents.
2. There is no clear gender difference in trainability.
3. Initial fitness level, quantified as $\dot{V}O_2$max ($ml \cdot kg^{-1} \cdot min^{-1}$), does not appear to be a major determinant of trainability in youngsters.
4. Young subjects appear to be physiologically adaptive to both interval and continuous training protocols and to programs using various modes of exercise.
5. There is some evidence that the magnitude of the training adaptation is related to the weekly training dose (frequency times duration of session), but the role of relative intensity is unclear.

Clearly, much more research is needed and should be focused in particular on (a) describing the dose-response relationship between training and change in $\dot{V}O_2$max, (b) examining the trainability of various sub-groups of youth, and (c) identifying the underlying physiological and biochemical mechanisms of the training adaptation in children.

## References

1. American Academy of Pediatrics: Physical fitness and the schools. *Pediatrics* 1987; 80:449–450.
2. American College of Sports Medicine: *Guidelines for Exercise Testing and Prescription,* 3rd ed. Philadelphia, Lea & Febiger, 1986.

3. American College of Sports Medicine: Opinion statement on physical fitness in children and youth. Med Sci Sports Exerc 1988; 20:422–423.
4. American College of Sports Medicine: Position statement on the recommended quantity and quality of exercise for developing and maintaining fitness in healthy adults. Med Sci Sports 1978; 10:vii–x.
5. Becker DM, Vaccaro P: Anaerobic threshold alterations caused by endurance training in young children. J Sports Med 1968; 23:445–449.
6. Committee on Exercise: Exercise Testing and Training of Apparently Healthy Individuals: A Handbook for Physicians. New York, American Heart Association, 1972.
7. Convertino VA, Brock PJ, Keil LC, et al: Exercise training-induced hypervolemia: Role of plasma albumin, renin and vasopressin. J Apply Physiol 1980; 48:655–699.
8. Corbin CB, Whitehead JR, Lovejon PY: Youth physical fitness awards. Quest 1988; 40:200–218.
9. Cunningham DA, Paterson DH, Blinkie CJR: The development of the cardiorespiratory system with growth and development, in Boileau RA (ed): Advances in Pediatric Sport Sciences, vol 1. Champaign, Ill, Human Kinetics, 1984.
10. Docherty D, Wenger HA, Collis ML: The effects of resistance training on aerobic and anaerobic power of young boys. Med Sci Sports Exerc 1987; 19:389–392.
11. Ekblom B: Effect of physical training in adolescent boys. J Appl Physiol 1969; 27:350–355.
12. Eriksson BO, Gollnick PD, Saltin B: Muscle metabolism and enzyme activities after training in boys 11–13 years old. Acta Physiol Scand 1973; 87:485–497.
13. Eriksson BO, Koch G: Effect of physical training on hemodynamic response during submaximal and maximal exercise in 11–14 year old boys. Acta Physiol Scand 1973; 87:27–39.
14. Gatch W, Byrd R: Endurance training and cardiovascular function in 9 and 10 year old boys. Arch Phys Med Rehabil 1979; 60:574–577.
15. Gilliam TB, Freedson PS: Effects of a 12 week school physical fitness program on peak $\dot{V}O_2$, body composition and blood lipids in 7–9 year old children. Int J Sports Med 1980; 1:73–78.
16. Hagberg JM, Goldring D, Ehsani AA, et al: Effect of exercise training on the blood pressure and hemodynamic features of hypertensive adolescents. Am J Cardiol 1983; 52:763–768.
17. Holloszy JO, Booth FW: Biochemical adaptations to endurance exercise in muscle. Ann Rev Physiol 1976; 38:273–291.
18. Kobayashi K, Kitamura K, Miura M, et al: Aerobic power as related to body growth and training in Japanese boys; a longitudinal study. J Appl Physiol 1978; 4:666–672.
19. Lussier L, Buskirk E: Effects of an endurance training regimen on assessment of work capacity in prepubertal children. Ann NY Acad Sci 1977; 301:734–747.
20. Massicotte DR, MacNab RB: Cardiorespiratory adaptation to training at specified intensities in children. Med Sci Sports Exerc 1979; 6:242–246.
21. Mirwald RL, Bailey DA: Maximal Aerobic Power. London, Sports Dynamics, 1986.
22. Pollock ML: How much exercise is enough? Physician Sportsmed 1978; 6:50–74.

23. Pollock ML: The quantification of endurance training programs, in Wilmore JH (ed): New York, Academic Press, *Exercise and Sport Sciences Reviews,* vol 1. 1973.
24. Rotstein A, Dotan R, Bar-Or O, et al: Effects of training on anaerobic threshold, maximal aerobic power and anaerobic performance of pre-adolescent boys. *Int J Sports Med* 1986; 7:281–286.
25. Rowland TW: Aerobic response to endurance training in prepubescent children: A critical analysis. *Med Sci Sports Exerc* 1985; 17:493–497.
26. Sady SP: Cardiorespiratory exercise training in children. *Clin Sports Med* 1986; 5:493–514.
27. Savage MP, Petratis MM, Thomson WH, et al: Exercise training effects on serum lipids of prepubescent boys and adult men. *Med Sci Sports Exerc* 1986; 18:197–204.
28. Scheuer J, Tipton LM: Cardiovascular adaptation to physical training. *Ann Rev Physiol* 1977; 39:221–251.
29. Stewart KJ, Gutin B: Effects of physical training on cardiorespiratory fitness in children. *Res Quart* 1976; 47:110–120.
30. Stransky AW, Mickelson RJ, Van Fleet C, et al: Effects of a swimming training regimen on hematological, cardiorespiratory and body composition changes in young females. *J Sports Med Phys Fitness* 1979; 19:347–354.
31. US Department of Health and Human Services: *Promoting Health/Preventing Disease: Objectives for the Nation.* Washington, US Government Printing Office, 1980.
32. Vaccaro P, Mahon A: Cardiorespiratory response to endurance training in children. *Sports Med* 1987; 4:352–363.
33. Van Dalen DB, Mitchell ED, Bennett BC: *A World History of Physical Education.* Englewood Cliffs, New Jersey, Prentice-Hall, Inc, 1953.
34. Weber G, Kartodihardjo W, Klissouras V: Growth and physical training with reference to heredity. *J Appl Physiol* 1976; 40:211–215.
35. Yoshida T, Ishiko I, Muraoka I: Effect of endurance training on cardiorespiratory function of 5 year old children. *Int J Sports Med* 1980; 1:91–94.

# Resistance Training for Youth

## Patty S. Freedson, Ph.D.

Associate Professor, University of Massachusetts, Department of Exercise Science, Amherst, Massachusetts

## Ann Ward, Ph.D.

Assistant Professor, Co-director, Exercise Physiology and Nutrition Laboratory, University of Massachusetts Medical Center, Division of Cardiovascular Medicine, Worcester, Massachusetts

## James M. Rippe, M.D.

Associate Professor, Director, Exercise Physiology and Nutrition Laboratory, University of Massachusetts Medical Center, Division of Cardiovascular Medicine, Worcester, Massachusetts

## Editor's Introduction

Another controversial area in youth sport is the issue of resistance training for children and youth. The authors employ a unique perspective as they address the issue. They summarize major points from recent position papers, and provide evidence from recent studies to support or refute the positions. They conclude with recommendations regarding the use of resistance exercise as a training modality for children and youth.

*Brian J. Sharkey, Ph.D.*

Resistance training for youth recently has become more popular as a means of enhancing fitness. While numerous studies examine the effects of resistance training on the muscular strength and endurance of adults, research regarding children is less prevalent. Despite this paucity of data, however, two position papers recently have been published concerning the potential positive and negative effects of resistance training and weight lifting for children.[1, 2] As few experimental studies examining the validity of some of the claims contained in these position papers have been published, researchers have begun to explore these issues in an effort to derive valid guidelines and principles.

This review will summarize the major points described in these position statements and provide evidence from the research literature which either supports or refutes the opinions described. To clarify these interpretations, this review first will define some of the more common terms employed in the resistance training literature. Based on the studies described and the interpretation of the results, several recommendations will be presented regarding the use of resistance exercise as a training modality for youth.

## Definition of Terms

Historically, resistance training has employed a variety of different techniques. Ten to 20 years ago, free weights and one's own body weight were the only types of resistance used in resistance training programs. Today, resistance training has taken on characteristics associated with high technology and may involve machine-based systems where weight plates, hydraulics, water, and/or cam systems provide the resistance. A computer system may even control the workout according to the individual's strength level and overall training goals. However, all of these programs produce the desired outcome of increased muscular strength and endurance.

The definitions provided below clarify the many different types of resistance training programs and the different types of contractions that can be done during resistance exercise:

1. Resistance training—regular exercise that involves repetitive movement against an opposing force.
2. Power lifting—a weight-lifting competition to determine the maximum amount of weight an individual can lift for a specific set of lifts.
3. Isometric contraction—muscle does not change in overall length during the contraction; muscle works against a force that is greater than the strength of the muscle; it is generally done at one angle within a range of motion.
4. Isotonic contraction—muscle works against a resistance that remains constant throughout a range of motion.
5. Concentric contraction—the muscle-shortening phase of an isotonic contraction, i.e., biceps shortening during a biceps flexion movement.
6. Eccentric contraction—the muscle-lengthening phase of an isotonic contraction, i.e., biceps lengthening during a biceps extension movement.
7. Isokinetic contraction—muscle works against a variable resistance that accommodates different strength levels of a given muscle or muscle group at the different points in a range of motion; speed of movement remains constant and there can be maximal overload to the muscle throughout the range of motion.

## Effects of Resistance Training on Strength in Prepubescent Children

The research studies examining the effects of resistance training in prepubescent youth have used predominantly machine-based circuit training with either weight plates, or pneumatic or hydraulic resistance. For young children, these techniques are the most practical since they are relatively safe, easy to use, and require no detailed instruction on proper lifting mechanics. On the other hand, most machine-based systems have been designed for adults. Therefore, small children may have difficulty executing the exercises properly because they do not fit the machines.

Several questions arise regarding resistance training in children. Is it necessary to have children participate in resistance training programs? Is the development of strength through specially designed programs needed for overall fitness development in youth? Don't children participate in adequate amounts of free play activity that promotes strength development? These are all logical questions, and the answers are not readily apparent. When the term overall fitness is applied to an adult, strength is definitely a component which is emphasized as part of "getting in shape." For example, it is known that if an adult does not maintain a certain level of physical activity, his or her capacity to perform work will decline with age. In contrast, in the context of fitness development, a child is an individual who is already fairly active and has not begun to experience any age-related decline in physical activity.

However, if one examines the descriptive research literature on health-related fitness test results for youth, some astounding findings emerge. For example, Part I of the National Children and Youth Fitness study[3] reveals a rather sad state of affairs for upper body strength in youth. This study reports that over 30% of 10- to 11-year-old boys and 60% of 10- to 18-year-old girls were unable to perform one chin-up. These results have led researchers to consider the use of alternative methods of assessing upper body strength in an effort to reduce the incidence of zero scores. More importantly, these results verify the fact that upper body strength among youth is poor. While it is necessary to develop and validate a test that allows a measurement of upper body strength to be obtained, these data strongly point to the need to develop appropriate and safe resistance training programs for youth in an effort to enhance muscular strength and endurance.

One of the first scientific studies to investigate the effects of resistance training on strength in prepubescent and pubescent boys was conducted by Vrijens.[4] The training was 8 weeks in duration and consisted of one set of 8 to 12 isotonic repetitions performed at 75% of one repetition maximum (RM) (1 RM = maximum load that can be lifted one time), three times per week. Strength changes were assessed isometrically using six different strength tests. Significant gains in all strength tests and lean body mass were observed among the pubescent children, whereas only increases in isometric strength were demonstrated by prepubescent children in the 6 tests. The differential effects of resistance training between the prepubescent and pubescent groups led to the conclusion that the hormonal changes that accompany maturation are necessary to elicit increases in muscle mass and strength. However, several subsequent investigations have found that resistance training can elicit strength gains in prepubescent children similar to those which have been observed in older children.

Pfeiffer and Francis[5] evaluated the effects of 9 weeks of resistance training performed three times per week using Universal equipment and free weights. Thirty-three prepubescent, pubescent, and postpubescent males completed the resistance training intervention and 31 similarly-aged children served as controls. The training intensity used the following system of progressive overload: three sets at each of four stations (two upper body and two lower body exercises) where set 1 was at 50% of 10 RM, set 2 was 75% of 10 RM, and set 3 was at 100% of 10 RM. These exercise stations specifically exercised the muscle groups that were evaluated in the strength testing. At five other stations, one set of each exercise was completed (three upper body exercises, one lower body exercise, and a sit-up station).

The upper and lower extremity flexor and extensor strength changes associated with the training were measured by determining maximum concentric torque (Cybex evaluation) at velocities of 30 degrees per second and 120 degrees per second (three trials at each velocity). Strength changes were expressed as a percent increase, and all strength scores were expressed relative to body weight. While all measures are not statistically significant between groups, flexor and extensor torque increased from 10.6% to 17.0% in the elbow and from 1.4% to 25.8% in the knee for the experimental group. In contrast to the Vrijens study,[4] no consistent differences were found in torque gains between the prepubescent, pubescent, and postpubescent children.

Sewall and Micheli[6] also showed prepubescent children to have significant gains in strength consequent to 9 weeks of pneumatic resistance training (Nautilus and Cam II). The training regimen was 3 days per week, for 25 to 30 minutes per session using a total of 10 subjects. Each participant completed three sets each on a thigh press, a chest press, and a back row machine, and intensity was changed progressively by increasing the resistance when the participant could complete 12 repetitions at a predetermined 10-RM level. Gains in knee and shoulder extension and flexion strength were measured with a cable tensiometer (isometric measure) which measured strength at only a single angle for each joint. Even though the mode of training was dynamic in nature, the static measures of strength increased an average of 43% in comparison to a control group (8 subjects) in which they increased 9.5% ($P<.05$ between groups). However, these results are somewhat misleading. An examination of the individual strength test results reveals that only shoulder flexion increased significantly more for the experimental group than for the control group. Thus, there were no significant differences between groups for knee extension, knee flexion, and shoulder extension.

Another training study which examined prepubertal boys (6 to 11 years of age) using Hydra-Fitness equipment (hydraulic resistance and only concentric contractions) as the training modality, demonstrated large improvements in strength and vertical jump.[7] In addition to the long training program in this study (14 weeks), the intensity of the workouts was greater, since the 10-station circuit was completed three times and each exercise was performed at maximal effort for 30 seconds. In this investigation, strength was measured isokinetically at 30 and 90 degrees per second for the concentric component of arm and leg flexion and extension. Only concentric torque changes were evaluated, since the training consisted only of concentric contractions.

Strength measures for the experimental group (16 subjects) increased significantly (18.6% for knee extension at 90 degrees per second), while those for the control group (10 subjects) generally remained within 6% of the pre-training baseline measures. Maximum oxygen consumption for the experimental group (ml/kg of body weight/min) increased significantly (13.8%) over the control group (decrease of 5.4%). Vertical jump increased by 2.2 cm (10.4%), which was significantly different than the control group, where a decrease of 3.0% was observed.

In a short-term training study, no significant improvements in anaerobic power were observed after 4 weeks of hydraulic resistance training (Hydra-Fitness equipment) in 10- to 14-year-old boys.[8] Training was performed three times per week and consisted of two sets of 20 seconds each of maximal effort with 20 seconds of rest between sets. The specific exercises included leg flexion/extension, arm abduction/adduction, thigh flexion/extension, military press/flexion, bench press/flexion, and cycle ergometry. The subjects were separated into three groups: control (n=11); experimental high velocity, low resistance training (n=11); and experimental low velocity, high resistance training (n=12). Anaerobic power of the legs, measured using a modified Wingate Test protocol, did not improve in either of the training groups. In contrast, aerobic power (ml/kg of body weight/min) improved significantly for the training groups by 17% to 18% even though the training was only 4 weeks long and was not the type typically associated with aerobic changes.

The apparent discrepancy between the results of Vrijens[4] and those of the other investigators[5–8] is due to the magnitude of the training load as well as to the methods employed to evaluate strength changes. That is, Vrijens' training program involved only one set performed three times per week for 8 weeks.[4] Although the training duration may not have been much longer in the other studies, the volume per training session was much greater. Specifically, the number of sets and/or repetitions and/or the intensity of the workouts was higher.[5–8] Moreover, Vrijens[4] used isometric strength measures which may not have been sensitive to more generalized strength gains in the prepubescent children.

The evidence is clearer that resistance training increases strength in pubescent children. As early as 1958, researchers demonstrated a 40% increase in the number of chin-ups completed and a 100% increase in the number of push-ups completed following an 8-week (3 days/week) resistance training program (12 to 17 year old boys, n=22).[9] More recently, Sailors and Berg[10] reported that an 8-week (3 days/week) resistance training program elicited 19% to 48% increases in muscular strength in 5 adolescent boys as measured by the maximum weight that could be lifted five times (5 RM).

In 1985, the National Strength and Conditioning Association (NSCA) published their "Position Paper on Prepubescent Strength Training."[1] This paper was an important contribution to the literature, particularly for the coach and young athlete, as it presented a series of recommendations based on a critical analysis of other opinion statements and careful interpretation of the research literature pertaining to resistance training for youth. What is clearly evident from this paper is that there are a very limited number of research studies that have examined the effects of resistance training on strength and other related physiological measures among prepubescent children. One of the factors that is partly responsible for the limited amount of research on this topic is the notion that prepubescent children cannot increase strength with resistance training because they lack adequate concentrations of circulating androgens. If this belief is correct, then it is not surprising that the consequences of resistance training among prepubescent children have not been examined thoroughly.

Interestingly, the opinion of the American Academy of Pediatrics' Committee on Sports Medicine is that prepubescent children engaged in weight training cannot increase strength because they lack sufficient androgens.[2] Apparently they base this opinion on the belief that it is necessary to increase the size of the muscle in order to increase strength, and that this can occur only in the presence of adequate levels of circulating androgens. However, there are several reports which clearly indicate that the muscle size to muscle strength relationship is not a direct cause and effect phenomenon, nor is muscle size precisely correlated with muscle strength.[11-13] In fact, Weltman et al.[7] investigated the effects of resistance training on prepubescent children with the hypothesis that these children could get stronger despite the fact that they lacked the androgens typically associated with the stimulus for muscle size gains. They suggested that gains in strength may be of neuromuscular origin. Although this study did not measure neuromuscular indices of strength, such as motor unit recruitment, it was proposed that the strength gains observed in the Weltman et al[7] investigation were mediated neurally, since the muscle size did not change and androgen levels were low. Further compelling evidence in opposition to the American Academy of Pediatrics' Opinion Statement is that most of the other investigations examining the effects of resistance training in prepubescent children also demonstrate significant gains in strength.[5-7]

In a more critical evaluation of the NSCA "Position Paper on Prepubescent Strength Training," the only data to support the "facts" presented in their paper relate to the effects of resistance training on strength development. The other supposed benefits and risks outlined are based on an interpretation of data not necessarily obtained from prepubescent children. For example, the position paper states that it is "well documented" that strength training reduces the risk for musculoskeletal injury in postpubescent children and adults. However, only one study is referenced to support this observation. Moreover, the study that is cited has some major experimental design problems that influence interpretation of the results. In this study, Hejna and Rosenberg[14] indicate that the injury rate among non–weight-trained athletes was 72.4% (20 out of 29 athletes were injured). In contrast, the injury rate for the weight-trained athletes was 26.2% (61 out of 232 athletes were injured). It cannot be determined how the subjects were placed into the different groups. Perhaps the control group (non–weight-trained) had a history of injury that was greater than that of the weight-trained athletes. In addition, the sample sizes between the groups were very different, making the percent differences in injury rates possibly misleading.

The belief that strength training reduces the risk of injury is intuitively logical. However, the data to support this position in regard to prepubescent children are not available. Thus, the statement concerning injury reduction certainly must be considered premature. The guidelines summarizing the factors that should be considered when designing and implementing a strength training program for prepubescent children are presented with safety in mind. For example, it is recommended that: (1) prepubescent children never train alone; (2) training sessions be preceded by a warm-up; (3) proper technique be maintained; and (4) emphasis be placed on high repetition (6 to 15 reps), low resistance workouts. These issues are important to minimize the risk of injury and to maximize enjoyment and participation for prepubescent children involved in resistance training programs.

## Recommendations for Resistance Training for Youth

Based on the evidence available in the literature, it is clear that muscular strength gains will occur among children who participate in a well-planned resistance training program. The exact mechanism that induces these changes is not totally clear. It appears to be, in part, neurally mediated since muscle size is not affected, particularly among prepubescent children. Whether or not strength training actually aids in reducing the incidence of musculoskeletal injury has not been established, but it certainly seems reasonable to predict that if a muscle or muscle group is stronger, its susceptibility to injury may be reduced. This hypothesis requires further investigation before a specific cause and effect can be confirmed.

The following points summarize guidelines that should be followed when implementing a resistance training program for children:

1. The focus of the resistance training should be on a high number of repetitions and low resistance. For example, a set should consist of 8 to 12 repetitions (8 to 12 RM) for upper body exercises and 15 to 20 repetitions (15 to 20 RM) for lower body exercises.[11] The best technique to establish the resistance that a child can lift the specified number of times (e.g., 12 repetitions) is trial and error. For example, if the prescribed regimen calls for a 12-RM set, a resistance should be set that is thought to allow the

child to lift 12 times. If that resistance is too light and the child can actually do 15 repetitions, the weight should be increased and the resistance re-evaluated.

2. If the mode of exercise is with hydraulic, isokinetic, or pneumatic devices, then it will not be necessary to establish appropriate resistances since these modes of exercise are designed so that maximal effort is maintained. In other words, the resistance offered accommodates the force applied. Although a maximal effort is required with this type of loading, there is no evidence available that indicates any increased risk of injury. Apparently the nature of the accommodating maximal effort is "safer" than the type of maximal effort required by the free weight 1 RM. It has been recommended that young children not participate in maximal efforts because of the increased risk of injury.[1]

3. As a training effect occurs, it is recommended that the overload be increased first by increasing the number of repetitions, then by increasing the absolute resistance. In other words, the number of repetitions should be increased to the maximum (e.g., if the repetition range is 8 to 12, the overload should be increased to 12 repetitions), and then the weight should be increased so that the number of repetitions is at the minimum level (e.g., 8 repetitions).[11]

4. It is recommended that 1 to 3 sets of approximately 6 to 10 different exercises be done in a workout where the muscle groups being exercised include both the upper and lower body in an alternating sequence. Two to 3 sessions per week is recommended with at least 1 day of rest between workouts.[11]

5. Each workout should be preceded by a warm-up that may include stretching exercises as well as unloaded or very lightly loaded resistance exercises.

6. Resistance training programs should be supervised closely and monitored carefully. Moreover, all participants should be instructed on the proper lifting techniques and breathing techniques (e.g., no breath-holding to minimize the risk of fainting). The safety of the participants should be of foremost concern.

Muscular strength and endurance are very significant parts of total fitness for people of all ages. Development of these areas should not be neglected for children, since exercise training studies clearly have demonstrated that significant improvements can be obtained. In addition, if the programs are designed properly and appropriate modes of resistance are employed, there does not seem to be an increased risk of injury. The development of muscular strength and endurance should begin to receive widespread attention as part of an overall effort to promote total fitness for youth.

## References

1. National Strength and Conditioning Association: Position paper on prepubescent strength training. *NSCA J* 1985; 7:27–31.

2. American Academy of Pediatrics: Weight training and weightlifting: Information for the pediatrician. *Physician Sportsmed* 1983; 11:157–161.
3. Ross JG, Gilbert GG: National children and youth fitness study. A summary of findings. *J Phys Ed Rec Dance* 1985; 56:45–50.
4. Vrijens J: Muscle strength development in the pre- and post-pubescent age. *Med Sport* 1978; 11:152–158.
5. Pfeiffer RD, Francis RS: Effects of strength training on muscle development in prepubescent, pubescent and postpubescent males. *Physician Sportsmed* 1986; 14:134–143.
6. Sewall L, Micheli LJ: Strength training for children. *J Pediatr Orthop* 1986; 6:143–146.
7. Weltman A, Janney C, Rians CB, et al: The effects of hydraulic resistance strength training in pre-pubescent males. *Med Sci Sports Exerc* 1986; 18:629–638.
8. Docherty D, Wenger HA, Collis ML: The effects of resistance training on aerobic and anaerobic power of young boys. *Med Sci Sports Exerc* 1987; 19:389–392.
9. Kusinitz I, Keeney CE: Effects of progressive weight training on health and physical fitness of adolescent boys. *Res Quart* 1958; 29:294–301.
10. Sailors M, Berg K: Comparison of responses to weight training in pubescent boys and men. *J Sports Med* 1987; 27:30–37.
11. Sale DG: Strength training in children, in Gisolfi C, Lamb, DR (eds): *Perspectives in Exercise Science and Sports Medicine: Youth, Exercise and Sport.* Indianapolis, Benchmark Press, Inc, 1989, pp 165–222.
12. Coyle EF, Feiring DC, Rotkis TC, et al: Specificity of power improvements through slow and fast isokinetic training. *J Appl Physiol Respir Environ Exerc Physiol* 1981; 51:1437–1442.
13. Hakkinen K, Komi PV: Electromyographic changes during strength training and detraining. *Med Sci Sports Exerc* 1983; 15:455–460.
14. Hejna WF, Rosenberg A, Buturusis DJ, et al: Prevention of sports injuries in high school students through strength training. *NSCA J* 1982; 4:28–31.

**Part II**

# *Medical Disorders*

Edited by
JOHN A. LOMBARDO, M.D.

# Pre-Participation Evaluation of the Young Athlete

## Keith Stanley, M.D.

Eastern Oklahoma Orthopedic and Sports Medicine Center, Tulsa, Oklahoma

## Editor's Introduction

The pre-participation evaluation of the young athlete is an exercise that faces all physicians involved in the care of athletes. There have been many variations of the evaluation from the locker room lineups to various sophisticated station examinations.

Dr. Stanley has very thoroughly reviewed the available literature on this topic. He presents it in a very practical manner which will be useful to any practitioner involved in sports medicine.

This represents yet another step towards a universally accepted pre-participation evaluation of athletes.

*John A. Lombardo, Ph.D.*

It is interesting to note that health care of the healthy adolescent population in the United States is largely crisis oriented. The only youths who have regular encounters with a physician generally are those with congenital or chronic medical illnesses (such as congenital heart disease, type I diabetes, mellitus and asthma). The only exceptions to this rule are the pre-participation physical examinations which are performed on the more than 20 million young people who are involved in organized athletics. As a result, interest in this examination is increasing among team physicians and the other health care professionals who are involved in the care of young athletes in this country.

The importance of the pre-participation physical examination was recognized by the American Medical Association's Committee on Medical Aspects of Sports as evidenced by their statement that every athlete has the right to a thorough pre-season evaluation.[1] While most physicians agree on the necessity of an examination, there are many controversies and conflicts regarding the content of the pre-participation evaluation and the best way in which to conduct it. As a result, this examination has undergone quite an evolution over the last several years. Many sports medicine physicians, including this author, remember the locker room line-up exam.

Fortunately, this has evolved into a better organized and even sports-specific examination. In many areas of the country, the examination now includes the expertise not only of primary care physicians but also of those in all specialties, both in and out of the sports medicine arena. Some athletic programs even include exercise physiologists, physical therapists, and athletic trainers to evaluate performance and maturity components.

In this chapter, I will attempt to synthesize the research and historical data that have altered the sports medicine physician's perspective on the purpose and utility of the pre-participation sports examination.

Several authors have offered statements concerning the purpose or goal of this examination.* Most agree that, in general terms, the focal purpose of the exam is to ensure the health and safety of the athlete. In his review, Jones[15] noted that examining and profiling young athletes involves gathering medical and physiological information that will help determine each child's suitability for participation in sports activities. Linder et al[18] state that the major purpose of the pre-participation examination is to screen for conditions that could predispose the athlete to injury or death. Evaluating health risks and relieving the school systems of the legal implications of sports participation by their students were applications of the exam noted by Rowland.[28] In Runyan's review,[29] he noted that some authors want the examination to serve as a comprehensive interval evaluation; however, this does not appear to be the prevailing attitude among most sports medicine physicians. In their statement, Strong and Linder[33] include the identification of conditions that need rehabilitation before sports participation as well as matching young athletes with an appropriate sport or position as important features of the exam. Lombardo[19] summarizes the purposes of the pre-participation examination very nicely in the following six points: (1) to detect additional risks; (2) to detect medical contraindications; (3) to indicate which sports are safe for the individual; (4) to serve as a limited general health screening; (5) to meet legal and insurance requirements; and (6) to evaluate maturation.

As can be seen from these statements, the purpose of the pre-participation sports examination has undergone significant transition. With the increasing interest in identifying conditions which require rehabilitation before performance and in obtaining performance measurements, it appears that the evolution of the pre-participation examination will continue for some time.

All states require that physical examinations be performed before young athletes participate in interscholastic sports in order to identify conditions that may increase the risk of injury.[9] Feinstein et al[11] conducted a survey of all 50 states and the District of Columbia. Out of the 45 replies that he received, he found that 35 states require a yearly examination, 3 states require an examination every 3 years, 1 state requires examination only once, and 6 did not specify their requirements.

Several authors now have spoken out in support of requiring only two

*See references 6, 14, 15, 18, 19, 28, 29, 31, 33, and 39.

comprehensive examinations, one to be performed in junior high and one in senior high, and annual medical history reviews. If the history indicates something of significance or if there is an injury, a medically specific examination then is recommended. Risser et al[27] found that, because of the low frequency of significant findings and unfavorable cost-benefit ratio of annual examinations, the University Interscholastic League recommended that the annual exam be required only once or twice in the secondary school years. In the American Academy of Pediatrics publication, Smith[31] proposes that examinations be performed every 2 years. Other authors support similar requirements.[19, 39] Wood[39] describes a pilot program in which examinations are done once in junior high and once in senior high, with the school nurse conducting annual reviews of the medical histories. The school nurse then refers athletes with significant interval histories to a physician. Therefore, while most states still require an annual examination, there is a growing body of data and an increasing number of sports medicine physicians advocating a reduction in the frequency of the pre-participation examination to twice during the secondary school years. Exceptions would be made for those athletes who experience an illness or injury which would require an updated examination.

Other data which support less frequent pre-participation examinations are those of Thompson et al,[36] who found that only 1.2% of 2,670 athletes had medical problems that excluded them from sports participation. During 2 consecutive years, Linder et al[18] found that none of 562 athletes were diagnosed with an exclusionary illness or injury the first year, and only 2 (0.3%) of 706 athletes were excluded from sports participation the following year. Out of 701 athletes in a study done by Goldberg et al,[12] only 1.3% were excluded from sports participation. Thus, because of the low frequency of significant findings, the impetus is to move away from the traditional annual pre-participation examination.

The pre-participation examination also has undergone a significant evolution in the manner in which it is conducted. The three most commonly identified means of conducting the examination are having it performed by the personal family physician, having it performed as a locker room examination, and having it performed through a station-type method. However, most sports medicine physicians feel that the locker room examination has no place in the evaluation of athletes. Although many authors point out that an examination performed by the family physician offers the advantages of continuity of care, a readily available complete medical history, and better doctor-athlete rapport,[5, 6, 19, 28, 33] there can be drawbacks to this type of examination. Lombardo[19] notes that the accuracy of this type of examination may be limited by the level of interest and knowledge of the private physician. Strong and Linder[33] indicate that the exam by the private physician may not be sports-oriented or sports-specific and all too often may be performed in a cursory manner.[33]

The group or station method appears to be the type favored by most sports medicine physicians. It is possible to include specialty physicians as well as flexibility and performance testing in this type of examination, and it also appears to be more sports oriented.[35] In addition, there is at least one study that would indicate that this type of examination is more sensitive in uncovering significant illness or injury.[5] DuRant et al[5] found that fewer diagnoses were recognized with single physician examinations than with multiple physicians examinations done in a station-type method. Multiple examiners found a higher percentage of abnormalities on 20 of 21 examination categories. The differences were statistically significant in six categories. These included diagnoses relating to the mouth, teeth, hips, thighs, knees, and ankles. They also noted that only 2.4% of athletes seen by a single physician were referred for further evaluation compared to 6.4% of those seen by multiple physicians. This study lends support to the station method of examination.

There is general agreement among sports physicians regarding the timing of the pre-participation examination. Most indicate that it is best to do the examinations or medical history reviews (if an institution is not doing annual examinations) 6 to 8 weeks prior to the beginning of the sports season.[17, 19, 31, 32, 33, 36] In most cases, this leaves adequate time for any additional evaluations that may be indicated. It also gives the athlete time to rehabilitate an injury or illness prior to the start of the season. Special cases may arise in which an athlete may need to be evaluated much earlier than 6 to 8 weeks prior to the start of the season. This would be true especially in cases of significant surgery involving the musculoskeletal system. Thus, it is important for the sports physician to have a close working relationship with the coaching staff and athletic trainer.

Obtaining a complete medical history is important in every area of medical care and this is no exception in the sports pre-participation examination. Runyan[29] indicates that the sports medical history should have a limited scope and should attempt to identify those conditions which are significant to sports participation. Taken in this manner, a medical history can be brief yet effective in identifying potential problems.

Ascertaining accurate information regarding an athlete's medical history can prove difficult. The athlete himself may neglect to indicate on the history form an illness or injury which he fears might exclude him from participation. He also may not deem significant something that may, in fact, be essential to his protection or rehabilitation. Another problem may lie in discrepancies between the medical history provided by the athlete and that provided by the parent. In a study by Risser et al,[27] only 39% of the athlete's histories agreed with those of their parents. Another problem that may sabotage the acquisition of a good medical history can be the inability of the athlete and/or his parents to read or understand the history form. With illiteracy as high as 25% to 30% in some areas, this can present a significant problem.[27] A solution may lie in having one station in the examination include a physician who takes the history.[18, 27] Smith[31] suggests that history-taking be assisted by either a physician, a nurse, or a trainer; Wood[39] utilized the school nurses to obtain the medical history in his program.

Other side issues may be important in the medical history. As Lombardo[19] indicates, it is very important to ascertain a history of chemical or substance abuse in a young athlete. He also notes that obtaining a menstrual history in female athletes may be critical in view of the growing concern regarding bone density and the prevention of osteoporosis in women. The medical history should also include questions concerning the potential existence of eating disorders.

Overall, most sports physicians agree that the medical history should be sports-specific and include certain targeted areas. Areas most often noted include musculoskeletal injuries, neurologic injuries, infectious diseases, cardiac diseases, pulmonary diseases, hospitalizations, medicine allergies, and surgeries.[5, 9, 29, 31, 33] In their study, Strong and Linder[33] indicated that the most frequently reported problems in the medical history were previous injury, hospitalization, and joint problems.

Many authors have formulated medical history forms that include those items which they feel are important.[5, 15, 17, 31, 32, 33] Feinstein et al.[11] found that 25 states have a standardized medical history questionnaire. While medical history forms do vary, they all have several areas that consistently appear to be viewed as significant by sports physicians. A history of sudden death or myocardial infarction in family members under the ageo of 50 years is found in most forms. This means of discovering an athlete with hypertrophic-obstructive cardiomyopathy[3, 8, 20, 22, 23, 24, 34] may be more sensitive even than the physical examination. The responses obtained to an inquiry regarding syncope or near-syncope, during exercise is deemed important. The ability to complete a quarter- or half-mile run without stopping is also questioned on most forms. The inclusion of questions concerning arrhythmias, murmurs, hypertension, and previous cardiac surgery on these forms is vital. All of these are necessary for proper screening of an athlete's cardiovascular medical history.

A neurological history is also critical, especially as it pertains to head and neck injuries. Since a neurologic deficit can occur from the cumulative effect of cerebral contusions, specific questions should be addressed to the athlete concerning any loss of consciousness associated with head injury or any history of diagnosed concussions. A history of a seizure disorder should prompt inquiries about medication, since the maintenance of good seizure control must be established.

Most forms contain inquiries about infectious diseases, but no specific diseases usually are mentioned. This places the onus on the examiner to be specific and inquisitive about infectious diseases.

The most significant history in regard to pulmonary disease in the athletic population would be that of asthma or exercise-induced bronchospasm. If the medical history is positive for either of these conditions, the examiner should inquire about any medications being used and their availability during practices and events should they be needed.

Inquiries should be made regarding medications being taken, medication allergies, and environmental allergies. One question that rarely is found on medical history forms for athletes is the presence of allergies to insect stings. In view of the life-threatening potential of these allergies, this should be included, especially for those athletes involved in outdoor sports.

Surgeries should be recorded; if any are recent, a proper release should be obtained from the surgeon of record to be included in the athlete's health record.

Any history of chronic illness should be elucidated. If such exists, and requires constant monitoring (such as is the case with diabetes mellitus), the medication history is necessary.

The musculoskeletal history is of utmost importance when evaluating the athlete. A history of sprains, strains, dislocations, or fractures involving the musculoskeletal system are reported often in the pre-participation examination. DuRant et al[5] found the most frequent problems discovered in the health history to be previous fractures (22.1%). Other injuries involving the musculoskeletal system comprised 20.9% of the responses. The examiner eliciting the medical history should indicate clearly any previous musculoskeletal injuries. This provides the physician doing the orthopedic examination the indication to give special attention to these areas of previous injury.

There are many other questions that may be included in the medical history. However, it should be kept in mind that the questionnaire should be sports-specific, easily understood, and constructed for efficient utility by the athlete and the examiner. Table 1 is a compilation of sports medical history questions that this author views as significant. While this list is not comprehensive, the questions listed should be found consistently on all medical history formats.

The importance of the medical history for sports participation is underscored by the results of two studies worthy of note. Risser et al.[27] found that 67% of all medical problems and 63% of all orthopedic problems were referred after being noted in the history. Goldberg et al[12] similarly found that 74% of significant medical and orthopedic problems were reported. Further, in Goldberg's study, 7 of 9 athletes excluded from participation would have been so excluded on the basis of the history alone.

Many have recommended that the pre-participation physical examination be sports-specific.[15, 17, 33] Since most significant findings on the sports pre-participation physical examination involve the musculoskeletal system, emphasis should be placed on this area of the examination.[5, 27, 28, 36] This will be addressed in more detail later. Another area of emphasis should be the cardiovascular examination, since most causes of sudden death are cardiac in origin[3, 8, 10, 23, 24] This subject will also be addressed in more detail.

Most examinations begin with measurements of height, weight, blood pressure, and pulse. Some also include body fat determination. Goldberg et al[12] found that 32% of the athletes in their study had excessive body fat. Blood pressure parameters as suggested by Smith[31] are <130/75 mm Hg for children aged 6 to 11 years and <140/85 mm Hg for those 12 years and older. As pointed out by Strong and Linder,[33] an athlete should not be labelled as hypertensive until three abnormal readings are obtained at different times. If a child is documented to be hypertensive, they further

## TABLE 1.
## Medical History Questions

1. Are you taking any medications?
2. Do you have any medication allergies?
3. Do you have any environmental allergies?
4. Do you have any allergies to insect stings?
5. Have you ever been hospitalized?
6. Have you ever had surgery?
7. Has any family member had sudden death or heart attack before age 50?
8. Have you had any heart disease, murmur, extra beats, or high blood pressure?
9. Have you ever been dizzy or passed out from exercise?
10. Have you ever been knocked out or had a concussion?
11. Have you ever had any joint injuries (fractures, sprains, strains, or dislocations)?

| _____ Neck | _____ Arm | _____ Thigh |
| _____ Back | _____ Hand | _____ Knee |
| _____ Shoulder | _____ Fingers | _____ Ankle |
| _____ Elbow | _____ Hip | |

12. Do you have any organs missing?
13. Do you have a chronic illness?
14. Have you ever participated in chemical or substance use?
15. Do you have any menstrual irregularities?
16. Have you ever induced vomiting, participated in binge eating or purged yourself?
17. Have you ever been disqualified from participation?
18. What is the date of your last tetanus injection?
19. Do you wear eye glasses, contact lenses, or dental appliances?
20. Do you have any history of a seizure disorder?

recommend testing the blood pressure response to exercise. They indicate that no data have been published to indicate that hypertension causes any direct morbidity or mortality during athletic participation. A rapid or irregular pulse should be correlated with the cardiovascular examination to determine its clinical significance.

Vision screening should be performed and an uncorrected vision of less than 20/40 should be referred.[31] This also should be the time to note whether corrective lenses have been prescribed already.

Certain findings in the head, eyes, ears, nose, and throat examination should be noted. Unequal or nonreactive pupils should be documented as this would be very important later should the athlete incur a head or neck injury. For athletes in water sports, the condition of the external auditory canals and tympanic membranes is important. Proper treatment and hygiene should be given to those who have chronic external otitis due to their constant water exposure. A new area of interest among young athletes is the sport of scuba diving. These young people require a more intense examination of the ear, nose, and throat[2, 4] since, as noted by Dembert and Keith,[4] most injuries sustained in scuba diving are related to barotrauma or decompression sickness. On inspection look for polyps, a deviated septum, or evidence of a necrotic or perforated septum that might indicate substance abuse. The inspection of the mouth should include the teeth. Dentition abnormalities are some of the findings reported most frequently on the physical examination.[33] Note should be made of any dental appliance that is being worn by the athlete as well.

A dermatologic assessment is vital, especially in those who are going to participate in contact or collision sports. As Lombardo[19] noted, clearance should not be given to those athletes demonstrating such dermatologic pathologies as herpes, scabies, louse infestations, or impetigo. Other dermatologic conditions such as acne and fungal dermatophytic infections also require referral for proper care.

Assessment of the lymphatics and abdomen is recommended also. The cervical supraclavicular, axillary, and inguinal lymph nodes should be checked for any enlargement or tenderness. The abdomen should be palpated for hepatomegaly or splenomegaly. Should any lymphadenopathy or organomegaly be discovered, referral should be initiated for further evaluation.

The genitourinary examination has, to a great extent, been conducted in males and neglected in females. Females with a significant menstrual history, such as primary or secondary amenorrhea, should be referred to their private physicians for further evaluation. A nurse or female physician may also need to check pubic hair and breast development to assess maturation. This will be discussed later. Examination of males should establish the presence or absence of a hernia and whether or not both testes are present and descended. Thompson et al[36] found three previously undiagnosed cryptorchid cases out of over 1,700 males examined. There were also three cases of inguinal hernia diagnosed. Strong and Linder[33] found that 6.5% of all abnormalities found on physical examination were related to the genital and hernia examination. If a hernia is present and additional risk would be incurred by continued sports participation, surgical correction should be performed before clearance is given.[19] The issue of participation by athletes who are missing a paired organ will be discussed below.

Since most catastrophic situations involving young athletes are related to sudden death and cardiovascular pathology, an indepth discussion of this topic is appropriate. The highly conditioned athlete is viewed as the epitome of health, and sudden death is such an alarming and unexpected event that it may cause overreaction in an entire community. Because of this, sports physicians and cardiologists have tried to search for the best screening methods to minimize the risk of this tragic occurrence.

However, cost containment is one major problem with an extensive cardiovascular screening examination. Another difficulty lies in how to target certain areas in the medical history and physical examination in order to have the most sensitive protocol. Maron et al[22] conducted a cardiovascular screening on 501 intercollegiate competitive athletes. The screening protocol included a personal and family history, a physical examination, and a 12-lead electrocardiogram. One hundred and two athletes had positive findings on one or more of the three parameters. Of the 90 who submitted to further evaluation, 75 (84%) had no definitive evidence of cardiovascular disease. Of the other 15, one had mild systemic hypertension and 14 had mild mitral valve prolapse. The authors concluded that performance of an electrocardiogram did not appreciably enhance the sensitivity of the informed history and physical examination. They noted further that it was responsible for a high number of false positive observations.

In a study of sudden death that included necropsy structure in highly-conditioned, competitive athletes, cardiovascular abnormalities were found in 28 of the 29 athletes (97%), and almost certainly were the cause of death in 22 of the athletes (76%).[23] In only 7 of the 29 patients was cardiac disease suspected and in only 2 of the 7 had the correct diagnosis been made. Table 2 lists the clinical complaints noted by family members of 8 of the athletes when questioned retrospectively. Table 3 lists the cardiac abnormalities that were found. Hypertrophic obstructive cardiomyopathy was found in 14 athletes and was the most common cause of death by far. Other diagnoses that were made in more than one athlete included anomalous origin of the left coronary artery from the right sinus of Valsalva, idiopathic concentric left ventricular hypertrophy, coronary heart disease, and ruptured aorta. Other authors mention other less common causes of sudden death such as prolonged QT syndrome, mitral valve prolapse, valvular heart disease, myocardial and pericardial diseases, sarcoidoses, and abnormalities in the cardiac conduction system.[3, 8, 20, 24, 34, 38] Thus far, no author on the subject of sudden death has recommended the inclusion of an electrocardiogram or echocardiogram in the screening of athletes. It appears that the most cost-effective screening comes from an informed medical history and physical examination.

---

## TABLE 2.
## Clinical Complaints of Athletes Suffering Sudden Death*

| Reported Symptoms | Number |
| --- | --- |
| Syncope | 3 |
| Presyncope | 1 |
| Chest pain | 2 |
| Periodic mild fatigue | 1 |
| Mild fatigue, presyncope, palpitations | 1 |

*Adapted from Maron BJ, Roberts WC, McAllister HA, et al: *Circulation* 1980; 62:218–229.

**TABLE 3.**
**Cardiac Abnormalities Found in Athletes Suffering**
**Sudden Death***

| Probable Cause of Death | Number |
| --- | --- |
| Hypertrophic cardiomyopathy | 14 |
| Idiopathic concentric LVH† | 5 |
| Anomalous origin of the left coronary artery | 3 |
| Atherosclerotic coronary disease | 3 |
| Ruptured aorta | 2 |
| Hypoplastic coronaries | 1 |
| No cardiovascular disease | 1 |

*Adapted from Maron BJ, Roberts WC, McAllister HA, et al: *Circulation* 1980; 62:218–229.
†LVH = left ventricular hypertrophy.

The cardiovascular examination should include inspection, palpation (especially of the femoral pulses and precordium), and auscultation of the heart sounds.[34] Strong and Steed[34] also note that unusual facies or body habitus which are characteristic of syndromes associated with cardiac defects should be recognized. Palpation of the brachial and femoral pulses should be done to rule out the presence of coarctation. A bifid pulse should be recognized as a possible abnormal finding consistent with hypertrophic cardiomyopathy. The carotid arteries and the precordium should be palpated for trills. Auscultation should be performed to identify $S_1$ and $S_2$ heart sounds. An $S_3$ may be a normal finding in young athletes, but an $S_4$ is always considered pathologic.[34] Murmurs should be identified as systolic or diastolic in origin. The intensity of a murmur itself may not be indicative of either a pathologic or non-pathologic state; the murmur associated with hypertrophic cardiomyopathy may be very soft.[23] Therefore, the intensity of a murmur should not be the only parameter by which one determines the necessity of referral for further evaluation. Most innocent murmurs should diminish with Valsalva; however, the murmur of hypertrophic cardiomyopathy increases in the sitting and standing positions, as well as with exercise. These parameters may help the examiner determine which athletes should be referred for further evaluation.

The auscultation of premature beats or frequent dysrhythmias also is an indication that further cardiac evaluation is needed. If the arrhythmia is suppressed with mild exercise, most likely it is benign. But if there is any question, referral for probable exercise testing and 24-hour Holter monitoring may be necessary. The cardiovascular examination should be emphasized during the sports pre-participation physical examination in order to attempt to identify those athletes who may be at risk for sudden death due to cardiovascular disease.

The musculoskeletal system is another area which should undergo close inspection during the pre-participation examination. Strong and Linder[33] found that 38.3% of abnormal findings on the physical examination were musculoskeletal in origin. Thompson et al[36] reported a much higher incidence of musculoskeletal problems in their series (67%). While the incidence of musculoskeletal abnormalities identified on a sports pre-participation physical examination may vary, they are still the findings which are most frequently identified and referred for further evaluation in every series. One exception is a study by Goldberg et al[12] in which 60 athletes were reported to have medical problems needing further consultation, 35 of whom had musculoskeletal problems. However, it should be noted that 40 of the athletes in the medical category were referred for proteinuria. The knees and ankles appear to be the most frequently injured joints in athletes. Linder et al[18] reported findings related to the knee in 6.9% and 8.8% of athletes and to the ankle in 2.1% and 2.5% in 2 consecutive years, respectively. DuRant et al[5] observed that in the multiple-examiner station examination method, more musculoskeletal problems were identified in more athletes (67%) than in the single-physician examination (5.4%). This illustrates the necessity of having an examining physician who is trained in musculoskeletal evaluation and understands a sports-specific examination.

Table 4 describes a functional orthopedic screening examination that has been recommended and is similar to that used by Thompson et al[36] in their series. This type of examination is very efficient in terms of both time and sensitivity in identifying problems. Any problem identified by the screening examination or by the medical history may require a more specific and in-depth evaluation. At the time of the examination it is important to identify problems that require rehabilitation so a program can be initiated which will have the athlete prepared in time for the sport season. Special emphasis should be placed on those athletes who have had previous surgery. If the surgery has been recent, it is necessary to coordinate the athlete's return to his sport with the surgeon of record.

In general, laboratory tests have been found to be an added expense with little return in the pre-participation examination. Urinalysis has not proved effective in identifying significant problems; in fact, it has created much anxiety because of the number of referrals it has prompted for further evaluation.[31] Hematocrit and hemoglobin determinations also have been found to be unnecessary; they may test normal even in athletes who are iron-deficient. Tissue iron depletion is best determined biochemically with serum ferritin levels. However, this should be reversed for those athletes who have indications for such evaluation (endurance athletes or female athletes with fatigue or diminished performance).

Currently, areas which are generating interest for inclusion in the sports pre-participation examination include maturation indexing, and physiologic testing such as endurance, agility, strength, flexibility, and body composition.[12, 15, 19, 30, 33]

Maturation indexing following the guidelines outlined by Tanner[35] is be-

## TABLE 4.
## Orthopedic Screening Examination*†

| Athletic Activity (Instructions)‡ | Observation |
| --- | --- |
| Stand facing examiner | Acromioclavicular joints; general habitus |
| Look at ceiling, floor, over both shoulders; touch ears to shoulders | Cervical spine motion |
| Shrug shoulders (examiner resists) | Trapezius strength |
| Abduct shoulders 90% (examiner resists at 90%) | Deltoid strength |
| Full external rotation of arms | Shoulder motion |
| Flex and extend elbows | Elbow motion |
| Arms at sides, elbows 90% flexed; pronate and supinate wrists | Elbow and wrist motion |
| Spread fingers; make fist | Hand or finger motion and deformities |
| Tighten (contract) quadriceps; relax quadriceps | Symmetry and knee effusion; ankle effusion |
| "Duck walk" four steps (away from examiner with buttocks on heels) | Hip, knee and ankle motion |
| Back to examiner | Shoulder symmetry; scoliosis |
| Knees straight, touch toes | Scoliosis, hip motion, hamstring tightness |
| Raise up on toes, raise heels | Calf symmetry, leg strength |

*From Smith NJ (ed): *Sports Medicine: Health Care for Young Athletes.* American Academy of Pediatrics, 1983. Used by permission.
†The orthopedic screening examination requires about 90 seconds. Time studies indicate it is most efficiently done one athlete at a time rather than in small groups. It is designed to reveal previous inadequately rehabilitated injuries or those few previously unrecognized orthopedic conditions that might be adversely affected by participation in a sports activity. Positive findings require a more extensive examination and/or history. A more detailed examination should not be attempted at the screening examination.
‡May require reflex hammer, tape measure, pin, and examination table.

ing recommended to profile athletes in an attempt to match them in competition with others who are at similar maturity levels. Proponents believe this will minimize the higher potential for injury which exists for those of a lesser maturity level.[13, 26] However, they also acknowledge that no data have been reported to indicate that such an increased risk exists. For the clinician, knowing that peak height velocities occur at Tanner stage 2 breast development in girls and at Tanner stage 4 genital development in boys may aid in predicting or even preventing certain injuries that occur with rapid growth.[15] This is true especially for injuries related to inflexibility or diminished agility.

In an effort to develop some type of screening method to aid in indexing maturity, Kreipe and Gewanter[16] used a handgrip strength measurement and a self-assessed Tanner Staging. They report that only 67 of 364 males (18%) had grip strength and self-assessed Tanner staging levels that were discordant. Tanner stage 3 was considered immature. The data indicated a break between Tanner stages 3 and 4 at about 55 pounds of grip as measured by a Jamar hand dynamometer. By their data, when self-assessed Tanner staging and grip strength were performed together to test for immaturity, the false negative rate was 5%. When testing for maturity, the false positive rate was 1%.

Maturity indexing may become a more important part of the pre-participation examination, especially if profiling becomes accepted more widely. This is probably very important to many young athletes. In his discussion about the uniqueness of young athletes, Martens[25] lists the six major reasons that young athletes drop out of sports. Two of these six reasons are not getting to play and being mismatched. Maturation assessment may

---

**TABLE 5.**
**American Academy of Pediatrics Sports Classification***

| | | Noncontact | | |
|---|---|---|---|---|
| **Contact/ Collision** | **Limited Contact/Impact** | **Strenuous** | **Moderately Strenuous** | **Non- Strenuous** |
| Boxing | Baseball | Aerobic dancing | Badminton | Archery |
| Field hockey | Basketball | Crew | Curling | Golf |
| Football | Bicycling | Fencing | Table tennis | Riflery |
| Ice hockey | Diving | Field | | |
| Lacrosse | Field | Discus | | |
| Martial arts | High jump | Javelin | | |
| Rodeo | Pole vault | Shot put | | |
| Soccer | Gymnastics | Running | | |
| Wrestling | Horseback riding | Swimming | | |
| | Skating | Tennis | | |
| | Ice | Track | | |
| | Roller | Weight lifting | | |
| | Skiing | | | |
| | Cross-country | | | |
| | Downhill | | | |
| | Water | | | |
| | Softball | | | |
| | Squash, handball | | | |
| | Volleyball | | | |

*From Dyment PG, Goldberg B, Haefele SB, et al: *Pediatrics* 1988; 81:737–739. Used by permission.

**TABLE 6.**
**American Academy of Pediatrics Recommendations on Sports Participation***

| | Contact/ Collision | Limited Contact Impact | Strenuous | Moderately Strenuous | Nonstrenuous |
|---|---|---|---|---|---|
| Atlantoaxial instability | No | No | Yes† | Yes | Yes |
| †Swimming: no butterfly, breast stroke, or diving starts | | | | | |
| Acute illnesses | † | † | † | † | † |
| †Needs individual assessment (contagiousness to others, risk of worsening illness) | | | | | |
| Cardiovascular | | | | | |
| Carditis | No | No | No | No | No |
| Hypertension | | | | | |
| Mild | Yes | Yes | Yes | Yes | Yes |
| Moderate | † | † | † | † | † |
| Severe | ‡ | ‡ | ‡ | ‡ | ‡ |
| Congenital heart disease | | | | | |
| †Needs individual assessment[2] | | | | | |
| ‡Patients with mild forms can be allowed a full range of physical activities; patients with moderate or severe forms, or who are postoperative, should be evaluated by a cardiologist before athletic participation[2] | | | | | |
| Eyes | | | | | |
| Absence or loss of function of one eye | † | † | † | † | † |
| Detached retina | ‡ | ‡ | ‡ | ‡ | ‡ |
| †Availability of American Society for Testing and Materials (ASTM)-approved eye guards may allow competitor to participate in most sports, but this must be judged on an individual basis.[3,4] | | | | | |
| ‡Consult ophthalmologist | | | | | |

| | | | | | |
|---|---|---|---|---|---|
| Inguinal hernia | Yes | Yes | Yes | Yes | Yes |
| Kidney: Absence of one | No | Yes | Yes | Yes | Yes |
| Liver: Enlarged | No | No | Yes | Yes | Yes |
| Musculoskeletal disorders | † | † | † | † | † |
| †Needs individual assessment | | | | | |
| Neurologic | | | | | |
| History of serious head or spine trauma, repeated concussions, or craniotomy | † | † | Yes | Yes | Yes |
| Convulsive disorder | | | | | |
| Well controlled | Yes | Yes | Yes | Yes | Yes |
| Poorly controlled | No | No | Yes‡ | Yes | Yes§ |
| †Needs individual assessment | | | | | |
| ‡No swimming or weight lifting | | | | | |
| §No archery or riflery | | | | | |
| Ovary: Absence of one | Yes | Yes | Yes | Yes | Yes |
| Respiratory | | | | | |
| Pulmonary insufficiency | † | † | † | † | Yes |
| Asthma | Yes | Yes | Yes | Yes | Yes |
| †May be allowed to compete if oxygenation remains satisfactory during a graded stress test | | | | | |
| Sickle cell trait | Yes | Yes | Yes | Yes | Yes |
| Skin: Boils, herpes, impetigo, scabies | † | † | Yes | Yes | Yes |
| †No gymnastics with mats, martial arts, wrestling, or contact sports until not contagious | | | | | |
| Spleen: Enlarged | No | No | No | Yes | Yes |
| Testicle: Absence or undescended | Yes† | Yes† | Yes | Yes | Yes |
| †Certain sports may require protective cup[3] | | | | | |

*From Dyment PG, Goldberg B, Haefele SB, et al: Pediatrics 1988; 81:737–739. Used by permission.

prove very helpful in screening the young athletes and placing them in a healthier sports environment.

Flexibility assessment is being used more in the preparticipation evaluation also. Goldberg et al[12] describe a flexibility screening technique. Some programs have performed goniometer measurements for selected joints and sit-and-reach measurements. The method described by Goldberg et al[12] is more comprehensive but may not fit into each program's framework of evaluation. As a result, this may be something the sports physician may want to have the coaching staff and athletic trainer conduct at another time, then assess the results with them at a later date.

Body composition already has been mentioned in the discussion on the physical examination. This can be done quickly by skin caliper measurement. This is important not only from the perspective of athletic performance but also may provide an opportunity for counseling an athlete about health issues that have a lifelong impact. This also may provide important information to wrestlers regarding how much weight loss is feasible and medically safe.

Strength and endurance measurements as well as agility assessments also are potentially valuable aspects of a pre-participation examination. However, each physician or school system may have to develop its own program in these areas, since many of these tests do not have well-defined standards. Except for the 12-minute or 1.5 mile run, standards for comparison may not be readily available.

The final step in the pre-participation examination is to classify the young athletes according to the safety of their participation. Most authors recommend three clearance options.[19, 33, 36] Clearance A permits unrestricted participation, clearance B permits participation after further evaluation and/or rehabilitation is completed, and clearance C defers clearance because of the detection of a high-risk medical contraindication to participation. The final results should be discussed with the athlete, his parents, and coaches if either clearance B or C is selected for that particular examination. Much has been written and debated about which sports are safe for young athletes with certain medical conditions. The American Academy of Pediatrics[7] recently published a statement classifying sports and listing recommendations for the participation of athletes with specific medical conditions in competitive sports (Tables 5 and 6). Sports are classified as contact or collision, limited contact or impact, and noncontact (including three levels: strenuous, moderately strenuous and nonstrenuous).

Sports participation by athletes who are missing one part of a paired organ is a controversial topic. Although many physicians and school districts have refused approval for participation in these cases the courts sometimes have intervened to allow the athlete to perform.[37] Thus, the ultimate decision may not rest with the physician in many cases. In cases of loss of vision in one eye, an approved eye protection device must be worn for participation in any sport that poses a risk to the eyes. In cases of an absent testicle, the risks should be discussed with the athlete and parents, and proper protection should be included in the athletic gear.[21] Athletes with a solitary kidney that demonstrates an abnormal anatomic variant (i.e., ectopic location or ureteropelvic junction abnormality) or any degree of obstruction or impairment of function according to Mendell et al[21] would not be allowed to participate in contact or collision sports.

It is evident, therefore, that inclusion or exclusion from participation in sports activities must be individualized. In tenuous cases there should be extensive discussion with the athlete, parents, coaches, school administrators, and physician before a decision is made.

In this discussion, this author has attempted to classify the goals and objectives of the pre-participation evaluation. It must be recognized that this examination does not replace regular, continuous care by an athlete's private physician, even though this currently is the view held by most athletes and parents, and even by some physicians.

The goal of the pre-participation examination should be to ensure as much as possible the health and safety of young athletes. The sensitivity design should be such that potential health risks and medical contraindications to sports participation by the athlete are identified. It should be regarded not as an examination designed to exclude young people from participation, but as an examination to include all young people who can participate safely in athletic endeavors. In addition, the examination should be sport-specific, designed not only for the athletic population as a whole, but emphasizing the sport or sports of choice. The examination also should convey a positive image of the physician and his role in the care of athletes. The athlete should be made comfortable in the relationship that may be built from this encounter. It is also a means by which to bring the physician, athletic trainer, and coaching staff together in a cooperative effort to provide a healthy, safe environment in which young athletes can compete. This also should be an opportunity for each professional involved to gain a better understanding of their roles in the care of the total person not just the athlete. Alienation of any of these components is not in the best interest of the young athlete.

The pre-participation evaluation is viewed by this author as a small, but significant, investment in our young people. Directly or indirectly, these evaluations impact upon their physical, psychological, and emotional development, and provide an opportunity for the physician to have a positive and rewarding influence on the lives of young athletes.

---

# References

1. *Medical Evaluation of the Athlete: A Guide,* revised ed. Chicago, American Medical Association, 1976.
2. Becker D, Parell GJ, Medical examination of the sport scuba diver, *Otolaryngol Head Neck Surg* 1983; 91:246–250.
3. Braden DS, Strong WB: Preparticipation screening for sudden cardiac death in high school and college athletes. *Physician Sportsmed* 1988; 16:128–40.
4. Dembert ML, Keith JF: Evaluating the potential pediatric scuba diver. *Am J Dis Child* 1986; 140:1135–1141.

5. DuRant R, Seymore C, Linder CW, et al: The preparticipation examination of athletes: Comparison of single and multiple examiners. Am J Dis Child 1985; 139:657–661.
6. Dyment PG: Another look at the sports preparticipation examination of the adolescent athlete. J Adolesc Health Care 1986; 7:130S–132S.
7. Dyment PG, Goldberg B, Haefele SB, et al: Recommendations for participation in competitive sports. Pediatrics 1988; 81:737–739.
8. Epstein SE, Maron BJ: Sudden death and the competitive athlete: Perspectives on preparticipation screening studies. J Am Coll Cardiol 1986; 7:220–230.
9. Esquivel MT, McCormick DP: Preparticipation sports evaluation, part 1: The station-method examination. Fam Pract Recert 1987; 9:41–60.
10. Esquivel MT, McCormick DP: Preparticipation sports evaluation, part 2: Recommendations for student participation. Fam Pract Recert 1987; 9:107–118.
11. Feinstein RA, Soilean EJ, Daniel WA: A national survey of preparticipation physical examination requirements. Physician Sports Med 1988; 16:51–59.
12. Goldberg B, Saranit A, Witman P, et al: Preparticipation sports assessment—an objective evaluation. Pediatrics 1980; 66:736–745.
13. Goldberg B, Boiardo R: Profiling children for sports participation. Clin Sports Med 1984; 3:153–169.
14. Hunter SC: Screening high school athletes. J Med Assoc G 1985; 74:482–484.
15. Jones R: The preparticipation, sport-specific athletic profile examination. Semin Adolesc Med 1987; 3:169–175.
16. Kreipe RE, Gewanter HL: Physical maturity screening for participation in sports. Pediatrics 1985; 75:1076–1080.
17. Kulund DN: The Injured Athlete. Philadelphia, JB Lippincott Co, 1982.
18. Linder CW, DuRant RH, Seklecki RM, et al: Preparticipation health screening of young athletes. Am J Sports Med 1981; 9:187–193.
19. Lombardo JA: Preparticipation physical evaluation. Prim Care 1984; 11:3–21.
20. Luckstead EF: Sudden death in sports. Pediatr Clin North Am 1982; 29:1355–1362.
21. Mandell J, Cromie WJ, Caldamore, et al: Sports-related genitourinary injuries in children. Clin Sports Med 1982; 1:483–493.
22. Maron BJ, Bodison SA, Wesley YE, et al: Results of screening a large group of intercollegiate competitive athletes for cardiovascular disease. J Am Coll Cardiol 1987; 10:1214–1221.
23. Maron BJ, Roberts WC, McAllister HA, et al: Sudden death in young athletes. Circulation 1980; 62:218–229.
24. Maron BJ, Epstein SE, Roberts WC: Causes of sudden death in competitive athletes. J Am Coll Cardiol 1986; 7:204–214.
25. Martens R: The uniqueness of the young athlete: Psychologic considerations. Am J Sports Med 1980; 8:382–385.
26. Nicholas JA: The value of sports profiling. Clin Sports Med 1984; 3:3–10.
27. Risser WL, Hoffman HM, Bellah G: Frequency of preparticipation sports examinations in secondary school athletes: Are the university interscholastic league guidelines appropriate? Tex Med 1985; 81:35–39.
28. Rowland TW: Preparticipation sports examination of the child and adolescent athlete: Changing views of an old ritual. Pediatrician 1986; 13:3–9.
29. Runyan DK: The pre-participation examination of the young athlete. Clin Pediatr (Phila) 1983; 22:674–679.

30. Smith NJ, Garrick JG: Pre-participation sports assessment. *Pediatrics* 1980; 66:803–806.
31. Smith NJ (ed): *Sports Medicine: Health Care for Young Athletes.* Evanston, Ill, American Academy of Pediatrics, 1983.
32. Strauss RJ (ed): *Sports Medicine.* Philadelphia, WB Saunders Co, 1984.
33. Strong WB, Linder CW: Preparticipation health evaluation for competitive sports. *Pediatr Rev* 1982; 4:113–121.
34. Strong WB, Steed D: Cardiovascular evaluation of the young athlete. *Pediat Clin North Am* 1982; 29:1325–1338.
35. Tanner JM: *Growth at Adolescence,* ed 2. Springfield, Charles C Thomas, 1962.
36. Thompson TR, Andrish JT, Bergfeld JA: A prospective study of preparticipation sports examinations of 2670 young athletes: Method and results. *Cleve Clin Quart* 1982; 49:226–233.
37. Tucker JB, Marron JT: The qualification-disqualification process in athletics. *Am Fam Physician* 1984; 29:149–154.
38. VanCamp SP: Exercise-related sudden death: Cardiovascular evaluation of exercises: Part 2. *Physician Sportsmed* 1988; 16:47–54.
39. Wood IR: A new approach to athletic physicals. *J Sch Health* 1987; 57:346–348.

# Cardiovascular Problems in the Young Athlete

## Richard Sterba, M.D.

Pediatric Cardiologist, The Cleveland Clinic Foundation, Cleveland, Ohio

### Editor's Introduction

The most frightening and saddest occurrence in sports is the sudden death of a young athlete. Most of these deaths are the result of cardiovascular malfunctions. In order to fulfill the physician's responsibility of ensuring the health and safety of the athlete, the physician must be familiar with the recognizable and avoidable causes of sudden death as well as other cardiovascular abnormalities.

Dr. Sterba presents a very practical review of the common cardiovascular problems which one may find in young athletes. Of prime importance are the areas on hypertrophic cardiomyopathy, congenital heart disease, and Marfan's syndrome. Even though these problems may not be common, their presence may be catastrophic.

Familiarity with these cardiovascular conditions is necessary for any primary care physician dealing with athletes.

*John A. Lombardo, M.D.*

Cardiovascular abnormalities in young athletes are usually congenital in origin. In the pediatric age group, the most competitive and aggressive participation in sports occurs at ages when repair of severe congenital heart defects should have been completed already. In fact, young athletes rarely have problems secondary to cardiovascular abnormalities. Congenital heart disease is rare, occurring in less than 1% of the population. In one half of these children the defect is so severe that they will probably never be able to participate in competitive situations. After corrective surgery for certain congenital heart defects (i.e., patent ductus arteriosus (PDA) ligation) some patients are considered cured. Other patients "develop" or "acquire" new problems after surgery (i.e., ventricular arrhythmias after repair of tetralogy of Fallot).

Sudden cardiac death can and unfortunately does occur, although it is rare. When it happens, the incidents are so newsworthy and spectacular that we tend to remember them in a very special manner, as in the recent cases of Flo Hyman, a United States woman volleyball player and "Pistol Pete" Maravich, a professional basketball player.

This discussion will cover pre-participation physical examinations, common congenital heart defects, postoperative congenital heart disease, and arrhythmias. I hope that it will aid physicians in determining safe levels of competition for athletes with known cardiovascular abnormalities and in uncovering athletes with previously undocumented cardiovascular problems.

## Pre-participation Examination

The best approach to cardiovascular disease in interscholastic athletes primarily involves preventing problems and imposing proper limitations on those athletes already diagnosed with problems. Most children with significant congenital heart disease are identified early in life. Their cardiovascular examinations are clearly abnormal. Occasionally there is a definite, strong family history suggesting genetic transmission of disease, as in Marfan's syndrome or hypertrophic cardiomyopathy. Most interscholastic athletes undergo yearly pre-participation medical evaluations which should uncover most significant cardiovascular abnormalities (Table 1). These evaluations should include a thorough history, with a checklist that includes questions concerning palpitations, chest pain with exertion, shortness of breath with exercise, or syncope at rest or with exercise. The family history should be obtained to rule out congenital problems, and should note such factors as siblings with unexpected deaths. Also, a history of early coronary artery disease in parents may mark patients with familial hypercholesterolemia who may be at risk for early myocardial infarction.

The examination should take place in a quiet and private area. The examiner should have the ability to auscultate the heart with the patient in multiple positions if needed. Most patients with congenital heart disease

---

**TABLE 1.**
**Pre-participation Evaluation**

History
    Syncope
    Chest pain with exercise
    Palpitations, tachycardias
    Family history of early coronary artery
       disease
Physical Examination
    Blood pressure
    Pulses
       1. Upper and lower extremity
    Auscultate
       1. Supine and upright
       2. Quiet and private room

---

have heart murmurs which are fairly typical of their underlying defect. Systolic murmurs will be the most common auscultatory abnormality noted, with a large percentage being of the functional, benign, or innocent type. A functional murmur is typically a mid-systolic ejection or crescendo-decrescendo type of murmur. The murmur can be heard at the left sternal border or at the apex of the heart. In the older patient, a pulmonary ejection functional murmur can be heard. Rarely, a functional murmur can be heard at the upper right sternal border. The murmur either disappears or significantly decreases in intensity when the patient stands up. Sometimes it will vary with respiration. With a functional murmur, one may opt not to pursue further studies and to allow participation. Of course, the examiner needs to have confidence in his ability to make the correct diagnosis; many patients with only a functional murmur are referred for further evaluation.

The murmur of the obstructive form of hypertrophic cardiomyopathy can be similar to a functional murmur. But the systolic murmur associated with this abnormality typically increases in the standing position and with the Valsalva maneuver, and decreases with the handgrip maneuver (Table 2). This is opposite of what is expected with a functional murmur, underlining the importance of evaluating patients in multiple positions to assure correct diagnoses.

Diastolic murmurs are always abnormal and athletes with these murmurs need to be referred for evaluation prior to participating in competition. Venous hums can be confused with both diastolic murmurs or continuous murmurs; these usually will disappear when the patient assumes a supine position. Compressing the jugular vein or having the patient turn his head also can cause the murmur to disappear totally. A true continuous murmur usually signifies a structural abnormality and merits referral.

Short, high-pitched sounds heard during diastole or systole are called clicks and typically are associated with valvular abnormalities of the heart. Stenosis of both semilunar valves can lead to an ejection type of systolic click. Mid-systolic clicks or multiple systolic clicks can be heard in mitral valve prolapse. Clicks secondary to semilunar valve stenosis or mitral valve prolapse are the most common types of clicks heard. Clicks also can be associated with rarer conditions, such as an aneurysm of a ventricular sep-

---

**TABLE 2.**
**Murmur Intensity***

|  | Valsalva | Handgrip | Upright |
|---|---|---|---|
| Functional | ↓ | ↑ → | ↓ |
| Idiopathic hypertrophic subaortic stenosis (IHSS) | ↑ | ↓ | ↑ |

*Upward arrow indicates an increase; downward arrow indicates decrease; horizontal arrow indicates no change.

tal defect or Ebstein's anomaly of the tricuspid valve. Patients who have clicks audible during examination should be referred to a center where echocardiography can be performed to make a correct diagnosis.

The examination also should include a blood pressure measured in the upper extremity, and palpation and comparison of upper extremity and lower extremity pulses. In muscular athletes, one should be careful to use an appropriately sized blood pressure cuff to assure accurate determination of the patient's blood pressure.

## Congenital Heart Disease

The pre-participation physical examination is important to protect the athlete from the rate occurrence of sudden death secondary to an underlying cardiovascular problem. It also should be used to protect the patient from increasing the progression of his underlying disease. Athletes with structural heart disease who are at risk for sudden death typically have some form of obstruction which limits their ability to increase cardiac output appropriately during exercise. The conditions of severe aortic or pulmonary stenosis (usually in conjunction with other significant congenital defects) fall into this category. Fortunately, these diagnoses are quite easy to make by auscultation alone, and catastrophes can be avoided in these patients. Patients with aortic or pulmonary stenosis may need surgical intervention prior to participation; the degree of participation will be limited for those who are not operative candidates.

Patients with hypertrophic cardiomyopathy need definite limits and should avoid high-intensity activities. These patients can develop left ventricular outflow tract obstruction with increasing activity or exertion. Patients both with and without outflow tract obstruction have a tendency towards significant, possibly fatal arrhythmias during periods of activity and exertion. In most studies looking at sudden death in young athletes, this diagnosis is the most common. Patients operated on for left ventricular outflow tract obstruction may still need limits on activities in the postoperative state because of the possibility of arrhythmias. Treatment with beta-blockers, and sometimes with antiarrhythmic agents, will be necessary.

Patients with Eisenmenger's syndrome or primary pulmonary hypertension are in another category where sudden death is common, even without exercise. These patients also have significant symptoms and usually abnormal physical findings of an increased pulmonary component of the second heart sound or cyanosis, which make the diagnosis relatively easy. They should not be allowed to participate in sports secondary to their underlying disease which makes them unable to increase their cardiac output significantly with exercise.

Marfan's syndrome is an inherited connective tissue disorder. The disease can affect the skeletal, ocular, and cardiovascular systems. Sudden deaths secondary to the rupture of a dilated aorta are known to occur. Marfan's syndrome can be suspected on the basis of a simple physical examination (Table 3). The patients are typically tall and thin. Many have scoliosis or a pectus deformity of the anterior chest wall. On cardiovascular examination, mitral valve prolapse or aortic regurgitation may be noted. Unfortunately, a dilated aorta may be silent on physical examination; for this reason, I recommend echocardiography to assess aortic involvement in patients whom I suspect may have Marfan's syndrome. If cardiovascular involvement is seen, the patient should be instructed to avoid contact sports and weight lifting, and possibly should be considered for therapy with beta-blockers. Theoretically, this medication decreases stress on the weakened walls of the aorta. Unfortunately, even if patients have a normal aorta on initial evaluation, they can develop the disease later in life. I recommend yearly follow-up echocardiograms and examinations on patients who continue to pursue sports which involve either contact or a high level of intensity.

Mitral valve prolapse is also a congenital heart defect and is thought to occur in about 10% of the general population. Patients with mitral valve prolapse can have a multitude of different findings present on their cardiovascular examination. They can have systolic clicks which can be either early systolic, mid-systolic, or multiple. The murmur can be a pansystolic murmur of mitral regurgitation or a late systolic murmur which has a character of mitral regurgitation and occurs after the mid-systolic click. Patients with mitral valve prolapse usually have an examination that is more positive in the standing position. If a click or murmur is audible in the supine position, the patient should be placed in the upright position because the murmur can intensify and lengthen. Most patients with mitral valve prolapse will be able to participate in athletics, as the mitral regurgitation seen in this defect is usually of a minimal degree and the heart size is normal. In patients with enlarged hearts or arrhythmias, limitations on the degree of participation may be necessary.

In 1984, a group of 40 physicians met to formulate recommendations

---

**TABLE 3.**
**Manifestations of Marfan's Syndrome**

---

Family History
Skeletal
   Kyphoscoliosis
   Pectus excavatum
Ocular
   Ectopia lentis
   Myopia
Cardiovascular
   Mitral valve prolapse
   Aortic root dilatation

---

for eligibility for competition in athletes who had a previous diagnosis of cardiovascular disease. The 16th Bethesda conference recommendations remain an excellent resource to help us decide on the appropriate level of competition in patients with many different types of cardiovascular abnormalities.

## Postoperative Congenital Heart Disease

In the 1980s and the 1990s many patients who survived and, in fact, have thrived after repair of their congenital heart defects will reach the age where competition and interscholastic sports may become practical. Earlier surgical repair has led to better results and, in some cases, essentially normal cardiovascular function. Children who have undergone PDA ligation, atrial septal defect closure, and perhaps even ventricular septal defect closure can participate in all activities within 6 months of surgical repair, as long as the chest x-ray and electrocardiogram have returned to normal. Twenty-four–hour ambulatory electrocardiographic monitoring should be considered in any patient who has an abnormal postoperative electrocardiogram and definitely should be performed in those patients who have had ventricular septal defect closure via ventriculotomy. In any of these postoperative situations, the finding of residual pulmonary hypertension will place significant limits on the degree of participation in athletics.

Patients who have had repair of tetralogy of Fallot often can participate in athletics. Repairs done early in life should decrease the amount of preoperative damage done to the myocardium secondary to hypoxia and/or the pressure load on the right ventricular. If the repair can be accomplished with a low right ventricular pressure (less than 40 mm Hg systolic), minimal shunting, and minimal cardiac enlargement, competition can be considered. Since late postoperative ventricular arrhythmias can be a problem in these patients, I recommend 24-hour ambulatory monitoring, as well as a stress test, before allowing participation in sports. These procedures should be repeated at yearly intervals to evaluate for ventricular arrhythmias.

Patients who have had either the Mustard or Senning procedure to correct transposition of the great vessels also have problems with arrhythmias. In these cases, sinus node dysfunction commonly is observed. Again, 24-hour electrocardiographic monitoring and stress testing is recommended. Exercise typically will not induce tachyarrhythmias, but the patient may show an abnormal chronotropic response to exercise which will help the managing physician in recommending a safe level of activity for the patient. Consideration of a pacemaker also may be made, depending on the heart rate response to exercise. After the Mustard or Senning procedure, the right ventricle is the determined systemic ventricle, and there is some concern over its capability for long-term function as a systemic pump. Echocardiography or stress ventriculography to assess right ventricular function may be helpful in some cases.

The Fontan procedure or modified Fontan procedure commonly is used to correct complex congenital heart defects where there is one functional ventricle. Postoperatively, patients may rely on right atrial contraction to provide forward flow through the pulmonary circulation. In most cases the response to exercise in these patients is abnormal. Careful pre-participation evaluation is needed to assess the level of exercise they can safely attain. Again, both supraventricular and ventricular arrhythmias are common and need to be evaluated before participation.

As we progress through the 1990s, more patients will fall into the category of corrected or postoperative congenital heart disease. The surgical results are improving and I suspect that long-term outcome for patients with more complex congenital heart disease will improve also. After careful evaluation, some will be able to participate in sports, and physicians need to keep updated on a yearly basis in order to screen these patients accurately.

## Coronary Artery Disease

Coronary artery abnormalities can be either acquired or congenital. Acquired coronary artery disease can be secondary to either Kawasaki disease or to hypercholesterolemia. Congenital coronary artery anomalies which may lead to myocardial ischemia during exercise are extremely uncommon, but catastrophic, abnormalities.

Approximately 10% to 20% of patients who develop Kawasaki disease (the mucocutaneous lymph node syndrome) will have coronary artery abnormalities noted by noninvasive techniques. Patients who have Kawasaki disease routinely undergo electrocardiography to look for abnormalities in myocardial perfusion and, in many cases, two-dimensional echocardiography is used to assess the presence of coronary artery aneurysms. In the majority of patients who develop coronary artery aneurysms there appears to be resolution of these abnormalities when the patients are reassessed with either echocardiography or angiography. This is a disease that has been recognized for only approximately 15 years, and it is not known whether patients who had Kawasaki disease as young infants will develop early coronary artery abnormalities and then ischemic problems with exercise. Although at this time I do not feel that a history of Kawasaki disease is a contraindication to sports participation, it is something that we will probably need to consider when taking histories as these young patients reach ages where competition in sports may be considered.

As stressed earlier in this chapter, the pre-participation physical examination is not complete without a detailed history. A young athlete may be ambiguous or incorrect when asked whether or not there is coronary artery disease or a history of early myocardial infarction in the family. Team physicians should consider whether or not questionnaires should be sent home for the family to fill out to ensure that accurate information is obtained, especially regarding familial hypocholesterolemia. This must be done yearly, or at least every 2 years, in the event that a parent develops early coronary artery disease during the athlete's time in high school. If there is a family history of high cholesterol, the athlete should have his cholesterol level measured. Although it would be unusual for athletes with elevated cholesterol levels to develop trouble in high school, one may consider performing a stress test just to ensure that there is absolutely no evidence of ischemia present.

Athletes who complain of chest pain during exercise need to be carefully evaluated to rule out underlying coronary artery pathology. The family history is extremely critical in such situations. Stress testing to look for ischemia should be considered also. Coronary artery anomalies, such as origin of the left coronary artery from the right sinus of Valsalva, have been noted in autopsy series on young athletes who have died suddenly. Unfortunately, there is no way to make this diagnosis based on physical examination or routine electrocardiography. Even with echocardiography the diagnosis can be difficult or impossible to make.

Patients with coronary artery anomalies will continue to be missed during the pre-participation physical examination, indicating once again how important a careful history is to uncover syncope or chest pain with exercise, which may be the only warning sign of such a significant problem. The case of Pete Maravich illustrates that even the best athletes can participate in athletics for a long period of time before a congenital anomaly may lead to a catastrophic event.

## Arrhythmias

Irregular heartbeats or palpitations are not an uncommon complaint in young patients. Twenty-four–hour Holter monitoring performed on large groups of normal teenagers have shown that between 10% and 25% have premature atrial or ventricular contractions recorded. A number of these premature beats are not noted by the individuals. Episodes of tachycardia which may be either ventricular or supraventricular in origin are much less common in this age group, with supraventricular tachyarrhythmias seen more often than ventricular tachyarrhythmias. Careful evaluation is needed in patients who complain of palpitations, abnormal types of tachycardia, or syncope with exercise. The physical examination needs to include careful ausculation to rule out the presence of any underlying structural cardiac disease. An electrocardiogram may be of help in defining silent abnormalities (such as Wolff-Parkinson-White syndrome), other types of ventricular preexcitation, or the long QT syndrome. Occasionally an extra heart beat recorded on a routine electrocardiogram (ECG) may help to determine what type of premature beats are present.

Premature beats, whether atrial or ventricular in origin, usually do not preclude participation in athletic events. In patients who have premature ventricular beats, one may wish to perform exercise testing to observe the response to exercise. Most benign premature ventricular contractions decrease in frequency with exercise; if this is the case, then the athlete should be allowed to participate in all types of competitive sports. If the premature ventricular beats increase in frequency with exercise but other noninvasive studies show that there is no underlying structural heart disease, competition may still be allowed, but may need to be limited in some instances. In patients who have premature ventricular beats and underlying structural heart disease or any evidence of cardiac dysfunction, significant limits should be placed on the athlete's participation. Treatment of the irregular rhythm and further invasive studies should be considered seriously. Myocarditis is a rare disease, but one which can present with a sensation of premature beats. Patients who have premature beats or ventricular dysfunction secondary to myocarditis should not be allowed to participate in sports until resolution of the abnormality is documented. Unfortunately, the only way to make the definite diagnosis of myocarditis is with an endomyocardial biopsy.

Paroxysmal supraventricular tachycardia is the most common cause of abnormal tachycardias in young patients. The physician first needs to differentiate between ventricular and supraventricular tachycardia when considering participation in athletics. Patients with paroxysmal supraventricular tachycardia usually can participate in all athletic activities, although medication may be needed to suppress the occurrence of tachycardia with exercise. Since hypotension and a less than optimal cardiac performance can be noted during episodes of paroxysmal supraventricular tachycardia, we recommend that the athlete be removed from competition during an episode of tachycardia. If the heart rate and rhythm returns to normal and the patient is asymptomatic, he may be allowed to return to the competition.

If a patient develops an episode of paroxysmal supraventricular tachycardia in a competitive situation, various vagal maneuvers can be used on the sideline in an attempt to terminate the tachycardia. The patient should be placed in the supine position and ideally have the feet positioned slightly above the level of the head. He may be instructed to perform a Valsalva maneuver, or the team physician may attempt carotid sinus massage. Ice which has been placed in a plastic bag and positioned over the patient's head or face may be used in an attempt to terminate the tachycardia. If the tachycardia cannot be terminated in a timely manner, referral should be made to an appropriate emergency care facility.

Ventricular tachycardia is uncommon in young athletes. Most patients with ventricular tachycardia will have some structural or mechanical abnormality of the heart. The majority of these patients will not be able to participate in highly competitive athletics, despite treatment with medication.

Wolff-Parkinson-White syndrome is an uncommon electrical abnormality of the heart in which an extra electrical connection is present between the atrium and ventricle. Patients with Wolff-Parkinson-White syndrome are prone to episodes of both paroxysmal supraventricular tachycardia and atrial fibrillation. The episodes of paroxysmal supraventricular tachycardia are quite similar to those described previously. Of more concern are the episodes of atrial fibrillation where there is a very rapid and uncontrolled ventricular response. Patients have been known to develop ventricular fibrillation and even experience sudden death. An athlete with Wolff-Parkinson-White syndrome and a history of tachycardia needs to undergo invasive electrophysiologic testing to see whether or not a rapid ventricular response to atrial fibrillation is present. If the ventricular response is controlled, participation in athletics can be allowed. Some patients may be controlled with medical therapy and then allowed to participate in sports, and some patients eventually may have to undergo a surgical procedure to ablate their accessory connection prior to participation.

Bradyarrhythmias can occur secondary to sinus node dysfunction or various degrees of atrioventricular block. Patients who have bradycardias may have significant limits on their ability to perform, secondary to an inadequate heart rate response to exercise. Stress testing can be used to evaluate the level of competition which can be expected and safely achieved. Some patients may benefit from placement of a pacemaker to allow their heart rate to respond normally throughout exercise. Pacemaker physiology at this time has improved to the point where a normal heart rate response to exercise can be expected in a majority of patients; current pacemakers have the ability to sense the atrial depolarization and pace the ventricle at an equal rate. In patients who have an abnormal chronotrophic response, placement of a rate-responsive pacemaker is now practical. Unfortunately, after placement of the pacemaker, most patients will not be able to participate in contact sports because of the possibility of injury or damage to the device.

## Conclusion

I have attempted to review some of the common cardiovascular abnormalities which occur in young athletes. These problems will continue to be present through the 1990s, but better and earlier management of congenital heart disease should allow many patients who would have been unable to participate in athletics previously to consider participation in highly competitive athletics now. Even patients who have undergone heart transplantation have been noted to participate in interscholastic activities without any limits. Arrhythmias are controlled much more easily with newer antiarrhythmic agents and standard and antitachycardia pacemakers now have the ability to control arrhythmias. Cardiovascular problems will remain a concern, but many strides have been made in improving the quality of life in these patients.

## Bibliography

1. Mitchell JH, Maron BJ, Epstein SE: 16th Bethesda conference: Cardiovascular abnormalities in the athlete: Recommendations regarding eligibility for competition. *J Am Coll Cardiol* 1985; 6:1189–1224.
2. Oppenheim EB: How to detect the young athlete at risk for sudden death. *Cardiovasc Rev Rep* 1987; 8:19–23.

3. Maron BJ, Epstein SE, Roberts WC: Causes of sudden death in competitive athletes. *J Am Coll Cardiol* 1986; 7:204–214.
4. Zipes DP, Cobb LA Jr, Garson A Jr, et al: Task Force VI: Arrhythmias. *J Am Coll Cardiol* 1985; 6:1225–32.
5. Braden DS, Strong WB: Preparticipation screening for sudden cardiac death in high school and college athletes. *Physician Sportsmed* 1988; 16:128–140.
6. Maron BJ, Roberts WC, McAllister HA, et al: Sudden death in young athletes. *Circulation* 1980; 62:218–229.
7. Driscoll DJ: Cardiovascular evaluation of the child and adolescent before participation in sports. *Mayo Clin Proc* 1985; 60:867–873.
8. Van Camp SP, Choi JH: Exercise and sudden death. *Physician Sportsmed* 1988; 16:49–52.

# Chronic Fatigue in the Young Athlete

## E. Randy Eichner, M.D.

Professor of Medicine, University of Oklahoma Health Sciences Center,
Oklahoma City, Oklahoma

## Editor's Introduction

One of the most common complaints that a physician might encounter in all patients is fatigue. This vague, nonspecific complaint is found not only in the general populace but also is a common complaint among athletes. Without a complete differential diagnosis, the work-up of a patient with chronic fatigue can be frustrating as well as costly.

Dr. Eichner presents a rational approach to the patient with chronic fatigue as a main complaint. He has not only reviewed the common causes of fatigue, but also has given an efficient and organized work-up of these patients. It is hoped that this will help the physician become comfortable and confident when approaching this problem.

*John A. Lombardo, M.D.*

Fatigue is a common complaint among young athletes. Usually, of course, it is benign and self-limiting. Sometimes, however, it becomes chronic and begins to generate increasing concern. Athletes, coaches, and parents alike begin to wonder whether the continuing problem stems from overtraining, psychological burnout, or underlying illness. Sooner or later, a physician is consulted.

A young athlete with chronic fatigue can pose a daunting and frustrating diagnostic and management challenge for the consulting physician. This challenge reflects not only the many potential causes of fatigue, but also the essence of the complaint itself. By its very nature, fatigue can be elusive. It is easy to feel, but hard to define, and impossible to see. Temporary fatigue, of course, is a part of life, even of young life. After a grueling competition, a sleepless night, or a relentless day, we are accustomed to fatigue, and we know that rest will "rejuvenate" us. Also, we know the profound but self-limited fatigue of "the flu." But compared with these common types of fatigue, chronic fatigue in young athletes can be both more subtle and more puzzling.

Different patients express fatigue in many ways. It may be verbalized as "I'm tired all the time," "I'm all in," "I have no energy, . . . no pep, . . .

no stamina," "My times are falling off," "I never seem to get enough sleep," "I can't concentrate," or "I've just lost interest," to name a few examples. These statements may reflect one common problem, or one athlete's fatigue may be another's boredom or burnout.

Fatigue also has many medical synonyms, such as tiredness, weariness, listlessness, lethargy, lassitude, and torpor, for example. With all this variation in expression, one wonders if athletes, parents, coaches, and doctors are always on the same wavelength when discussing "fatigue."

What, then, is fatigue? To the muscle physiologist, fatigue is the failure to sustain the expected or required muscular force. But physicians define it more broadly. Most physicians would agree that fatigue is a subjective condition wherein patients feel tired before they begin activities, lack the energy to accomplish tasks that require sustained effort and attention, and become abnormally exhausted after normal activities.

Even if fatigue can be defined, it cannot be reliably measured. In the final analysis, therefore, fatigue is in the mind of the fatigued.

This chapter reviews the most common causes of chronic fatigue in the young athlete. Other recent exemplary reviews of fatigue in adolescents should also be consulted to contrast and complement the material covered here.[1-3]

## Infection

Infection, especially viral infection, is often considered as a possible cause of chronic fatigue in young athletes. The most common viral infections, however, do not present primarily as chronic fatigue in otherwise healthy youngsters. The common cold, for example, often caused by the rhinovirus, is easily recognized and produces fatigue for only a few days. Similarly, influenza, with its high fever, myalgias, hacking cough, and seasonal occurrence, is also easy to recognize and rarely causes fatigue for longer than a week or two. Mycoplasmal pneumonia, too, is usually a subacute illness that does not remain undiagnosed very long.

## Infectious Mononucleosis

Infectious mononucleosis can cause chronic fatigue in the young athlete. Consider the following case reports:

A 15-year-old middle distance runner complained of loss of stamina and inability to manage his normal training schedule. His competition performance had deteriorated also. The problem had been preceded by a mild infection of the upper respiratory tract and a sore throat that were not serious enough for him to have consulted a doctor. Examination showed several small supraclavicular lymph nodes. Atypical mononuclear cells were visible in a blood film, and a screening test for infectious mononucleosis (Monospot) gave positive results. Training was temporarily reduced, and he had regained his form after 4 months.[4]

An 18-year-old cross-country runner presented with loss of stamina and an inability to maintain his former training schedule. He had experienced no recent symptoms of the upper respiratory tract. Physical examination gave negative results, but he had a raised aspartate transaminase activity of 57 IU/L (normal range 12–42), which suggested mild hepatitis. A Monospot test gave positive results, indicating recent infectious mononucleosis. Six months later he still complained of tiredness and aching legs and had not been able to repeat previous performances.[4]

Although these two cases suggest that incipient or insidious infectious mononucleosis can produce fatigue in an athlete, it is more common for chronic fatigue to follow an otherwise typical, florid case of mononucleosis. Mononucleosis typically presents with a 3- to 5-day prodrome of headache, malaise, fatigue, anorexia, and myalgia, followed by a 5- to 15-day syndrome of moderate fever with sweats, sore throat, and tender, enlarged cervical lymph nodes. Lymphadenopathy actually is generalized, and an enlarged spleen becomes palpable by the second week in up to 75% of cases. The pharyngitis is usually the incapacitating feature.

Typical laboratory findings include modest leukocytosis, lymphocytosis, and atypical lymphocytes (10% to 20% of all leukocytes). Transient, mild neutropenia and thrombocytopenia are common, but autoimmune hemolytic anemia is rare. Abnormal liver chemistries, reflecting mild hepatitis, are the rule, but severe hepatitis is very rare.

These clinical and laboratory features should lead to serologic diagnosis with a rapid slide test such as the Monospot. The Monospot and most similar tests are sensitive and accurate 95% to 98% of the time. Most patients will have a positive test by the end of the third week of illness, but up to 10% of adults (and a higher percentage of children) will have negative results repeatedly. Most patients who have apparent mononucleosis but negative serologic tests probably have other viral illnesses, such as cytomegalovirus disease.

No specific therapy exists for mononucleosis, but supportive therapy usually suffices. Analgesics, antipyretics, and hydration are indicated. Lozenges, saltwater gargles, and viscous xylocaine can ease throat pain and dysphagia. The role of corticosteroid therapy is controversial; the emerging consensus is that corticosteroids are indicated only for impending airway obstruction (from large tonsils), immune cytopenias, severe hepatitis, neurological complications, or extreme fever, pharyngitis, and malaise.[5]

Activity should be individualized, but most patients are much better within 1 week, so there is no basis for strict bedrest. In one college study, bedrest did not shorten symptoms, and moderate activity as desired seemed to hasten recovery rather than impede it. Convalescence occurs gradually, with some waxing and waning of fatigue, but most patients are back to normal within 4 to 8 weeks. The highly trained athlete, however, may not regain top fitness for 3 months or more.

Some patients remain fatigued for months after a bout of mononucleosis. Research has shown, however, that the course of mononucleosis is influenced by personality. In West Point cadets, for example, the combination of high motivation but low academic performance predicts the development of symptoms from the infection, whereas the state of psychological health predicts the rate of recovery. Other studies have correlated slow recovery from infectious mononucleosis with depression.

In fact, we have long known that depression-prone persons convalesce slowly. For example, delayed recovery from Asian influenza in 1957 was more common in a subset of patients previously shown to be depression-prone. Similarly, in a 1959 study of patients convalescing from brucellosis, objective clinical and laboratory findings could not distinguish patients who had recovered from those who, years later, still had "chronic brucellosis" in the form of fatigue, headaches, and myalgias. Psychological testing, however, linked the delay in recovery with emotional disturbance, especially depression.[6]

## Other Viral Infections

As mentioned earlier, cytomegalovirus infections can mimic infectious mononucleosis. Probably more common as a cause of chronic fatigue in young athletes, however, is viral hepatitis—especially the sporadic, community cases of non-A, non-B hepatitis.

The case has been made for yet other viral infections as a cause of chronic fatigue in athletes. The earlier report of the two teenage runners with infectious mononucleosis, for example, included two other young athletes with "viral infections," from a total of 12 athletes the author had seen in 1 year. (All 12 had complained of "loss of form," and had "no features suggesting an underlying medical cause.") In both cases, however, the diagnosis of viral infection was based solely on elevated viral titers, specifically, titers to Coxsackie B2 of 1/512 and to Coxsackie B3 of 1/256, respectively.[4]

A recent prospective study, however, points out the limitations of using viral titers alone to attribute chronic fatigue to viral illness. Elite track and field athletes vying for the Scottish Athletic Team were monitored for evidence of viral infection during winter training. Their athletic form was assessed subjectively and also semi-objectively by scaled questionnaires. Among 68 athletes, 47 (68%) reported one or more upper respiratory tract infections and 41 (59%) reported a change of more than one scale unit in performance.

Fifty-four (79%) of the athletes had elevated antibody titers against one or more of the 14 viruses in the screening panel. Serological evidence of past infection with Coxsackie B 1–5 was present in 31 athletes (46%), but only one had evidence of recent infection as reflected by IgM antibody titer. This athlete was performing well and, in the group as a whole, loss of form did not correlate with high viral titers.

The authors concluded that loss of form was unrelated to subclinical viral infection, and that elevated viral titers should be interpreted with great caution among athletes complaining of poor performance.[7]

## Postviral Fatigue Syndrome: Fact or Fancy?

A recent review on viruses and sports performance accepts postviral fatigue syndrome as a possible cause of poor athletic performance.[8] Indeed, our national outbreak of the chronic fatigue syndrome, which in 1985 seemed to spring forth fully formed, like Athena from the brow of Zeus, was initially ascribed to chronic infection with the Epstein-Barr virus (EBV), the cause of infectious mononucleosis.[6] And young athletes have been included among the victims of the "chronic EBV fatigue syndrome," as in the reported cases of 6 women cyclists, aged 18 to 29 years, on the United States Cycling Federation national team.[9] But does the EBV cause fatigue that can last for months or years? In normal persons, it probably does not. As recently reviewed,[6] the chronic fatigue syndrome is not new, but old. It has occurred in dozens of outbreaks dating back to the 1930s. And the rationales for chronic fatigue, like the rituals of quackery, mirror the times. Current times reflect concern about chronic viral infections (e.g., AIDS), so today we tend to ascribe chronic fatigue to viruses.

Instead, the lastest research suggests that the chronic fatigue syndrome often stems from psychological roots, and cycles according to the mood of the patient.[6] Because of the poor correlation between chronic fatigue and EBV titers, and the poor response of the syndrome to acyclovir therapy,[10] most experts no longer think the EBV causes the chronic fatigue syndrome. Indeed, some experts think today's chronic fatigue syndrome, in adults at least, is merely "depression with a new face." The same may apply to some cases of chronic fatigue in young athletes. This is discussed further under "Psychological Problems."

## Anemia

Anemia, even of a mild degree, can cause chronic fatigue in young athletes, but the fatigue is expressed in a special pattern. In the throes of depression, for example, the patient feels fatigued even upon arising in the morning. He or she "gets up tired." In contrast, in the recovery phase of mononucleosis (and that of other viral infections), the typical patient is not fatigued in the morning, but later in the day. He "poops out" as the day wears on, and needs an afternoon nap.

With anemia, the pattern of fatigue is different yet in that it occurs only during effort. The athlete generally feels normal all day until, that is, he or she works out. With mild anemia, the fatigue occurs only during all-out exertion, such as racing. Typical symptoms include labored breathing, "heavy" limbs, early sweating, and (from accelerated accumulation of blood lactate) burning muscles, "tying up," nausea, and perhaps retching.

The most common cause of anemia in young athletes, as in the general population, is iron deficiency. In women, the cause may be physiologic; iron loss via menses may exceed iron gain from the diet. In teenage men, the cause may also be physiologic; iron use in the "growth spurt" may exceed iron supply from the diet. Among mature men, however, iron deficiency anemia should be considered tantamount to gastrointestinal blood loss. Athleticism itself, especially distance racing, can trigger or potentiate gastrointestinal bleeding in certain individuals; the sites and mechanisms of bleeding remain unclear but seem to be diverse.[11]

The definition of mild anemia in athletes is complicated by the fact that the endurance athlete has an expanded plasma volume that dilutes the hemoglobin concentration to cause a mild pseudoanemia. Thus, a hemoglobin level of 13.5 gm/dl may be normal for an elite male marathon runner. A level below 13 gm/dl in a male athlete, however, is usually a true anemia. The corresponding value for a female athlete is less certain, but is probably between 11 and 12 gm/dl. With iron deficiency anemia, the mean red cell volume (MCV) is decreased and the plasma ferritin is under 12 μg/L.

Of course, an individual athlete can be anemic despite a hemoglobin level within the normal range for the general population. For example, if a female athlete's hemoglobin normally is 14 gm/dl, she is probably anemic at 13 gm/dl and definitely anemic at 12 gm/dl. Such as anemia, even though very mild, impairs peak performance. When in doubt, then, an empiric trial of iron (ferrous sulfate, 325 mg three times a day for 1 to 2 months) is prudent. The final proof of iron deficiency anemia is a rise in hemoglobin level with iron therapy.

Iron depletion (manifested by a low plasma ferritin) without anemia probably does not cause chronic fatigue or impair athletic performance. The notion that it does arose from misinterpreted animal research and placebo responses in famous runners. This created a myth of the existence of iron-deficient muscles in the absence of anemia. For example, elite marathon runners normally have lower plasma ferritin levels than the general population. Because of hemodilution and transfer of stored iron into expanded muscle and red cell compartments, a ferritin of 20 to 30 μg/L may be normal for a male marathon runner. Despite this low ferritin value, in the absence of anemia, his performance remains normal.

The best proof that performance remains normal in the presence of low ferritin levels comes from a study in which iron deficiency was induced by venesection. Over a period of 5 weeks, nine men were bled an average of 3.5 L. For the next 4 weeks, they were severely iron-deficient (mean serum ferritin 7 μg/L) and mildly anemic (mean hemoglobin 11 gm/dl). At the ninth week, anemia was obviated by transfusion. At this point, mean maximal aerobic power and running endurance were unchanged from baseline, and muscle enzyme activities also were normal.[12] In short, low ferritin without anemia does not cause fatigue.

## Psychological Problems

### Burnout

Psychological burnout can frustrate elite athletes, and chronic fatigue can be a cardinal symptom of this burnout. Athletes, especially female athletes, often retire from their sport during their mid-teens, long before they have reached their physical and psychological prime. This seems especially common among elite gymnasts, swimmers, and divers, who may already have trained for many years by their mid-teens. Why do elite adolescent athletes burn out? Consider the following case:

A 12-year-old girl is seen by her family physician because of physical and emotional exhaustion. A swimming star, she has captured every state record for her age group. Her father, not her coach, is her major motivator. He is president of her swim club, and has taken time off work to take her to many national meets, where she now ranks in the top 10 in her age group. Six months before a junior Olympic championship for which she has trained rigorously the past 2 years, her competitive times have fallen off. Her school performance has also deteriorated, as has her interaction with both peers and family. She seems to have undergone some involutional depression. She claims she does not want to swim anymore, and that it is not fun. She feels she is being separated from her peers by her success and her demanding father. [13]

Athletic burnout has been defined as a condition produced by working too hard for too long under too much pressure. It is characterized by a progressive loss of idealism, energy, and purpose, and a feeling of being locked into a routine, along with physical and emotional exhaustion.

Burnout may be progressive, with three broad stages. In the early stage, the athlete experiences growing fatigue, loss of enthusiasm, irritability or anger, and diverse somatic complaints. In the intermediate stage, the athlete is often withdrawn and sullen, and complains of severe fatigue, frequent colds, and appetite and weight changes. In the advanced stage, the athlete, by now convinced that he is just not good enough, is cynical, alienated, and sometimes obnoxious. Escapist behavior is common, as well as sudden, dramatic changes in values and beliefs. [3]

Who is most susceptible to burnout? Psychologists point to four traits that characterize athletes at risk: perfectionism, high energy level, orientation toward others, and lack of assertiveness. Ironically, these quiet, intense, sensitive, energetic, perfectionistic athletes are just the sort that coaches tend to like best.

How can burnout be prevented? Coaches can help athletes to combat five common de-motivators. [3] To combat the law of diminishing returns from ever-higher levels of training, coaches can heighten the athlete's awareness of subtle gains. To meet the teenager's growing need for self-determinism, coaches can foster independence and responsibility. To adjust for the athlete's awareness of the increasing physical price (the growing list of aches and pains) the coach can modulate workouts. To keep the athlete from setting goals so high they cannot possibly be achieved, the coach can emphasize broader goals, as well as the many gains from being an athlete. Finally, to adjust to the teenager's growing awareness of the social price, coaches can free time for fun and emphasize that elite athleticism and an enjoyable social life are not mutually exclusive.

## Depression

Burnout merges into depression. Everyone feels "blue" at certain trying times of his life. Indeed, such a response is normal. But someone who cannot "snap out of it" within 2 weeks may be suffering from the illness called depression. And a key feature of depression is chronic fatigue.

Depression is the most common and treatable of all mental illnesses. One in 4 women and 1 in 10 men can expect to develop it during their lifetimes. At any one time, 1 person in 20 is depressed. And the incidence of depression is increasing fastest among the young. Depression is not unusual in the teen years, and it now occurs most often among 25- to 44-year-olds, a shift from the years before World War II, when it most often struck people in their fifties.[6]

The American Psychiatric Association stresses that nearly everyone suffering from depression has pervasive feelings of sadness, helplessness, and hopelessness. Probably, professional help should be sought if the athlete has had four or more of the following symptoms continually for more than 2 weeks: change of appetite, with major weight loss or gain, though not dieting; change in sleeping patterns—too much or too little; waking at least 2 hours earlier than normal in the morning, feeling sad, and moving slowly; loss of interest or pleasure in activities formerly enjoyed; fatigue or loss of energy; feeling worthless or inappropriately guilty; irritability and inability to concentrate, decide, or think; or recurring thoughts of death or suicide.

Unfortunately, only one in five victims of depression seeks help. Most fail to recognize a pattern and instead attribute the physical symptoms to "a virus," the sleeping and eating problems to "stress," and the emotional problems to lack of sleep or improper eating. Any athlete who is chronically fatigued should consider whether he or she is depressed. With therapy (counseling and medications) 80% to 90% of depressed persons can be cured.

## Overtraining and Other Lifestyle Facets

Everyone seems to agree that overtraining causes chronic fatigue, but no one seems to know exactly what overtraining is. To be sure, it contains elements of burnout or depression. But it also contains elements of muscle damage and "underfueling."

The chronic fatigue, or "staleness," that seems to parallel "overtraining" is noted especially among elite college swimmers, where the yearly incidence of staleness may approach 10%, and among elite distance runners, where the career prevalence may approach 60%. Morgan et al. have examined the link of chronic fatigue with burnout or mood disturbance by administering to 400 swimmers the Profile of Mood Scores, a scaled self-rating of tension, depression, anger, vigor, fatigue, and confusion.

Results showed that mood disturbance increases in a dose-dependent fashion with step-wise increases in training load, and that reductions in training load are accompanied by improvements in mood scores. Also, in a study of an intensive, 10-day regimen of overtraining, in which 12 male college swimmers had their daily training distance suddenly doubled, the mood scores predicted with 90% certainty which swimmers showed adverse physiological signs of overtraining and which did not.[14] In other words, the athlete's mood somehow reflects the chronic fatigue evoked by overtraining.

This study of overtraining also emphasized the role of muscle dysfunction. Four of 12 swimmers could not tolerate the heavier training demands, and were forced to swim at significantly slower speeds during the training sessions. These men were found to have significantly reduced muscle glycogen stores, which was the result of their abnormally low carbohydrate intake. Thus, some swimmers may experience chronic muscular fatigue because they do not eat sufficient carbohydrates to match the energy demands of heavy training.[15]

The same might be said of elite distance runners. In a survey of 93 elite female runners, fewer than half of them ate sufficient calories for optimal performance.[16] Similarly, in a nutritional survey of 51 highly trained women runners, caloric intakes generally appeared low for women running 10 miles a day.[17]

It might be noted here that the eating disorders of anorexia nervosa and bulimia typically do not present as chronic fatigue. Although anorexia nervosa can impair cardiac function and thereby reduce peak exercise capacity,[18] the athlete suffering from this disorder (typically a ballet dancer, gymnast, or distance runner) usually manifests not chronic fatigue, but the opposite problem; she is hyperactive, and does not act fatigued even when, by all rights, she should be.[19]

Pathogenic weight-control behavior in the "low-weight sports," however, could plausibly contribute to chronic fatigue in athletes. Some athletes use extraordinary means to reduce body fat in an effort to improve performance. One survey of 182 female college athletes, for example, revealed that 32% practiced at least one pathogenic weight-control behavior daily for at least 1 month. These included self-induced vomiting, binges more than twice weekly, and the use of laxatives, diet pills, and/or diuretics. Such practices were most common in gymnasts and distance runners.[20]

Subsequent surveys among ballet dancers, swimmers, and wrestlers have yielded similar results.[21] It seems likely, therefore, that drastic weight-loss measures contribute to fatigue in certain hard-training athletes.

Muscle damage, too, may be a part of the fatigue of overtraining. As previously reviewed, overtraining causes muscle soreness and ultrastructural muscle damage, and may trigger the acute phase response, an age-old biological host-defense response to injury that itself may induce sleepiness and fatigue.[22] In a sense, the acute phase response, arguably a key feature of overtraining, is the "body's doctor," whose prescription is to slow down, rest, and heal.

Other lifestyle facets potentially can contribute to chronic fatigue in young athletes. Lack of sleep is one of these. Research shows that total sleep hours per week decrease steadily between the ages of 12 and 18 years.[23] Many teenage athletes probably train and compete on too little sleep. Excessive caffeine may also complicate things. Caffeine can foster fatigue by creating peaks and troughs in alertness and by disrupting sleep. Jet lag also can cause fatigue by interfering with key bodily rhythms. In fact, each athlete has a unique circadian rhythm, or "body clock," and trying to train or compete at the "wrong time" of day can produce a sense of fatigue. When all else is equal, the "lark" will win the morning race, but the "owl" will win the evening race.[24]

## Ergolytic Drugs

We hear too much these days about ergogenic drugs, but too little about "ergolytic drugs." Ergolytic drugs sap energy and promote fatigue, especially during all-out exertion. I have already mentioned the possible "ergolytic" roles of caffeine and diuretics. Indeed, it is well known that diuretics, by reducing plasma volume, can curb athletic performance, reducing strength and endurance in wrestlers, and slowing running times in distance racers.[25]

Some young athletes use other drugs that cause fatigue, not so much at rest, but during all-out exertion. Alcohol, for example, slows sprinting and middle-distance running. Marijuana, like alcohol, makes the heart work harder and curtails the ability for all-out exercise. The same is true of smokeless tobacco, commonly used by baseball and football players. Cocaine has been shown to be ergolytic in a recent animal model, in addition to the beta-adrenergic blockers, especially nonselective blockers, commonly used to treat hypertension. All of these drugs can contribute to fatigue during athletic performance.[26]

## Endocrine Disorders

Thyroid disorders can cause chronic fatigue in athletes. Margaret Groos, for example, had suffered a severe slump before placing first in the 1988 U.S. women's Olympic marathon trials. In late 1984, after finishing fifth in that year's Olympic trials, she developed terrifying symptoms, including a pulse rate that went to 250 when she tried to run. She was so fatigued that she could not run even a single mile in less than 8 minutes. After 10 months of suffering, hyperthyroidism (Graves' disease) was diagnosed, and she was cured with radioactive iodine.

Hypothyroidism can cause fatigue also, so thryoid function tests are in order when evaluating an athlete who complains of chronic fatigue. Other endocrine disorders are also possible culprits. Addison's disease should be considered in the adolescent with unexplained fatigue, anorexia, nausea, postural hypotension, and weight loss. Although rare, it has been implicated as a cause of sudden collapse and death during exercise. Juvenile diabetes mellitus, too, which commonly begins in the teen years, can cause chronic fatigue. Typically, however, other symptoms predominate: thirst, polyuria, weight loss, blurred vision, and irritability.

## Respiratory Disorders

Paradoxically, exercise-induced asthma can be an unrecognized cause of fatigue during athleticism. Classically, of course, it comes to light because of the characteristic wheezing, chest tightness, and breathlessness. Sometimes, however, its manifestations can be subtle, as in children, for example, coughing in class after recess. Even high school athletes may not necessarily be aware that they have exercise-induced asthma.

For example, there is a case of a basketball player who saw a physician because of sneezing during the hay fever season.[27] Although he was not aware he had it, an exercise test showed severe exercise-induced asthma. When his asthma was treated, he suddenly realized that "the second quarter of the game did not have to be a wipeout." He had thought that "everybody got this tight and this down."

Hyperventilation does not cause chronic fatigue, but it does cause early fatigue during the game. One physician described hyperventilation episodes in ten high school athletes as they played soccer, hockey, or tennis. The main symptoms were anxiety, tingling of the fingers and mouth, and an inability to catch their breath.[28]

Inhaling ozone can also cause early fatigue during exercise. When highly trained endurance athletes, for example, are exposed to low concentrations of ozone, running and cycling endurance is reduced.[29, 30] Ozone-sensitive athletes may not be able to perform maximally even at the lower end of the first-stage smog alert. At the upper end of the first-stage alert, virtually all endurance athletes will suffer undue fatigue during all-out competition.

If athletes train in indoor facilities when the polyurethane track is being constructed, toxic vapors (ethyl acetate and toluene) can cause wheezing, coughing, breathlessness, and early fatigue.[31]

Finally, seasonal allergic rhinitis, if severe enough, can cause malaise and mild fatigue, which can be compounded on occasion by a secondary bacterial sinusitis.

## Heart Disorders

In young athletes, structural heart disease, usually congenital, is a common cause of exercise-related sudden death,[32] but not of chronic fatigue. Hypertrophic cardiomyopathy most commonly causes no symptoms, but may cause atypical chest pain, dyspnea, palpitations, and near-syncope.[33] Mitral valve prolapse can cause nonexertional chest pain, palpitations, and dizziness, but more often this disorder is asymptomatic and does not curb athleticism.[34] Myocarditis, presumably viral, is a recognized cause of exercise-related sudden death,[35] but whether this tragic event is routinely heralded by chronic fatigue is unknown.

Tachyarrhythmias are a rare cause of fatigue during athleticism. For example, a 16-year-old boy in excellent health had been running 2 to 3 miles a day until 2 weeks before he saw his physician, complaining of light-headedness, palpitations, and breathlessness after running 1 mile. The electrocardiogram revealed atrial flutter with an atrial rate of 250. In an exercise test, he developed a 1:1 ventricular response, and stopped early because of weakness and palpitations. No underlying heart disease was apparent. After DC cardioversion, he remained in normal sinus rhythm and was exercising normally 5 months later.[36]

## Miscellaneous Conditions

Finally, one must consider a miscellaneous group of disorders that are rare causes of chronic fatigue in young athletes. Crohn's disease often begins in adolescence, with fatigue, abdominal pain, bloody diarrhea, fever, and weight loss. Several prominent athletes have overcome Crohn's disease and resumed active sports careers. The same applies to Hodgkin's disease and certain other cancers that presented initially as performance-sapping fatigue in young athletes.

Neuromuscular disease, myasthenia gravis or multiple sclerosis, for example, could conceivably present as chronic fatigue in a young athlete, as could chronic renal disease.[1, 2] Finally, in young female athletes with new-onset fatigue, a possible cause is pregnancy.[37]

## References

1. Rowland TW: Exercise fatigue in adolescents: Diagnosis of athlete burnout. Phys Sportsmed 1986; 14:69–77.
2. Cavanaugh RM Jr: Evaluating adolescents with fatigue. Am Fam Physician 1987; 35:163–168.
3. Feigley DA: Psychological burnout in high-level athletes. Phys Sportsmed 1984; 12:109–119.
4. Roberts JA: Loss of form in young athletes due to viral infection. Br Med J 1985; 290:357–358.

5. Eichner ER: Infectious mononucleosis: Recognition and management in athletes. *Phys Sportsmed* 1987; 15:61–69.
6. Eichner ER: Chronic fatigue syndrome. *Phys Sportsmed* 1989; 17:142–152.
7. Roberts JA, Wilson JA, Clements GB: Viral infections and sports performance: A prospective study. *Br J Sports Med* 1988; 22:161–162.
8. Roberts JA: Viral illnesses and sports performance. *Sports Med* 1986; 3:296–303.
9. Eichner ER: Chronic fatigue syndrome: How vulnerable are athletes? *Phys Sportsmed* 1989; 17:157–160.
10. Strauss SE, Dale JK, Tobi M, et al: Acyclovir treatment of the chronic fatigue syndrome: Lack of efficacy in a placebo-controlled trial. *N Engl J Med* 1988; 319:1692–1698.
11. Eichner ER: Gastrointestinal bleeding in athletes. *Phys Sportsmed* 1989; 17:128–142.
12. Celsing F, Blomstrand E, Werner B, et al: Effects of iron deficiency on endurance and muscle enzyme activity in man. *Med Sci Sports Exerc* 1986; 18:156–161.
13. McKeag DB, Brody H, Hough DO: Medical ethics in sport. *Phys Sportsmed* 1984; 12:145–150.
14. Morgan WP, Costill DL, Flynn MG, et al: Mood disturbance following increased training in swimmers. *Med Sci Sports Exerc* 1988; 20:408–414.
15. Costill DL, Flynn MG, Kirwan JP, et al: Effects of repeated days of intensified training on muscle glycogen and swimming performance. *Med Sci Sports Exerc* 1988; 20:249–254.
16. Clark N: Elite women runners: What do they eat? *Boston Running News* April, 1987, pp 14–16.
17. Deuster PA, Kyle SB, Moser PB, et al: Nutritional survey of highly trained women runners. *Am J Clin Nutr* 1986; 45:954–962.
18. Moodie DS, Salcedo E: Cardiac function in adolescents and young adults with anorexia nervosa. *J Adolesc Health Care* 1983; 4:9–14.
19. Weight LM, Noakes TD: Is running an analog of anorexia?: A survey of the incidence of eating disorders in female distance runners. *Med Sci Sports Exerc* 1987; 19:213–217.
20. Rosen LW, McKeag DB, Hough DO, et al: Pathogenic weight-control behavior in female athletes. *Phys Sportsmed* 1986; 14:79–86.
21. Brownell KD, Steen SN, Wilmore JH: Weight regulation practices in athletes: Analysis of metabolic and health effects. *Med Sci Sports Exerc* 1987; 19:546–556.
22. Eichner ER: The marathon: Is more less? *Phys Sportsmed* 1986; 14:183–187.
23. Levy D, Gray-Donald K, Leech J, et al: Sleep patterns and problems in adolescents. *J Adolesc Health Care* 1986; 7:386–389.
24. Eichner ER: Circadian timekeepers in sports. *Phys Sportsmed* 1988; 16:78–86.
25. Armstrong LE, Costill DL, Fink WJ: Influence of diuretic-induced dehydration on competitive running performance. *Med Sci Sports Exerc* 1985; 17:456–461.
26. Eichner ER: Ergolytic drugs. *Sports Sci Exchange* 1989; 2:1–4.
27. Miller RK: Exercise and asthma. *Phys Sportsmed* 1984; 12:59–77.
28. Karofsky PS: Hyperventilation syndrome in adolescent athletes. *Phys Sportsmed* 1987; 15:133–138.
29. Adams WC, Schelegle ES: Ozone and high ventilation effects on pulmonary function and endurance performance. *J Appl Physiol* 1983; 55:805–812.

114 / E.R. Eichner

30. Schelegle ES, Adams WC: Reduced exercise time in competitive simulations consequent to low level ozone exposure. *Med Sci Sports Exerc* 1986; 18:408–414.
31. Larson DC: Toxic vapor exposure and aerobic exercise. *Phys Sportsmed* 1985; 13:76–83.
32. Van Camp SP: Exercise-related sudden death: Risks and causes. *Phys Sportsmed* 1988; 16:97–112.
33. Cantwell JD: Hypertrophic cardiomyopathy and the athlete. *Phys Sportsmed* 1984; 12:111–121.
34. McFaul RC: Mitral valve prolapse in young patients. *Phys Sportsmed* 1987; 15:194–198.
35. Thompson PD: Cardiovascular hazards of physical activity. *Exerc Sport Sci Rev* 1982; 10:208–235.
36. Blair TP, Baker WP: Atrial fibrillation and flutter in athletes. *Phys Sportsmed* 1985; 13:57–71.
37. Cohen GC, Prior JC, Vigna Y, et al: Intense exercise during the first two trimesters of unapparent pregnancy. *Phys Sportsmed* 1989; 17:87–93.

# Psychosocial Development in the Young Athlete

## Kathleen A. Ellickson, Ph.D.

Department of Psychiatry, Ohio State University College of Medicine, University Hospitals Clinic, Columbus, Ohio

## Editor's Introduction

The role of sports in the psychosocial development of youth is an area in which it is not difficult to find individuals willing to enter discussion. However, one of the problems is that there is not a great deal of conclusive evidence of these effects. Questions such as:

1. Does participation in athletics help in the development of positive psychosocial characteristics, or were these characteristics present prior to participation?
2. What are the positive and negative influences of competition on development?
3. How much parental and adult supervision is beneficial, and when does it become intrusive?

These and other questions will be addressed by Dr. Ellickson in this chapter. However, this area is truly in its early stages and is fertile ground for further research.

*John A. Lombardo, M.D.*

Psychosocial development refers to the problems of social adaptation which the individual faces as he or she grows up within a wide range of human relationships.[1] Successful psychosocial development leads to a mature adult who enjoys a general adjustment to life. That is, the mature adult is one who "attains reasonable happiness, contributes to the happiness of others, deals adequately with the normal vicissitudes of life, and enters into and sustains mutually gratifying and rewarding relationships with other people in his or her life."[2]

The challenge for adults who are conscious of the importance of early psychosocial development to success in later years is to find appropriate experiences that will foster healthy personality development in their children.[3] Historically, community organizations have been thought to provide appropriate psychosocial experiences for the young, and many types of activities have flourished.

Organized athletic programs for children have multiplied over the last decade[4] and, while it is beyond the scope of this chapter to examine the many reasons behind this trend, sport is a socially sanctioned activity of considerable interest to many communities.[5] A conservative estimate is that 50,000,000 children in the United States between the ages of 6 and 16 years participate in organized youth sport(s).[6] Thus, sport is a pervasive force which children encounter during their development. A variety of features which make sport theoretically beneficial to the psychosocial development of the child, as well as those potentially damaging aspects of organized sport, will be reviewed in this chapter.

## Sport and Psychosocial Health

A controversy has surrounded the impact that sport has on the psychosocial development of young people. Proponents cite a number of features which support the beneficence of organized athletics for children, while critics offer an equally long list of complaints. However, it is impossible to settle the debate between those who claim sport is beneficial to the psychosocial development of children and those who claim sport is harmful. While there is a considerable body of literature addressing psychosocial development in the young athlete, the majority of this work represents atheoretical treatises and cross-sectional or correlational studies. For instance, children involved in sport are typically found to possess a variety of positive psychosocial characteristics, including higher self-confidence, better emotional control, greater extroversion, and an increased ability to cooperate with others.[5] However, the temporal sequence between these qualities and athletic participation is still uncertain. In other words, it is impossible to determine whether the positive characteristics observed in children who participate in sport are a result of their athletic involvement (*consequence* of the sport) or act as a selection mechanism (*antecedent* of sport involvement) propelling the individual to become involved in sport.

## Organizational Position Stands on Children in Sport

Organizations which focus on sport or have a division devoted to sport, such as the American Psychological Association, North American Society for the Psychology of Sport and Physical Activity, American Association for Applied Sport Psychology, and United States Olympic Committee, have yet to formulate formal position statements on organized, competitive sport for children. However, The President's Council on Physical Fitness and Sports, the International Council on Children and Sports, the Canadian Association of Applied Sport Sciences, and the Sport Psychology Model developed by the Swedish government have adopted position stands guiding the involvement of children's participation in sports.

The stands taken by these organizations in order to foster positive psychosocial development in the young athlete are summarized in the following selected statements:

1. Access to sport participation should be available for all children regardless of ability, age or gender.
2. Organized programs should emphasize opportunities for socialization and the development of leadership skills.
3. Cooperation and fair play should be promoted.
4. Intensive training in a sport specialization should be avoided while there is still a lack of information on the consequences of such training on the child's growth and development.
5. Practice and competition should be geared to the child's needs, not directed by the needs of adults.
6. Sport programs should be available for handicapped individuals.
7. There should be a commitment to a physically healthy lifestyle through sport activities which provide a release for the stresses of daily living.

## Stress and Anxiety in Youth Sport

A major topic of debate concerning children's participation in sport is the notion of stress. Proponents of organized sport for the young maintain that stress is a positive element, because it helps children learn to deal with unpleasant situations outside of the athletic arena. Critics of organized sport for children, however, insist that not only is stress harmful to the developing self-esteem of the child, but it is a major factor in attrition rates.

Extensive literature exists demonstrating an increase in state anxiety for athletes in precompetition settings.[7-10, 35] The assumption by many has been that anxiety is unhealthy and to be avoided, however, elevated anxiety levels prior to an event requiring active participation do not necessarily imply that the event is detrimental to the young athlete.

For example, Spielberger[11] has challenged the view that stress and anxiety are synonymous states or emotions. Rather, he maintains that stress is a complex psychobiological process which includes three elements: a stimulus variable (stressor), a cognitive appraisal of the stimulus variable, and a response. The stressor may be any stimulus situation, such as altitude, heat, cold, exercise, competition, fans, coaches, and so forth. A cognitive appraisal of the stressor is then made. If the stressor is viewed as harmful or threatening, the perception may be followed by an anxious response. However, based not only on the perception of the stressor but also on the individual's perceived ability to cope with the stressor, a variety of responses may result. An anxiety response has two dimensions: intensity and direction. The intensity of the anxiety can be monitored through physiologic measures such as heart rate, blood pressure, electromyography (EMG), and galvanic skin response (GSR), as well as through measures of self-reported anxiety. The individual's cognitive appraisal of the stressor will lead him to approach or avoid the stressor. Thus, Spielberger's model makes it clear that stressors cannot be avoided or controlled, since they occur in the external environment, and that they are not inherently "good" or "bad." Their meaning is influenced by the individual's aptitude, ability, coping skills, and past experience, as well as by the perceived danger in the situation. The individual can become aware of his perceptions of the stress, and thereby of his emotional response to the stressful environmental factors. Selye[12] has written, "You should not and can not avoid stress, because to eliminate it completely would mean to destroy life itself. If you make no more demands on your body you are dead." Developing higher tolerance levels for stress may in fact be the best strategy to learn.

Railo[13] has suggested that sport may act as a protective agent against the development of psychosocial disorders in children who are experiencing stress or failure in other areas of their life. For instance, a child from a chaotic family may find security in the structure of the team setting; a child with a learning disability may find the success on the playing field not found in the classroom; or a child with a physical limitation may feel a sense of competence and pride for the first time through participation in an adapted sport program.[14-18]

In an attempt to obtain a reference point to compare the anxiety found in sport, Railo[5] asked boys to assess the amount of anxiety they felt in regard to both sport and school. And, as he states, "Fifty-four percent of the boys said that the pressure to succeed was greater in school than in sport, while only 16% felt the opposite."

Railo found that only 5% of the boys in his study experienced stress in the form of extremely angry or abusive parents or coaches. In these few situations, the child perceived the adult to be dissatisfied with the athlete's effort or performance. In the majority of cases, however, the boys were characterized by a positive attitude toward their sporting experience.

Children encounter many activities on a daily basis which evoke potentially high levels of anxiety. Sport may be one such activity, but it is not the only evaluative situation in which children participate. Simon and Martens[19] examined pre-event anxiety levels among 9- to 14-year-old boys participating in required school activities (academic tests and physical education classes), band solos and band group competitions, and athletics. They found that pre-performance anxiety levels did not differ significantly between required school activities and athletics. Band soloists, however, experienced the greatest pre-performance anxiety.

Brown[20] observed that participation on a team was not overly stressful for junior and senior high school students. However, the inability to make a sport team was more stressful to the child than the death of a grandparent, suspension from school, or a parent losing his or her job.

While there is only limited data that demonstrate this advantage equivocally, the possibility that sport may increase a child's tolerance for uncontrollable negative environmental factors deserves further study.

## Intrusive Adults

A frequent criticism among observers of children's sport is the notion that adults often create an unfavorable environment, thereby making it impossible for young competitors to learn new skills and test their physical and emotional natures. Although no studies empirically substantiate the claim that the exaggerated meaning that adults may attribute to organized sport for children creates a dangerous mental health issue for the child, one view among psychologists and behavioral scientists is that adults often manipulate the sport experience to meet their own psychosocial needs rather than allow the activity to be child-oriented.[4, 6, 21, 22]

For example, correlational data suggest that a relationship exists between parents' dissatisfaction with their own working experience and the intensity of projective identification with their child's athletic success. Anecdotal evidence supports the view that performance success in children compensates for frustrated or otherwise unrealized achievement strivings in their parents.[3] When the emphasis in children's sport is placed on performance success, rather than participation for all, a variety of potential problems arise for which children are unprepared to cope.

Children may be more motivated to participate in activities which they believe will gain their parents' love and approval or secure peer acceptance than in winning a game or succeeding in an extrinsic manner.[1] Children who believe that their sense of worth is dependent upon their performance success may feel devalued and unlovable if they experience performance failure. Freeman[23] states, "Children who expect too much of themselves begin to develop a sense of failure to the extent that they may give up trying." Low self-esteem and poor body image are recognized as negative assumptions of melancholic children.[24, 25]

Sport programs which belittle the unskilled child and exalt the "star" performers are also considered to be harmful to the psychosocial development of the participants.[4] Children denied the opportunity for sport participation at an early age may never pursue the chance to enjoy fun and affiliation with peers while exercising their physical and mental energy.

The psychosocial development of the child with exceptional talent may be more problematic than that of the clumsy child, for a variety of reasons. The elite child may be the target of exaggerated adult expectations. For instance, despite the fact that only 2% of boys competing in high school basketball and 4% of participants in high school football make varsity NCAA competition in college, adults may instill their dreams of elite competition in the young athlete. Talented performers may be encouraged to develop their athletic talent at the expense of their educational and personal development. Sport may come to possess disproportionate value to the child who is totally dependent upon it for his or her feelings of self-worth.

In summary, adults involved in children's sport are often thought to misunderstand the young athlete's emotional, educational, and interpersonal needs. Further study is needed in this area, since reliance on anecdotal evidence leaves many issues unresolved.

## Sport and Juvenile Delinquency

The relationship between sport and juvenile delinquency has been of interest to social scientists for more than a century. During the 1850s, English public schools, tired of loitering and drunkenness among their pupils, turned to sport as a mechanism of social control.[26] The idea that sport involvement would fill the student's leisure time, and thereby replace unacceptable behaviors with socially sanctioned ones, had great intuitive appeal.

A number of theories have been advanced to explain the beneficial relationship between sport and delinquent youth. Spencer[27] advanced the idea that delinquent behavior was an attempt at tension-reduction. A child who did not work off his excess energy would reach a bursting point as the energy built. Expending the energy in a wholesome way through sport negated the need to expend it in a deviant way. Several theorists have proposed that violence and vandalism among children and adolescents result from boredom. The notion that "the boy who steals second isn't stealing autos"[28] underscores this view. Conceptually, a child who achieves recognition and achievement in sport is less likely to seek deviant settings for goal satisfaction.

The empirical evidence on sport and delinquency is not conclusive. Since Shafer's[29] original investigation, a few studies have reported no significant relationship between participation in sport and juvenile delinquency, while the majority of studies have reported a negative relationship. Patterns of behavior do seem to exist, however, and while the degree of difference is not the same across studies, the results support the general conclusion that athletes tend to be less delinquent than comparable nonathletes.[30] The negative correlation is strongest among children classified as low socioeconomic athletes who engage in delinquent behavior significantly less than do children classified as low socioeconomic nonathletes.

Whilst the research tends to support the view that a negative relationship exists between sport and juvenile delinquency, the data are descriptive and correlational, making an explanation problematic.

## Attrition

An extensive empirical literature exists describing the relationship between overtraining and staleness in elite adult athletes,[31, 32] but no such systematic inquiry has been conducted with elite young athletes. Despite the absence of data, there exist widely held beliefs that attrition rates in young athletes are a result of increased training demands or increased performance expectations.

Spontaneous, active play is almost universal among children, but participation in organized sport does not typically occur until approximately age 6 years. As Brown[20] observed, participation in competitive youth sport steadily declines after age 12 years and, while many investigations suggest reasons for this trend, more questions than answers still remain. Brown concluded that the strongest indictment against organized sport for children is their "mass exodus" away from sport when they are no longer eligible for Little League.

Some children may drop out of sport due to the competitive emphasis of the programs, but many children seem to thrive on the excitement and challenge of athletic participation and competition. As a child becomes older, the intensity of his training regimen is likely to increase, involving more hours per week devoted to practice and competition. Rowley[33] advanced the idea that for a child to continue in sport he must make personal sacrifices, but his family must also make enormous commitments in terms of time and money, and must be available to fulfill a variety of supportive roles. If the family is reluctant or unwilling to provide transportation and financial assistance as well as to alter the domestic schedule (such as accepting flexible meal times) to accommodate the child, he will not be able to continue in sport, regardless of his personal commitment to participation.

## Summary

The function of sport in the psychosocial development of the young athlete may be inferred only from the state of the existing literature in this area. While the general principle of a sound mind in a sound body continues to receive support,[34] little is known about specifics. Nevertheless, since many believe that an active lifestyle is important and that the patterns of behavior, attitudes, and beliefs that are developed in childhood continue into the senior years, organized sport for children will most likely continue to be promoted. To ensure that young athletes enjoy a reasonably positive experience in sport, the emphasis in athletic programs should be on the individual differences of each child and the opportunity for participation for all children. Sport should not be so dominant an activity to the family (or the community) that the child learns to judge his worth as a person by his physical abilities or worth to the team. Positive as well as negative features exist in sport. The psychosocial development of the young athlete will therefore, to a large extent, be a function of the values promoted by the team to which he belongs.

## Acknowledgments

The author expresses appreciation to William P. Morgan and Patrick J. O'Connor for their thoughtful and constructive comments.

# References

1. Erikson EH: *Childhood and Society*, 2nd ed. New York, Norton, 1963.
2. Kaplan HI, Sadock BJ: *Comprehensive Textbook of Psychiatry*, 4th ed. Baltimore, Williams & Wilkins, 1985.
3. Elkind D: *The Hurried Child*. Reading, Massachusetts, Addison-Wesley, 1988.
4. Orenstein DM: Exercise and the young. *Compr Ther* 1985; 11:38–41.
5. Railo WS: The relationship of sport in childhood and adolescence to mental and social health. *Scand J Soc Med (Suppl)* 1982; 29:135–145.
6. Ogilvie B: The orthopedist's role in children's sports. *Orthop Clin North Am* 1983; 14:361–373.
7. Ellickson KA: Precompetition anxiety states in college athletes. *J Appl Sport Psychol*, submitted.
8. Hanson DL: Cardiac response to participation in Little League baseball competition as determined by telemetry. *Res Quart* 1967; 38:384–388.
9. Morgan WP, Hammer WM: Influence of competitive wrestling upon state anxiety. *Med Sci Sports Exerc* 1974; 6:68–81.
10. Scanlon TK, Passer MW: Factors related to competitive stress among male youth sport participants. *Med Sci Sports Exerc* 1978; 10:103–108.
11. Spielberger CD: Stress, emotions, and health, in Morgan WP, Goldston SE (eds): *Exercise and Mental Health*. Washington, Hemisphere, 1982.
12. Selye H: *Stress Without Distress*. Philadelphia, JB Lippincott & Co, 1974.
13. Railo WD, Unestahl LV: The Scandinavian practice of sport, in *Coach, Athlete, and the Sport Psychologist*. Champaign, Ill, Human Kinetics, 1979, pp 248–271.
14. Edlund LD, French RW, Herbst JJ et al: Effects of a swimming program on children with cystic fibrosis. *Am J Disabl Child* 1986; 140:80–83.
15. Kern L, Koegel RL, Dyer K, et al: The effects of physical exercise on self stimulation and appropriate responding in autistic children. *J Autism Dev Disord* 12(4):399–419.
16. Orenstein DM: Exercise and cystic fibrosis. *Phys Sportsmed* 1983; 11:57–63.
17. Strauss GD, Osher A, Wang CI, et al: Variable weight training in cystic fibrosis. *Chest* 1987; 92:273–276.
18. Watters RG: Decreasing self stimulating behaviors with physical exercise in a group of autistic boys. *J Autism Dev Disord* 1980; 10:379–387.
19. Simon JA, Martens R: Children's anxiety in sport and nonsport evaluative activities. *J Sport Psychol* 1979; 1:160.
20. Brown RD: Exercise and mental health in the pediatric population. *Clin Sports Med* 1982; 1:515–527.
21. Feltz DL: The relevance of youth sports for clinical child psychology. *Clin Psychol* 1986; 39:74–77.
22. Ogilvie B: The child athlete: Psychological implications of participation in sport. *Ann Politic Soc Sci* 1979; 445:47–58.
23. Freeman J: Emotional problems of the gifted child. *J Child Psychol Psychiatry* 1983; 24:481–485.
24. Kashani JV, Husain A, Shekin W, et al: Current perspectives on childhood depression. *Am J Psychiatry* 1981; 138:143–153.
25. Pfeffer CR: Suicidal behavior of children: A review with implications for research and practice. *Am J Psychiatry* 1981; 138:154–159.
26. McIntosh PC: An historical review of sport and social control. *Int Rev Sport Sociol* 1971; 6:5–6.

27. Spencer H: *Principles of Psychology.* New York, Appleton, 1873.
28. Fichter JH: *Parochial School: A Sociological Study.* Garden City, New York, Anchor Books, 1961.
29. Shafer WE: Participation in interscholastic athletics and delinquency. *Soc Probl* 1959; 17:40–47.
30. Segrave JO: Sport and juvenile delinquency. *Exerc Sport Sci Rev* 1983; 11:181–209.
31. Morgan WP: Selected psychological factors limiting performance: A mental health model, in Clarke DH, Eckerts HM (eds): *Limits of Human Performance.* Champaign, Illinois, Human Kinetics, 1985, pp 70–80.
32. Morgan WP, Brown DR, Raglin JS, et al: Psychological monitoring of over-training and staleness. *Br J Sports Med* 1987; 21:107–114.
33. Rowley S: Psychological effects of intensive training in young athletes. *J Child Psychol Psychiatry* 1987; 28:371–377.
34. Morgan WP: *Coping with stress: The potential and limits of exercise intervention (A state-of-the-art workshop). Final report.* Rockville, Maryland, National Institute of Mental Health, 1984.
35. Morgan WP, Ellickson KA: Health, anxiety, and physical exercise, in Spielberger CD, Hackbarth D (eds): *Anxiety in Sport: An International Perspective.* New York, Hemisphere Publishing Company, 1987.

**Part III**

# *Sports Traumatology*

Edited by
WILLIAM A. GRANA, M.D.

# Acute and Chronic Injury: Its Effect on Growth in the Young Athlete

## William A. Herndon, M.D.

Associate Professor, Department of Orthopedic Surgery, University of Oklahoma
College of Medicine, Oklahoma City, Oklahoma

## Editor's Introduction

This chapter reviews the pathophysiology of growth center injury due to acute and chronic trauma. This material is an update of our current file of knowledge and points out the many questions which remain to be answered. We have long recognized the potential problems with acute trauma and now there is the possibility of overuse problems as well, as more and more children participate in endurance and high-performance activity.

*William A. Grana, M.D.*

There is a general consensus that children and adolescents are now involved in the fitness trend that has developed in this country. In addition, they are becoming more actively involved in organized sports.[1] This trend, when it occurred in adults, led to an increase in both acute and chronic musculoskeletal injuries. These injuries have usually been attributed to factors such as overtraining, underconditioning, overuse, and poor technique.[2,3] More recently, an increasing incidence of sports-related injuries in children and adolescents has been reported.[2-15] Although the evidence to date is mostly anecdotal and studies are often contradictory, there is no evidence that the incidence of acute traumatic injuries has increased. In fact, it is likely that fractures, dislocations, contusions, and sprains are as common in play activities and unsupervised sports as they are in organized sports activities.[3,16,17] However, the chronic injuries that have always been seen in the adult recreational athlete are now being documented more frequently in the younger age group and it has been postulated that the immature skeleton is susceptible to this type of injury.[3]

Any discussion of injuries in the young athlete must address several questions. Is this apparent increase in the injury rate really due to a peculiar susceptibility of the growing child to musculoskeletal injury or are the injuries just being reported more frequently? What are the differences between the adult overuse syndromes and those of the younger age group?

Should some sports be avoided in the growing athlete or can some of the injuries be prevented?

For the purposes of this discussion, acute and chronic injuries will be discussed separately with an emphasis on injuries seen most frequently in athletic endeavors. Acute and chronic injuries of the bone and growth plate, joint-ligament complex, and muscle-tendon-bone unit will be covered.

## Growth

Ten percent to 15% of all childhood injuries involve the skeleton and 15% of those involve the physeal region.[18] In addition, acute and chronic injuries of muscles, tendons, and ligaments are frequently seen in this age group. The unique characteristics of these various injuries are determined by both the process and interactions of the growth of bone and the other musculoskeletal tissues. An understanding of growth is therefore necessary for adequate prevention, treatment, and rehabilitation of these injuries.

Growth of the musculoskeletal system is extremely complex and not completely understood. The timing, rate, magnitude, and duration of growth, as well as the onset of periods of rapid growth, are genetically determined and under hormonal control. A complex interaction of nutrition, growth hormone, testosterone, insulin, and thyroid hormone as well as other factors is responsible for the ultimate size and shape of each individual's musculoskeletal system. Additionally, various mechanical forces may be involved (i.e., disuse, paralysis).

The entire skeleton is formed initially as a condensation of mesenchymal tissue. Each bone then forms in one of two ways. Bones such as the skull and facial bones ossify directly from the collagenous model (membranous bone formation). The remaining bones are first formed as a cartilaginous model and then ossify in a progressive fashion with the formation of growth plates at the ends of the bones (enchondral bone formation). Subsequent bone formation may occur by either type of ossification, membranous bone formation from the periosteum or enchondral bone formation from the growth plate. The majority of bones are formed initially by enchondral bone formation but the majority of bone mass is achieved by membranous bone formation.

Enchondral ossification is becoming better understood at a cellular and subcellular level. It occurs in three different anatomic regions: at the physis (pressure epiphysis), at the base of hyaline articular cartilage, and at the apophysis (traction epiphysis). The majority of growth in length occurs in the physis. Growth and remodelling of the joint surfaces occurs at the junction of the articular cartilage and subchondral bone. At the apophyses certain major muscle groups attach to bone. Each of these anatomic regions is subject to either acute or chronic injury with resultant possible alteration in growth. In each place the sequence of growth occurs as described below.

The zones of the growth plates are well known to all orthopaedists (Fig 1). Matrix production occurs in the zone of resting cells (reserve zone).

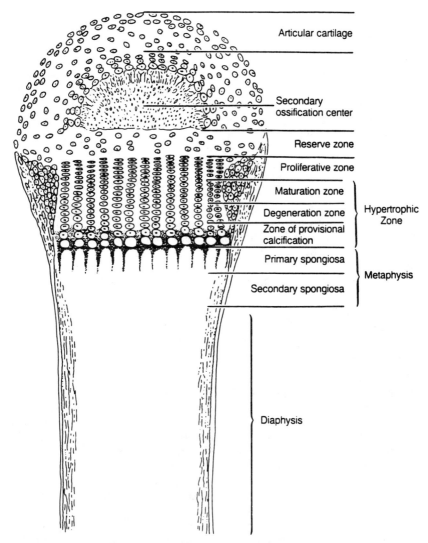

**FIG 1.**
Anatomy of the growth plate.

Growth in length actually occurs in the zone of proliferation where the cells replicate and synthesize matrix. In the zone of hypertrophy, cells imbibe water, increase in size at the expense of the matrix, and subsequently die. Matrix calcification then proceeds at the lower end of the hypertrophic zone (provisional calcification). Finally, in the metaphysis, vascularization leads to deposition of woven bone on the calcified columns (primary trabeculae). The primary trabeculae are then internally remodelled to secondary trabeculae while external remodelling produces the shape of the bone.

Soft tissue growth is not as well described and understood. It is likely that the newborn infant has his full complement of muscle fibers so that muscle volume is increased by adding myofilaments (hypertrophy of fibers), while muscle length is increased by adding sarcomeres to the ends of fibers.[19, 20, 21] However, there is some evidence that the number of muscle fibers may increase with exercise.[22] Growth in muscle volume and length is primarily under hormonal control. Proper muscle growth, however, has been shown to be dependent upon the presence of tension in the muscle,[23] indicating that mechanical factors are also important. Growth in the length of muscles and tendons occurs near the musculotendinous junction, an area that functions somewhat like a "growth plate."[24] Ligamentous growth occurs throughout the length of the ligament.[24, 25] Both ligaments and tendons probably grow by adding fibers.

While there is some evidence that children can increase muscle strength to some extent with directed exercise,[26] muscle size cannot be increased without the necessary hormonal stimulation that comes with puberty. Micheli[3] believes that a muscle-tendon imbalance occurs during the growth spurt. He postulates that muscle length lags behind bone growth, producing a relative muscle tightness and a subsequent decrease in flexibility. This is conjectural, but there is some evidence that flexibility decreases as adolescence is reached.[27-29]

## Acute Injuries of the Bone and Growth Plate

There are significant differences in the biomechanical properties of immature and mature skeletons.[18] Children's bones are in a dynamic state of constant growth and remodelling, while adults' bones change in a much slower fashion in response to the stress placed upon them. Differences in biomechanical properties make fractures less common in adults, generally occurring after much greater trauma. In addition, modes of bone failure are different. Torus fractures, greenstick fractures, and plastic deformation (bowing) of bones are seen in children but not in adults. The growth plate is a weak area and is responsible for unique fracture patterns with potentially serious sequelae.

The response to skeletal injury is also different in the younger age group. Fractures heal much faster and nonunion or delayed union is usually not a problem. In addition, remodelling occurs to a much greater extent in children. Fractures closer to the joint and in the plane of motion of the joint remodel best, while significant rotational deformities do not remodel well. Overgrowth may occur during the process of healing, particularly in femur fractures.

While metaphyseal and diaphyseal fractures are more common in the immature skeleton, there is no evidence that they occur more frequently in organized athletics than in play activities or unorganized sports. In addition, with proper management, these injuries usually do not affect future growth.

## Growth Plate Injuries

A significant percentage of children's fractures involve the growth plate, a factor which complicates treatment and may lead to sequelae. The physis is a biomechanically weak area. A force that causes a sprain in an adult often causes a physeal fracture in a child. Apparent joint instability in the skeletally immature patient is usually due to disruption through the growth plate. This is most commonly seen about the knee, so that an unstable knee in a patient with open growth plates must have stress radiographs taken. Unique fracture patterns may be seen at certain locations when the physis is in the process of closing. An example is the Tillaux fracture, an avulsion of the epiphysis of the lateral distal tibia. The distal tibia growth plate begins to close medially, creating a weak area laterally that is susceptible to avulsion. The corresponding adult injury would be a tibiofibular syndesmotic disruption.

Although numerous classifications of growth plate injuries have been described, the one in greatest clinical use is that proposed by Salter and Harris in 1963.[30] Growth plate injuries are divided into five types that are well known to all orthopaedists (Fig 2). In type I injuries, the epiphysis is separated from the metaphysis. This injury typically occurs in very young children and is almost never associated with growth arrest. In type II injuries, the fracture proceeds through the growth plate and exists on the metaphyseal side of the bone. It is the most frequent type of physeal injury and may or may not lead to growth arrest. When it occurs in the distal femur, up to 36% of patients[31, 32] may develop complete or partial growth arrest. Type III injuries are intra-articular. The fracture line extends from the periphery of the physis transversely across the plate and exits through the epiphysis into the joint. Anatomical reduction is required to prevent growth arrest as well as to provide adequate joint congruity. Type IV injuries extend from the metaphysis vertically across the growth plate to exit into the joint. There is a high incidence of growth arrest if the fracture is not anatomically reduced. The type V injury is controversial and some authors question whether or not it exists.[33] It is believed to be a crushing injury to the plate that is only identified after growth arrest has occurred.

In summary, the unique biomechanical properties of children's bones make them more susceptible to acute injury than are adults' bones. The pattern of injury is different; the presence of growth with the possibility of its alteration may lead to serious problems following healing. However, there is no evidence that organized participation in sports or the training process involved makes the immature athlete any more susceptible to these injuries than his friend who does not participate.

## Acute Injuries to the Joint

Joint injuries include sprains, dislocations, and intra-articular fractures. The overwhelming majority of intra-articular fractures in this age group are

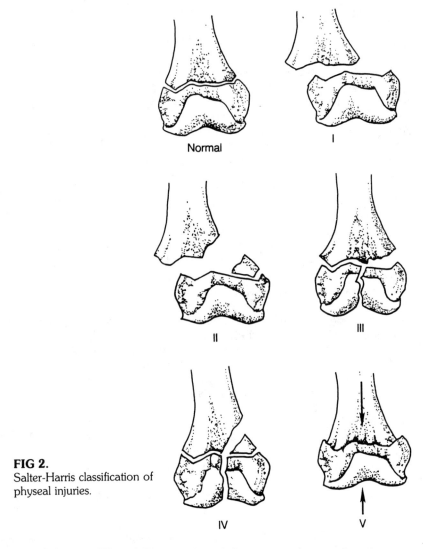

**FIG 2.**
Salter-Harris classification of physeal injuries.

Salter-Harris type III and IV injuries and these were discussed in the preceding section. Ligament injuries (sprains and dislocations) are unusual in the child. Their incidence increases with age as the growth plates close and the biomechanics of the ligament-bone complex approach those of the adult.

The treatment of sprains and dislocations in this age group is the same as with adults and consists of initial rest and stabilization followed by mobilization and strengthening. Once again, these injuries are rare in children and there is nothing to suggest that athletic participation increases their incidence.

## Tibial Spine Avulsion

A study by Noyes[34] has demonstrated that injury to the anterior cruciate ligament complex in adults depends on the rate of loading. Faster loading rates result in ligament rupture, while slower rates result in bone avulsion. Injury to this complex also occurs in children. Because immature bone is weaker than the anterior cruciate ligament, avulsion of the intercondylar eminence of the tibia occurs rather than ligament disruption. However, the mechanism of injury is the same as that which in adults would result in anterior cruciate ligament disruption. This can be seen in athletic injuries, but the most common mechanism of injury is a fall from a bicycle.[35] The injury has been classified into three types based on the degree of displacement. Treatment is most often nonoperative. The knee should be fully extended and a cylinder cast applied. If the reduction is not satisfactory, then open reduction is required. In our experience, even perfect anatomical reduction often leads to mild cruciate ligament laxity. This leads us to believe that some degree of ligament disruption occurs as the spine is avulsed.

## Acute Injuries to the Muscle-Tendon-Bone Complex

Contusions and strains occur in this age group and treatment is essentially the same as for adults. Apophyseal injuries, however, are peculiar to children and adolescents. The apophysis is a traction epiphysis to which major muscle groups are attached. It is the weak link in the muscle-tendon-bone structure and may be avulsed by a sudden strong muscle pull. The most commonly injured apophyses are the medial epicondyle about the elbow, the anterior superior iliac spine, the anterior inferior iliac spine and ischial tuberosity about the pelvis, and the tibial tubercle about the knee. Micheli[3] feels that growing children become less flexible during the growth spurt and he attributes many of the overuse problems to the relative tightness that subsequently occurs. These avulsions commonly occur during athletic activities and may represent poor conditioning and/or poor flexibility. Some may represent the end stage of chronic overuse. It is therefore possible that a program designed to improve conditioning and flexibility could lessen the incidence of these injuries. In the adult, the comparable injury is a severe muscle strain or tear or a tendon rupture. It is likely that the growth process does not change the incidence of the problem but rather is responsible for a different manifestation of the same injury seen in adults.

These injuries usually result in closure of the growth plate, but the injuries typically occur near the end of growth so that the significant problems associated with early closure of the pressure epiphyses are not seen.

## Avulsion of the Medial Epicondyle

This injury commonly occurs in the younger adolescent and is often associated with the act of throwing. It represents an avulsion of the epicondyle by the medial collateral ligaments and the flexor pronator mass of muscles that arise from that region. It may be associated with a dislocated elbow and can also result in medial instability of the elbow joint (Fig 3). In some instances this injury may be the end result of chronic overuse of the elbow (Little League elbow syndrome), which will be discussed later.

Treatment depends on the amount of displacement of the fragment. Nondisplaced or minimally displaced fractures usually require a short period of immobilization followed by early range of motion. Displaced injuries have done very nicely with open reduction and internal fixation in our hands.[36] Entrapment of the fragment in the elbow joint requires open reduction. The fracture heals either with a fibrous union or with a bony union, thereby closing the apophysis. It is usually asymptomatic, although loss of full extension of the elbow may be seen.

## Avulsion of the Ischial Tuberosity

This injury is seen frequently in adolescents and young adults and results from a sudden stretch or pull of the hamstring muscles (Fig 4). The ischial apophysis may not close until the age of 25 years, so the injury represents

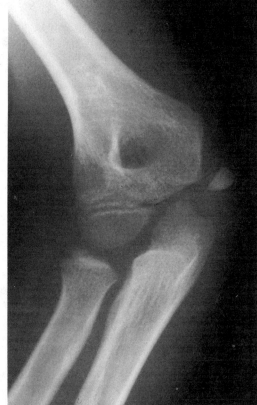

**FIG 3.**
Acute avulsion of the medial epicondyle sustained in a fall on an outstretched arm.

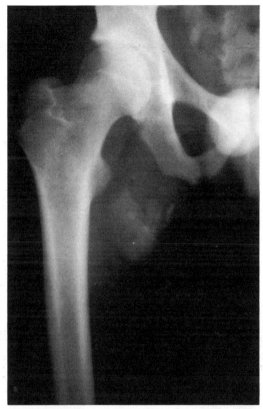

**FIG 4.**
Ischial tuberosity avulsion
sustained when broad
jumping.

an acute avulsion of the apophysis. The fragment is usually not displaced very far since it is held in place by the intact sacrotuberous ligament. Treatment is usually symptomatic and consists of initial bedrest followed by protected weight bearing for 3 to 4 weeks. Occasionally these injuries may heal with an abundant amount of callus that may require surgical removal.

## Avulsion of the Anterior Superior Iliac Spine

This results from an overpull of the sartorius muscle when the hip is in forced extension with the knee flexed. It occurs in adolescence, frequently during participation in athletics. Treatment consisting of rest and protected weight bearing for 2 to 4 weeks is usually all that is required.

## Avulsion of the Anterior Inferior Iliac Spine

Overpull of the straight head of the rectus femoris when the hip is extended and the knee is forcibly flexed produces this injury. It is often seen with kicking (as in football or soccer) and occurs less frequently than anterior superior iliac spine avulsion. The reflected head of the rectus remains intact and prevents significant displacement. Treatment is the same as with anterior superior iliac spine injuries.

## Avulsion of the Tibial Tubercle

This injury results from overpull of the quadriceps mechanism. It may occur without warning or it may represent one end of the spectrum of Osgood-Schlatter disease. The avulsion may range from separation of the tibial tubercle in its distal portion to severe intra-articular fracture of the proximal tibia (Fig 5). The most widely used classification of this injury is that of Ogden et al:[37] type I involves the distal portion of the apophysis; type II is a more proximal fracture that occurs between the tubercle apophysis and the proximal tibial epiphysis; and type III is a severe injury that passes into the knee joint through the proximal tibial epiphysis.

Treatment depends on the type of fracture and the degree of displacement that occurred. An anatomic reduction should be obtained. This usually requires open reduction and internal fixation. A potential complication

**FIG 5.**
Type III tibial tubercle avulsion.

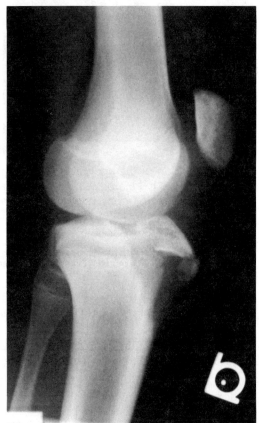

is premature closure of the anterior portion of the proximal tibial growth plate with subsequent genu recurvatum. It is generally not of concern, however, since this injury almost always occurs near skeletal maturity.

## Chronic Injuries in the Growing Athlete

Some authors[3, 4, 7] have indicated that greater involvement in organized sports has created a new series of "overuse" injuries in the skeletally immature athlete. Boland[38] has defined these injuries as "a chronic inflammatory condition caused by repeated microtrauma from a repetitive activity." Micheli[3] believes that the etiology of most of these injuries can be traced to one of seven "risk" factors. He lists these factors as (1) training errors; (2) muscle-tendon imbalance; (3) anatomic malalignment; (4) improper footwear; (5) poor playing surface; (6) associated disease of the lower extremity; and finally (7) growth, in particular the growth spurt.

Overtraining can occur in the young athlete, just as in the adult, and may be responsible for the development of chronic injuries from repetitive microtrauma. There is no evidence that children or adolescents are more susceptible to these problems. Satisfactory studies are not available, but it is likely that this age group can participate in long-distance running and other aerobic training from both a physiological and musculoskeletal standpoint.[39] However, problems with temperature regulation as well as possible psychological problems associated with very long distance running have led the American Academy of Pediatrics[40] to advise against the participation of children in competitive long-distance events.

Muscle-tendon imbalance occurs because of an inadequacy in strength or flexibility. Training for one sport or event may create this problem. Micheli[3] believes that early recognition of this potential problem and the institution of a correct program of exercise will be preventative.

Skeletal malalignment will have an effect on performance and the occurrence of injuries regardless of age. This is perhaps most apparent about the knee, but angular or rotational deformities may create symptoms in any joint of the lower extremities.

Problems with footwear and poor playing surfaces are self-explanatory and are usually easily recognizable and correctable. Associated disease states (i.e., arthritis, severe leg length discrepancy, congenital abnormalities, etc.) are also easily recognizable and may preclude participation in certain activities or sports.

The final risk factor listed by Micheli[3] is growth. He states, "There is clinical and some biomechanical evidence that the growth cartilage, particularly the growing articular cartilage, is less resistant to repetitive microtrauma than is adult cartilage." This statement is difficult to substantiate. The articles he cites[41, 42] seem to refer to sequelae following slipped capital femoral epiphyses rather than athletically induced injuries. Micheli states a second reason that growth can cause problems as follows: "During periods of rapid growth, the growth spurts, there can be a real increase in muscle-tendon tightness about the joints, loss of flexibility, and an enhanced environment for overuse injury." This concept, based on the premise that the growth in length of muscle is secondary to the growth in length of bone, is appealing and would help to explain the apophyseal injuries that are seen during adolescence.

In summary, it appears that the same problems that have caused overuse injuries in the older age group cause similar problems (although often with different manifestations) in the younger age group. Whether or not growth increases the juvenile athlete's susceptibility to these injuries is controversial.

## Chronic Injuries of the Bone and Growth Plate

### Stress Fractures

Stress fractures occur in the child just as in the adult—they are the result of repetitive stress on the bone.[2, 43, 44] As in adults, these fractures are usually the result of "overtraining." The most common sites are in the lower extremities (tibia and fibula), although cases of upper extremity stress fractures have been reported. The spine is another site of frequent overuse injury. Although there may be a hereditary predisposition, spondylolysis has frequently been attributed to a stress fracture of the pars interarticularis. It is seen characteristically in football linemen and female gymnasts.

The radiologic changes of stress fractures may take 2 to 3 weeks to appear and may be confused with bone malignancy, so diagnosis requires a high index of suspicion and a great deal of care. In the absence of definitive radiographic findings, persistent pain related to activity should prompt a search for a stress fracture. Nuclear scintigraphy can be particularly helpful in this regard. The injury responds to rest and cessation of the offending activity. Prevention requires a proper training regimen.

Stress fractures should not result in serious growth sequelae unless they remain undiagnosed to the point where a complete fracture occurs. For example, a femoral neck fracture would have the possible sequelae of nonunion, malunion, or avascular necrosis.

Chronic injuries to the growth plate have not been frequently reported. The most common example appears to be the syndrome of "Little League shoulder." It probably represents a stress fracture of the proximal humeral epiphysis from repetitive throwing by an immature athlete.[45, 46] The injury responds to rest and growth problems have not been reported.

Recent reports[47, 48] have described stress injury of the distal radius and ulna in gymnasts. No growth problem occurred in the single case reported in the first paper but the authors recommended against the use of dowel grips in gymnastics.[47] The second series[48] included 21 gymnasts (17 males and 4 females). The authors found delayed skeletal maturity in these athletes and suggested that these injuries may represent stress fractures of the physis, which is widest and weakest during the growth spurt.

## Chronic Injuries of the Joint-Ligament Complex

### Osteochondritis Dissecans

Osteochondritis dissecans occurs with descending frequency in the knee, elbow, and ankle. The etiology in children is not certain, but it is probably related to either direct or indirect trauma with associated disruption of the subchondral blood supply.[49, 50] Micheli feels that many of these lesions are due to overuse and he uses the occurrence of osteochondritic lesions in young baseball pitchers as a prime example. This has been reported frequently and is considered by some authors as part of the syndrome of Little League elbow.[3, 50–52] These authors have noted changes that include irregularity and fragmentation of the lateral humeral condyle, at times associated with loose body formation (Fig 6). Chronic pain and swelling develops and loose body symptoms may occur. With longstanding cases, enlargement of the capitellum and radial head are often seen and degenerative arthritis may develop. Treatment consists of rest and cessation of the throwing activity. Loose body removal may be required. Development of this condition probably precludes serious involvement in a throwing sport.

The knee is the most common site of involvement of osteochondritis dissecans. Symptoms there are nonspecific. Mild aching pain associated with mild swelling may be seen. In advanced cases, separation of the fragment may have occurred, producing loose body symptoms. Occasionally this condition is found incidentally and there have been reports of familial occurrence, suggesting that there may be a hereditary or constitutional pre-

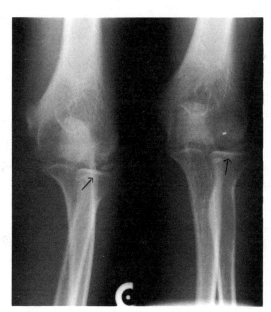

**FIG 6.**
Irregularity of the lateral condyle associated with loose body formation in a 13 year-old male who had been pitching since the age of 4 years old.

disposition.[49] Radiographs demonstrate a subchondral fragment of bone with a surrounding radiolucent area, usually on the lateral aspect of the medial femoral condyle. Conservative treatment consisting of limiting activity, sometimes with periods of immobilization, usually results in healing unless a loose body has developed.

Osteochondral lesions of the talus were reviewed by Canale.[53] All lateral lesions were associated with trauma but some medial lesions were not. It is difficult to say whether or not any of the medial or lateral lesions were truly overuse injuries.

In summary, the hypothesis that overuse is an etiology of osteochondritis dissecans is best substantiated in the elbow. The evidence in the case of the knee and ankle is not clear. There is no question however, that osteochondritic lesions of any of the joints can be seen without a definite history of repetitive microtrauma.

## Patellofemoral Pain

The most common overuse injury about the knee involves the patellofemoral joint and the remainder of the extensor mechanism. Many different etiologies have been implicated in the so-called patellofemoral pain syndrome. There is a spectrum of severity of this disease with a basic syndrome consisting of aching knee pain accompanied by occasional swelling at one end and frank recurrent dislocation of the patella at the other. The milder forms probably represent an imbalance in the muscular and ligamentous structures of the patellofemoral complex, while the more severe forms probably have some degree of anatomic malalignment of the extensor mechanism.

The most common symptom of chronic patellofemoral pain syndrome is aching knee pain, either with activity or at rest. Pain when climbing or descending stairs or with prolonged knee flexion from sitting may be seen also. Other symptoms include giving out or buckling of the knee, recurrent swelling, and crepitus. Examination may reveal an effusion, decreased motion, patellofemoral crepitus with motion, and a positive patellar apprehension sign. Extensor mechanism malalignment should be searched for.

Treatment should be directed toward restoring the muscular ligamentous imbalance. Most patients respond to a program designed to strengthen the medial quadriceps mechanism and stretch the tight lateral ligamentous structures (iliotibial band). If that program is unsuccessful, a lateral release[54] may be required. Rarely, more extensive operative extensor realignment may be required.

## Chronic Injuries of the Muscle-Tendon-Bone Unit

Injuries to this complex are the most common overuse injuries seen in all age groups. Symptoms are inflammatory in nature and may well be caused by a relative imbalance in strength and flexibility. In adults, injuries occur because of underconditioning, while the problems in children have been attributed to an imbalance created by growth.[3]

This type of overuse injury is not limited to the immature athlete. This author frequently sees these problems develop secondary to play activity in non-athletes encountered in a busy pediatric orthopaedic clinic. This is probably analogous to the adult who develops symptoms after "overdoing it" during a weekend recreational activity. As in adults, the most effective cure for these injuries in children is prevention. Proper conditioning and coaching should prevent the majority of these symptoms in the absence of serious malalignment problems. As with all athletic endeavors, emphasis should be placed on flexibility and strengthening with the realization that the rapidly growing athlete may actually require more work on flexibility than does his adult counterpart.

## Tendinitis

Tendinitis is unusual in this age group. Usually, symptoms occur at the apophyses rather than at the tendons. The most common tendinitis seen in our clinic is posterior tibial tendon tendinitis and this is usually seen in the patient with pronated feet. Symptoms usually respond to rest, occasional immobilization, and occasional orthotics.

## Little League Elbow

Biomechanically, the throwing action places tremendous compression forces across the lateral side of the joint and tension forces across the medial side of the joint. Although osteochondritic lesions of the capitellum and/or radial head occur as discussed previously, injury to the medial side of the joint is more common.[55–57] The recognition of this entity represents an instance where an overuse injury has led to significant rule changes in a sport. Since the incidence of these injuries has been found to be proportional to the amount of throwing in which a player engages[51] rules have been made limiting the amount and duration of throwing allowed in Little League baseball.

Recurrent tension forces across the medial side of the joint by the flexor pronator mass of forearm muscles produces a chronic apophyseal injury. Early changes may include aching pain, tenderness, swelling, and erythema over the medial epicondyle. Radiographically, fragmentation or mild separation of the apophysis may be seen. At times, a complete avulsion fracture may occur. Treatment consists of rest and cessation of pitching followed by gradual resumption of activity. Proper conditioning and coaching will help prevent further episodes, but often a change in playing position is necessary.

## Iliac Apophysitis

Anterior and posterior iliac apophysitis was first described by Clancy in 1976.[58] It occurred in a group of middle- and long-distance adolescent runners. It was presumed to be due to repetitive trauma to the anterior or posterior iliac crest (Fig 7). Anteriorly, the abdominal obliques, tensor fascia, and gluteus medius were implicated, as were the gluteus maximus and

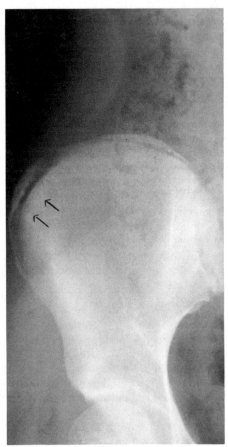

**FIG 7.**
Radiographic changes of iliac
apophysitis in a 14-year-old female
athlete.

latissimus dorsi posteriorly. The condition was a significant cause of disability to these athletes and resolved with 4 to 6 weeks of rest.

## Osgood-Schlatter Disease

This is one of the most common knee complaints seen in a busy pediatric orthopaedic practice. It occurs in older children and adolescents and is more common in males. It represents an inflammatory response to overpull of the extensor mechanism at its insertion into the tibial tubercle.[59] It may be seen with any athletic endeavor or in children and adolescents participating in play activity. Symptoms include pain and tenderness directly over the tibial tubercle, often with enlargement of the tubercle. The symptoms are aggravated by running and jumping. Radiographs may be normal, but often show enlargement and fragmentation of the tubercle.

Treatment consists of rest, activity modification, anti-inflammatory agents, and a regimen of quadriceps muscle stretching and isometric strengthening. A program of heat before activity and ice afterwards has been helpful. Excision of the boney fragments is not indicated before growth is completed, and then only very rarely. Cast immobilization should be avoided if possible.

## Calcaneal Apophysitis

The gastro-soleus inserts into the calcaneal apophysis. Overuse of this complex produces an inflammatory response at the insertion of the Achilles tendon into the calcaneal apophysis.[60] Patients complain of heel pain with activity, and examination often reveals heel cord tightness, swelling, and local tenderness. Radiographs are usually normal. In the past, increase in density and fragmentation of the apophysis have led to a diagnosis of Sever's disease. These represent normal findings in most cases and may be seen in asymptomatic individuals. Management consists of rest, stretching, occasional anti-inflammatory agents, and occasional immobilization. With symptomatic treatment, athletic participation can usually continue.

## Summary

It has been established that involvement in sports does not present any greater risk of acute musculoskeletal injury than participation in playground activities. Acute fractures are, however, more common in the young athlete with open physes than in the adult athlete. This is due to the biomechanical differences between the immature and mature musculoskeletal systems. While certain fractures may cause serious growth disturbances, the usual circumstances are that these injuries heal quickly with no sequelae.

The occurrence of overuse syndromes in the younger age group seems to be increasing. This has paralleled a similar increase in these injuries in the adult population and for the most part can be attributed to the same factors. Data are not available to tell whether or not these injuries are more common in children and adolescents involved in sports than in the nonathletic individual of the same age group.

It has been postulated that the growth spurt, by causing a relative musculotendinous tightness, is partially responsible for the occurrence of these injuries. In fact, whether or not this tightness actually occurs has not been demonstrated. While the manifestations of overuse injury are different in the immature skeleton, a true increase in risk has not been proven. The majority of overuse injuries in this age group do not result in permanent sequelae and, in fact, readily respond to rest, changes in training or equipment, and a stretching and strengthening program.

Training for and participation in athletics is safe for the immature individual. As with adults, proper supervision and instruction will result in fewer injuries. Recognition of higher-risk situations followed by modification of activity (such as limiting the number of innings pitched per week) has been shown to be effective. To date, no evidence has been shown which would preclude participation in sports for this age group.

# References

1. Stanitski CL: Pediatric sports injuries. *Adv Orthop Surg* 1985; 9:53–57.
2. Micheli LJ, Santopietro F, Gerbino P, et al: Etiologic assessment of overuse stress fractures in athletes. *Nova Scotia Med Bull* 1980; 59:43–47.
3. Micheli LJ: Overuse injuries in children's sports: The growth factor. *Orthop Clin North Am* 1983; 14:337–360.
4. Kozak B, Lord RM: Overuse injury in the young athlete: Reasons for concern. *Phys Sports Med* 1983; 11:116–122.
5. Chandy TA, Grana WA: Secondary school athletic injury in boys and girls: A three-year study. *Phys Sports Med* 1985; 13:107–111.
6. Grana WA: Little League sports: Are they safe? *Orthop Trans* 1979; 3:88.
7. Wilkins KE: The uniqueness of the young athlete: Musculoskeletal injuries. *Am J Sports Med* 1980; 8:377–382.
8. Caine DJ, Lindner KJ: Growth plate injury: A threat to young distance runners. *Phys Sports Med* 1984; 12:118–124.
9. Larson RL: Epiphyseal injuries in the adolescent athlete. *Orthop Clin North Am* 1973; 4:839–851.
10. Goldberg B, Rosenthal PP, Nicholas JA: Injuries in youth football. *Phys Sportsmed* 1984; 12:122–130.
11. Dehaven KE: Athletic injuries in adolescents. *Pediatr Ann* 1978; 7:704–714.
12. Roser LA, Clawson DK: Football injuries in the very young athlete. *Clin Orthop* 1970; 69:219–223.
13. Goldberg B, Whitman PA, Gleim GW, et al: Children's sports injuries: Are they avoidable? *Phys Sports Med* 1979; 7:93–101.
14. Chambers RB: Orthopaedic injuries in athletes (ages 6 to 17). *Am J Sports Med* 1979; 7:195–197.
15. Micheli LJ, Gerbino PJ: The epidemiology of children's sports injuries. *Orthop Trans* 1979; 3:88.
16. Jackson DW, Jarrett H, Bailey D, et al: Injury prediction in the young athlete: A preliminary report. *Am J Sports Med* 1978; 6:6–14.
17. Larson RL, McMahan RO: The epiphyses and the childhood athlete. *JAMA* 1966; 196:99–104.
18. Ogden JA: The uniqueness of growing bones in fractures in children, in Rockwood CA, Wilkins KE, King RE (eds): *Fractures in Children.* Philadelphia, JB Lippincott, 1984, pp 1–86.
19. Tawa NE, Goldberg AI: Proteins and amino acid metabolism in muscle, in Engel AG, Banker BQ (eds): *Myology.* New York, McGraw-Hill, 1986, pp 721–743.
20. Astrom KE, Adams RD: Pathological changes in disorders of skeletal muscle as studied with the light microscope, in Walton J (ed): *Disorders of Voluntary Muscle,* 5th ed. New York, Churchill Livingstone, 1988, pp 153–209.
21. Ziv I, Blackburn N, Rang M, et al: Muscle growth in normal and spastic mice. *Dev Med Child Neurol* 1984; 26:94–99.
22. Gonyea W, Erickson GL, Bonde Peterson F: Effect of exercise on muscle growth and hypertrophy. *Acta Physiol Scand* 1977; 99:105–109.
23. Williams PE, Goldspink G: Longitudinal growth of striated muscle fibres. *J Cell Sci* 1971; 9:751–767.
24. Dahners LE, Mueller P: Longitudinal ligamentous growth occurs throughout the ligament. *Orthop Trans* 1987; 11:264.
25. Frank L, Bodie D, Anderson M, et al: Growth of a ligament. *Orthop Trans* 1987; 11:264–265.

26. Sewall L, Micheli LJ: Strength training for children. *J Pediatr Orthop* 1986; 6:143–146.
27. Kendall HO, Kendall FP: Normal flexibility according to age groups. *J Bone Joint Surg* 1948; 30A:690–695.
28. Leighton JR: Flexibility characteristics of males ten to eighteen years of age. *Arch Phys Med Rehabil* 1956; 37:494–499.
29. Leighton JR: Flexibility characteristics of males six-to-ten years of age. *JAPMR* 1964; 18:19–25.
30. Salter RB, Harris WR: Injuries involving the epiphyseal plate. *J Bone Joint Surg* 1963; 45A:587–622.
31. Stephens DL, Louis DS, Louis E: Traumatic separation of the distal femoral epiphyseal cartilage plate. *J Bone Joint Surg* 1974; 56A:1383–1390.
32. Lombardo SJ, Harvey JP Jr: Fractures of the distal femoral epiphyses. Factors influencing prognosis: A review of the thirty-four cases. *J Bone Joint Surg* 1977; 59A:742–751.
33. Peterson HA, Burkhart SS: Compression injury of the epiphyseal growth plate: Fact or fiction? *J Pediatr Orthop* 1981; 1:377–388.
34. Noyes FR, Delucas JL, Torvik PJ: Biomechanics of anterior cruciate ligament failure: An analysis of strain-rate sensitivity and mechanisms of failure in primates. *J Bone Joint Surg* 1974; 56A:236–253.
35. Meyers MH, McKeever FM: Fracture of the intercondylar emence of the tibia. *J Bone Joint Surg* 1959; 41A:209–222.
36. Hines RF, Herndon WA, Evans JP: Operative treatment of medial epicondyle fractures in children. *Clin Orthop* 1987; 223:170–174.
37. Ogden JA, Tross RB, Murphy MJ: Fractures of the tibial tuberosity in adolescents. *J Bone Joint Surg* 1980; 62A:205–215.
38. Boland AL: Upper-extremity injuries: Overuse syndromes of the shoulder, in Cantu RL (ed): *The Exercising Adult.* Lexington, Mass, Collamore Press, 1982, pp 115–120.
39. Rowland TW, Walsh C: Characteristics of child distance runner. *Phys Sports Med* 1985; 13:45–53.
40. American Academy of Pediatrics: Risks in long-distance running for children. *Phys Sports Med* 1983; 11:116–122.
41. Murray RO, Duncan C: Athletic activity in adolescence as an etiological factor in degenerative hip disease. *J Bone Joint Surg* 1971; 53B:406–419.
42. Stulberg SD, Cordell LD, Harris WH, et al: Unrecognized childhood hip disease: A main cause of idiopathic osteoarthritis of the hip, in *The Hip: Proceedings of the Third Open Scientific Meeting of the Hip Society,* vol 3. St Louis, CV Mosby, 1975, pp 212–228.
43. Devas MB: Stress fractures in children. *J Bone Joint Surg* 1963; 45B:528–541.
44. Walter NE, Wolf MD: Stress fractures in young athletes. *Am J Sports Med* 1977; 5:165–170.
45. Cahill BR, Tullos HS, Fain RH: Little League shoulder. *J Sports Med* 1974; 2:150–153.
46. Barnett LS: Little League shoulder syndrome: Proximal humeral epiphyseolysis in adolescent baseball pitchers. *J Bone Joint Surg* 1985; 67A:495–496.
47. Yong-Hing K, Wedge JH, Bowen CVA: Chronic injury to the distal ulnar and radial growth plates in an adolescent gymnast. A case report. *J Bone Joint Surg* 1988; 70A:1087–1089.
48. Carter SR, Aldridge MJ: Stress injury of the distal radial growth plate. *J Bone Joint Surg* 1988; 70B:834–836.

49. Griffin PP: The lower limb, in Lovell WW, Winter RB (eds): *Pediatric Ortho-paedics*. Philadelphia, JB Lippincott, 1986, pp 865–893.
50. Micheli LJ: Overuse injuries in children, in Lovell WW, Winter RB (eds): *Pediatric Orthopaedics*. Philadelphia, JB Lippincott, 1986, pp 1103–1120.
51. Adams JE: Injury to the throwing arm. *Calif Med* 1964; 102:127–132.
52. Lipscomb A: Baseball pitching injuries in growing athletes. *J Sports Med* 1975; 3:25–34.
53. Canale TS, Belding RH: Osteochondral lesions of the talus. *J Bone Joint Surg* 1980; 62A:97–102.
54. Micheli LJ, Stanitski CL: Lateral patellar retinacular release. *Am J Sports Med* 1981; 9:330–336.
55. Gugenheim JJ, Stanley RF, Woods GW, et al: Little League survey: The Houston study. *Am J Sports Med* 1976; 4:189–199.
56. Larson RL, Singer KM, Bergstrom R, et al: Little League survey: The Eugene study. *Am J Sports Med* 1976; 4:201–209.
57. Torg JS, Pollack H, Sweterlitsch P: The effect of competitive pitching on the shoulders and elbows of preadolescent baseball players. *Pediatrics* 1972; 49:267–272.
58. Clancy WG, Foltz AS: Iliac apophysitis and stress fractures in adolescent runners. *Am J Sports Med* 1976; 4:214–218.
59. Ogden JA, Southwick WO: Osgood-Schlatter's disease and tibial tuberosity development. *Clin Orthop* 1976; 116:180–189.
60. Micheli LJ, Ireland ML: Prevention and management of calcaneal apophysitis in children: An overuse syndrome. *J Pediatr Orthop* 1987; 7:34–38.

# Update on Elbow Injuries in the Young Athlete

## Kenneth M. Singer, M.D.

Clinical Instructor in Orthopaedic Surgery, University of Oregon Health Sciences Center, Eugene, Oregon

## Daniel O'Neill, M.D.

Director, Plymouth Sports and Orthopaedic Clinic, Plymouth, New Hampshire

### Editor's Introduction

More than 10 years ago, Dr. Singer participated in a classic study of elbow pain in the Little League athlete. In this chapter, he gives a reprise of these problems and other concerns in the pediatric athlete. Because there are many growth centers about the elbow with rather late closure, the potential for growth deformity is a risk in the young athlete. Awareness and appropriate evaluation are the best safeguards to prevent these problems.

*William A. Grana, M.D.*

The spectrum of injuries in skeletally immature athletes is different from that of their adult counterparts. Children are now often involved in *organized* sports activities, with scheduled practice sessions and competitions. They are encouraged by parents and coaches to achieve excellence by practice and repetition. They are becoming better athletes at an earlier age, and now indeed can run faster, jump higher, and throw farther than the generations preceding them. Skill levels have increased, and so has the risk of injury, both the acute and overuse types. In addition, more girls are participating than ever before, which increases the size of the population at risk. It is, therefore, understandable that injuries in the young athlete have increased in prevalence and complexity.

The elbow, with its six growth centers, fragile articular cartilage, and immature muscle and ligament attachments, is sandwiched in a vulnerable position between the weight of the body and the fulcrum of the hand. Although injuries occur in children by the same mechanism as in adults, the injury pattern in the child and adolescent is different.

Initially, it was baseball that demonstrated how susceptible the immature elbow is to injury,[1, 2] but it is apparent that gymnastic,[3] tennis, and even field events[4] and wrestling are also of concern. In fact, any sports activity poses the risk of an acute injury, and any activity that involves repetition

**147**

can cause overuse injuries in the area of the elbow. These injuries range from skeletal abnormalities such as epiphyseal fractures or osteochondritis of the capitellum, to soft tissue problems such as ligament injuries and tendinitis. They may be caused by an individual traumatic event, such as a fall or a forceful throw, or may occur as a result of repetitive stresses that are cumulative, as is the case with osteochondritis or tendinitis.

Coaches and parents of children involved in organized sports activities must be educated to be cognizant of the potential seriousness of symptoms involving the elbow, and physicians caring for skeletally immature individuals participating in organized sports today must remain vigilant for articular and epiphyseal injuries that are often difficult to detect and treat.

## Anatomy

The stability of the elbow joint is derived from both the osseous and soft tissue structures.

The combination of osseous and ligamentous components of the elbow forms a relatively tightly constrained hinge joint. The proximal ligament/capsular complex attaches circumferentially around the distal humeral metaphysis and distal humeral epiphyses, and particularly at the epicondyles. The distal capsular attachments are on the metaphysis of the radius and ulna, and because of these attachment sites, forces directed to the elbow will tend to be transmitted to the supracondylar humeral area or to the proximal forearm. When the child falls on his outstretched hand, supracondylar or proximal radius and ulnar fractures are more likely to occur, because the attachment sites of the ligament/capsular complex are weaker than the complex itself.

The epiphyses are also a site of relative weakness, and if the forces involve the elbow joint itself, epiphyseal fractures result. As the child matures into adolescence, the bones become stronger than the soft tissues, and dislocations or severe ligament injuries, which are rare in the child, are more apt to occur.[5]

There is much variation in the radiographic appearance of the elbow in the child and adolescent because of the numerous ossification centers. The average ages of the appearance and closure of these centers are seen in Table 1.[6] Because of the variability, radiographs are often difficult to interpret, and when abnormalities are suspected, it is often advisable for even the experienced practitioner to obtain comparison views of the normal side.

Some unusual ossification situations are worth noting. The proximal portion of the ulna is formed by the olecranon epiphysis. The secondary center of ossification appears at approximately age 10 years, and may occasionally be bipartite. The epiphysis of the radial head, which ossifies earlier (ages 5 to 7 years) and fuses at ages 16 to 18 years, has an intracapsular blood supply, similar to the femoral head, and thus is at risk for avascular necrosis should trauma occur to the epiphyseal plate.

**TABLE 1.**
**Ages of Appearance and Fusion for Secondary Ossification Centers About the Elbow***

| | Approximate Age of Appearance (Years) | | Approximate Age of Fusion (Years) | |
| --- | --- | --- | --- | --- |
| | Males | Females | Males | Females |
| Capitellum | 2 | 2 | 14.5 | 13 |
| Radial head | 5 | 4.5 | 16 | 14 |
| Medial epicondyle | 7 | 5 | 17 | 14 |
| Lateral epicondyle | 11 | 10 | 15 | 12.5 |
| Trochlea | 9 | 8 | 13 | 11.5 |
| Olecranon | 10 | 8 | 16 | 14 |

*From Pappas AM: *Clin Orthop* 1982; 164:30–41. Used by permission.

The ligamentous stability of the elbow assumes clinical importance after epiphyseal closure.[7] On the lateral side, the lateral collateral ligament complex extends from the lateral epicondyle to the annular ligament, usually with some fibers going from the lateral epicondyle directly to the ulna posteriorly (Fig 1). The lateral collateral ligament provides, at most, only 10% of the stability to varus stress, with the joint articulation providing the majority of the stability. The anconeus possibly functions as a lateral collateral ligament as well.

The structures imparting stability to the medial side of the elbow are of much greater clinical importance (Fig 2). The posterior oblique ligament, or the posterior bundle[8] of the medial ligament, extends from the posterior aspect of the medial epicondyle of the humerus to the posterior half of the olecranon, and functions to resist valgus stress only with the elbow flexed. It is, in fact, absent in many primates. The anterior oblique ligament, or the anterior bundle,[8] is the major medial stabilizer and is essential to valgus stability. It consists of two sets of fibers, one taut in flexion and the other taut in extension. The anterior oblique ligament extends from the medial epicondyle distally and anteriorly to the medial aspect of the ulna just below the coronoid process. With the elbow in extension, valgus stress is resisted by the osseous structures, with the olecranon firmly stabilized in the olecranon fossa of the humerus. Valgus stress is enhanced in flexion by the common flexor muscles and the anterior joint capsule.[8]

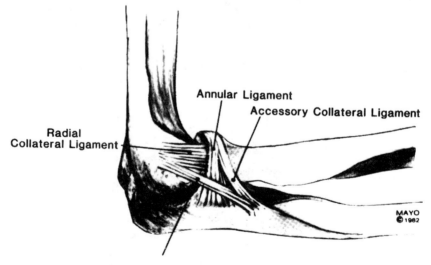

Annular Ligament

Accessory Collateral Ligament

Radial
Collateral Ligament

MAYO
© 1982

Lateral Ulnar Collateral Ligament

**FIG 1.**
Anatomy of the lateral side of the elbow showing the broad radial collateral ligament inserting into the annular ligament and the ulna. (From Morrey BF [ed]: *The Elbow and Its Disorders.* Philadelphia, Penn, WB Saunders Co., 1985. Used by permission.)

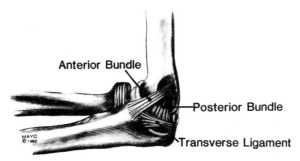

**FIG 2.**
The ligaments of the medial side of the elbow depicting the components of the medial collateral ligament. (From Morrey BF [ed]: *The Elbow and Its Disorders.* Philadelphia, Penn, WB Saunders Co., 1985. Used by permission.)

As flexion increases, the capsule and ligaments account for progressively more of the medial stability.

## Mechanism of the Throwing Motion

A complex series of events must be set in motion in order to forcefully throw an object, be it for speed, distance, or accuracy. If one understands the stresses placed on the elbow during throwing, it becomes easier to understand the spectrum of injuries that occur.[9, 12]

The overhand throwing motion, used in pitching a baseball, serving a tennis ball, or throwing a javelin, derives energy that originates from the powerful muscles of the legs and trunk, and then involves in succession the muscles of the shoulder, arm, forearm, and finally the hand. The throwing motion can be divided into distinct phases (Fig 3).

The initial phases of the throwing motion place the arm in a preparatory position for throwing, and are referred to as the wind-up and cocking phases. These motions bring the shoulder into a position of external rotation, abduction, and extension, and bring the elbow into flexion. They are essentially static phases, and place no stresses of note on the elbow. By the end of the cocking phase, the body is turned 90 degrees to the direction being thrown, the weight transfer has started to the front foot, the ball is poised as far back as it will ever be, ready to begin its propulsion forward, and the shoulder has started forward. The shoulder adductors, internal rotators, and flexors are all preloaded, ready to begin their strong contractions.

The acceleration phase is the most forceful part of throwing. During the early portion of the acceleration phase, the shoulder propels the arm forward and, because of the inertia of the aftercoming arm, the elbow is forced into valgus and extension. It is during this phase that the lateral side of the elbow is subjected to high compression forces, and these are distributed to the radial head, the capitellum, and the intervening articular carti-

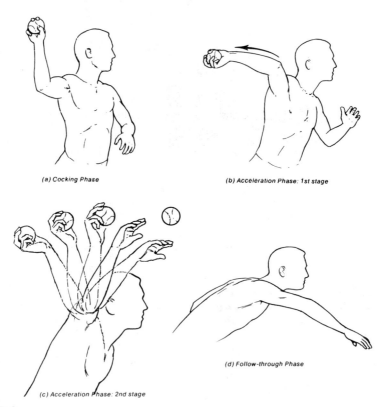

(a) Cocking Phase

(b) Acceleration Phase: 1st stage

(c) Acceleration Phase: 2nd stage

(d) Follow-through Phase

**FIG 3.**
The phases of the throwing motion (Courtesy of Dr. G. William Woods. Used by permission.)

lage. The structures on the medial side are placed under tension as the arm is forced into valgus, and this produces stretching of the medial capsule, the medial ligaments, and the origin of the forearm flexor muscles.

At the point of ball release, the wrist flexors contract forcefully, adding to the stresses on the medial ligament, the forearm flexor muscles, and the medial humeral epicondyle.

Also during the acceleration phase, the elbow is extended rapidly by a strong contraction of the triceps, exposing the muscle, its tendon, and its attachment at the olecranon to injury. Very large forces occur during this phase, and angular velocities averaging 4,595 degrees/sec have been reported in professional pitchers.[10]

The ball is released during the late acceleration phase, usually at the level of the ear, and the arm continues into the deceleration or follow-through phase. During this phase, the arm is decelerated rapidly. The elbow flexors contract to brake the extending elbow, and the ligamentous and boney components must absorb the forces that are not dampened by the eccentric muscle contractions. The olecranon strikes the supracondylar fossa of the humerus as the ultimate endpoint of extension, causing impingement at impact.

In addition to the valgus and extension forces, if the athlete is throwing a fast ball or a screw ball, the elbow is snapped into pronation and radial deviation, and if he is throwing a curve ball, forceful supination and ulnar deviation will occur, adding additional stresses to the elbow. When a youngster attempts to throw a breaking ball and does so incorrectly, he may snap the wrist forcefully, increasing the muscle forces on the medial side of the elbow. However, when electromyography (EMG) analyses have been performed on experienced pitchers while they were throwing breaking balls correctly, no increase in the use of the flexor muscles has been demonstrated.[11]

While stresses placed across the elbow joint are particularly illustrated in the baseball pitcher,[12] the same general principles apply to similar motions, such as those that occur in tennis,[13] volleyball, and javelin throwing. There are differences noted in each specific sport which change the injury pattern and characteristics, but in each the throwing motion can be broken down into the same phases for analysis.

## Specific Elbow Injuries

Injuries to the elbow occurring as a result of throwing will occur to the medial, lateral, or posterior aspect of the elbow depending on the mechanism of injury.

## Medial Tension Injuries

The most common injuries to occur in young throwers occur on the medial side of the elbow. They may occur as a result of an acute episode resulting from a single throw, or, more often, because of chronic overuse or repetitive stress placed on the elbow by throwing. The pathologic entities consist of flexor muscle strains, changes in or avulsion of the ossification center of the medial epicondyle, medial elbow ligament sprains, or ulnar neuropathy. The severity will vary from mild elbow sprains and strains to the more serious avulsion fracture of the medial epicondyle or occasionally acute rupture of the medial ligament or flexor muscle origin.

Common physical findings include pain and tenderness at the medial side of the elbow, and the precise site of the tenderness will identify the involved anatomical structure. If it is at the medial epicondyle, radiographic changes may occur (Fig 4).

The treatment of most medial tension entities is primarily symptomatic. If the problem is chronic, rest, ice, and aspirin usually will resolve it quickly. In acute sprains or strains, particularly if swelling is present, a short period of immobilization will speed recovery. In the rare instance where the epi-

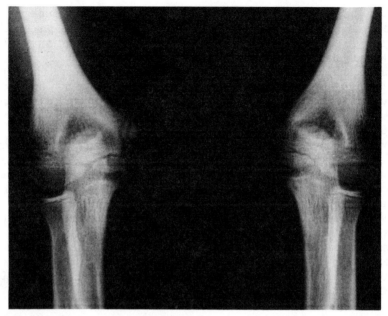

**FIG 4.**
An 11-year-old Little League pitcher presented with a 3-week history of mild pain on the medial side of the elbow. X-rays of the elbows show enlargement and fragmentation of the medial epicondylar epiphysis as compared with the normal side.

condyle has been avulsed (Fig 5), or the flexor muscle mass ruptured, surgical repair may be necessary (Fig 6).

Medial symptoms also may be caused by muscle tears. Late cocking, acceleration, and follow-through all put significant direct valgus stress on the medial aspect of the elbow, which is magnified by the indirect forces caused by the severe acceleration and deceleration forces at the wrist and elbow because of the strong forearm flexor muscle contraction.[14] Pain is caused by micro-tears at or near the medial epicondyle in the origin or substance of the flexor pronator group or in the medial ligament itself. If the flexor muscle mass or flexor tendon is involved, maximum tenderness is usually present in the proximal forearm and is increased with forced wrist flexion. Repetitive injury followed by repair of these micro-tears with fibrous tissue may be the cause of the mild flexion contracture sometimes seen in adolescent pitchers.

Medial elbow pain is quite common, particularly in pitchers, and the frequency seems to increase with experience and growth. Generally speaking, medial tension injuries are benign. Most medial tension injuries respond well to treatment, and the athletes are usually able to return to throwing with no residual problems.[15]

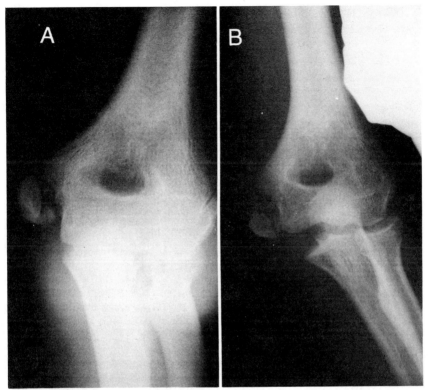

**FIG 5.**
A 14-year-old boy presented with acute disabling pain on the medial side of the elbow following a single forceful throw. X-rays **(A)** showed an avulsion fracture of the medial epicondyle of the humerus, and **(B)** a stress view showed that this is an unstable epiphyseal fracture.

## Lateral Compression Injuries

Injuries to the lateral side of the elbow are potentially more serious, as they result from compression of the intra-articular structures. The most common is an osteochondrosis, known as Panner's disease (Fig 7), or osteochondritis dissecans of the capitellum, which may result in a loose body in the elbow (Fig 8). Osteochondritis dissecans of the radial head may also occur, but it is quite rare.

It has been postulated that Panner's disease is a distinct and separate entity from osteochondritis dissecans.[16] The distinguishing features are that Panner's disease is most commonly seen in males in younger age groups (mean 5 to 7 years), at which time fragmentation and deformity of the entire ossific nucleus of the capitellum occurs, and the capitellum subse-

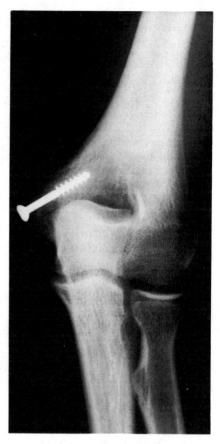

**FIG 6.**
The avulsion fracture has healed after
having been reattached with a single
screw.

quently reconstitutes itself without damaging the joint surface. This theory
postulates that Panner's disease is not a precursor of osteochondritis dissecans, which does damage the joint surface.

It is unlikely that such a theory is correct. There may be an entity of
asymmetrical ossification, much as is seen in the knee, which is self-limited;
however, true osteochondrosis or osteochondritis dissecans must be considered a potentially serious problem. It occurs as a result of repetitive
trauma to an epiphysis at a time when the capitellum is supplied by only
one or two vessels which do not communicate with other vascular systems,
thus functioning as end arteries and making the capitellum vulnerable.[3]

Osteochondritis may present either insidiously with increasing pain with
use, or as a single traumatic event. If an acute injury or catching is the initial symptom, it frequently indicates that a loose body or chondral separation has occurred.

Physical examination will localize the site of tenderness, and reveal
whether there is an effusion or limitation of motion. Radiographs are essential. If the child presents with gradually increasing elbow pain, no limi-

tation of motion or effusion, and normal x-rays, he or she may be treated with rest, sports restriction, and salicylates. If the pain quickly resolves, resumption of sports is allowed. The child should not be allowed to return to sports until all pain and tenderness have subsided, and there is a normal range of elbow motion and normal strength in the arm.

If the onset is sudden, or if there is associated clicking, catching, limitation of motion, or effusion, a careful search must be made for osteochondritis dissecans and a loose fragment. The loose portion may be all articular cartilage, and may not be visible on x-ray, so the clinician's suspicions must prevail. If symptoms are difficult to diagnose, and they persist, nuclear bone scans, tomography, or even arthroscopy may be necessary to resolve the issue.

Osteochondritis of the capitellum and radial head without loose body symptoms should be treated with prolonged rest. The elbow should be splinted as long as synovitis is present. Serial radiographs may be used to

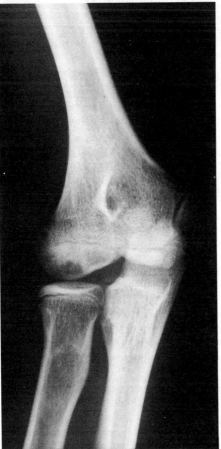

**FIG 7.**
X-ray of the elbow of an 11-year-old female gymnast with elbow pain. Note the radiolucency of the capitellum, indicating osteochondritis dissecans.

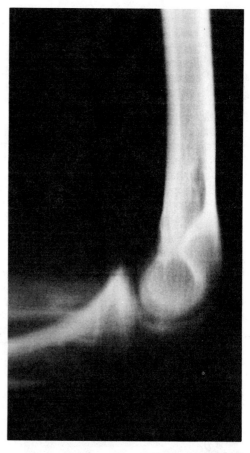

**FIG 8.**
Lateral tomogram which shows a
loose body (arrow) in the anterior
aspect of the elbow of an
11-year-old elite gymnast with a
history of several weeks of elbow
pain and a 2-day history of the
elbow catching.

follow the course of the lesion, but it should be remembered that complete
radiographic resolution may never occur. Sports, and particularly throwing,
should not be allowed for a minimum of 12 weeks. Then, if symptoms
have resolved, the athlete can be allowed to return to activity, but we recommend that he not return to repetitive throwing positions, such as pitching or catching.[17]

If a loose body is present, it should be removed either with arthroscopy
or arthrotomy, and the source should be documented carefully. Occasionally a loose body will form and no articular source can be found at arthrotomy. If such is the case, removal is all that is necessary, and the long-term
prognosis is good. Usually, however, the source will be found on the capitellum or, less commonly, on the radial head. Such individuals will never
have a normal elbow, and should be counseled against returning to high-
demand throwing. Any young athlete who has had an articular cartilage
defect is at risk to develop post-traumatic arthritis of the elbow, and while it
may not occur until mid-adult life, it can be quite disabling. After having
the loose body removed, most athletes will become asymptomatic and will

be able to continue in active athletics; many who have returned to pitching have developed significant long-term problems.

Lateral elbow symptoms in a young athlete are always a reason for serious concern. Fortunately, however, lateral compression injuries are much less common than medial tension injuries.

## Posterior Injuries

Posterior injuries, in our experience, are more common in the older throwing athlete and are relatively uncommon in the presence of open epiphyses. Posterior impingement can give rise to irritation of the olecranon, and can eventually cause spurs or loose bodies to form in the posterior compartment. As the young athlete becomes older and more muscular, triceps tendinitis may occur, and this may be difficult to differentiate from olecranon impingement.

In the child, olecranon apophysitis may occur, although it is uncommon.[18] Its features are similar to apophysitis of the tibial tubercle, with progressive pain with activity, tenderness and swelling over the olecranon apophysis, and fragmentation seen on x-ray (Fig 9). Treatment is based entirely on symptoms, and a good result may be expected.

In the adolescent, posterior impingement can incite synovitis of the ole-

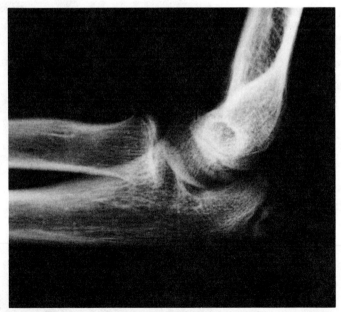

**FIG 9.**
X-ray of a 9-year-old gymnast who had a 6-week history of posterior elbow pain with tenderness only over the olecranon. The radiographic findings of fragmentation of the olecranon epiphysis are typical for osteochondrosis of the olecranon epiphysis.

cranon fossa or growth plate disturbances.[19, 20] The growth plate of the olecranon normally fuses around the age of 16 years. However, we have observed delayed union as a result of baseball, tennis, and diving. This patient is most likely to present with pain and stiffness, particularly at terminal extension. The diagnosis can be confirmed by the localized tenderness along with typical radiographic evidence of either a widened growth plate compared to the uninvolved extremity or a nonunion of the growth plate after the normal side has closed. Nonsurgical treatment of patients may be successsful in alleviating symptoms if the epiphyses are open.

Stress fractures may occur in the olecranon, either after the olecranon epiphysis has closed (and proceed to nonunion) or before it has closed (resulting in a nonunion of the epiphysis) (Fig 10).[21] Surgical correction will be required in these instances (Fig 11).

## Nerve Injuries

Injuries to the ulnar nerve usually consist of a traction neuritis, and usually are the result of longstanding chronic irritation. Therefore, ulnar neuropa-

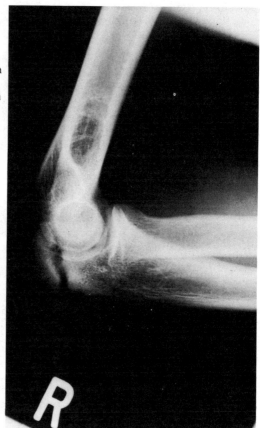

**FIG 10.**
Nonunion of a stress fracture of the olecranon epiphysis in a 16-year-old competitive diver who had persistent elbow pain for several months. The olecranon epiphysis on the opposite side had closed.

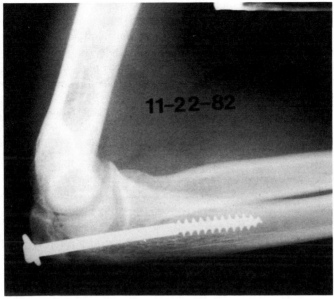

**FIG 11.**
Healing of the nonunion of the olecranon epiphysis 10 weeks after internal fixation. The fracture continued to complete union, the screw was removed, and the athlete returned to competitive diving with no symptoms.

thy is not often seen prior to adulthood. When it does occur in adolescence, it usually responds well to rest and anti-inflammatory agents.

Rarely, the ulnar nerve will traumatically sublux from the cubital tunnel as a result of a single throwing event, resulting in a rupture of the restraining ligament. Once this has occurred, recurrent subluxation with forceful throwing may become a significant problem, and may require cessation of throwing or anterior transposition of the ulnar nerve.[22, 23]

---

## Sports-Specific Injuries

### Baseball

"Little League elbow" was first described in 1960 by Brogdon and Crow[1] as pain, tenderness, and swelling of the medial aspect of the elbow, associated with radiographic findings of fragmentation and separation of the medial humeral epicondyle in skeletally immature baseball pitchers.

In 1965, Adams[2] published his series calling attention to the entities that occur to the immature elbows of baseball players as a result of pitching. Subsequently, the term "Little League elbow" became commonly used to refer to all entities involving the elbow in young baseball players, predominately pitchers. The sports medicine community became concerned, and rightly so, as it witnessed an epidemic of similar injuries, some quite serious, resulting from an activity that was intended to be fun and safe for youngsters.

Subsequent surveys in Houston, Texas,[24] and Eugene, Oregon,[25] provided data that confirmed the existence of radiographic changes occurring on the medial side of the elbows in Little League pitchers, but did not substantiate that these changes were detrimental. In neither survey were lateral compression injuries—osteochondrosis of the capitellum or radial head—detected. Subsequently, more recent studies have demonstrated that at the current time, with the safeguards and rule changes in place, the medial side changes are for the most part benign, and the lateral compression injuries very rare.[26]

However, such was not the case in a study of over 2,500 baseball players in Japan.[27] Approximately half of these youngsters aged 9 to 12 years had elbow symptoms. Radiographic abnormalities were found in 19% of the children, and of those with x-ray changes, 89% had medial abnormalities, 15% had lateral abnormalities, and 5% had posterior lesions. Of the entire group, 452 (17.6%) had medial changes and 52 (2%) had osteochondritis dissecans of the capitellum. Radiographic abnormalities were found in direct relation to the amount of throwing performed, with 38% found in pitchers, 32% in catchers, 13% in infielders, and 8% in outfielders.

Little League rules now specify the number of innings one child is allowed to pitch each week and the rest periods necessary between pitching appearances. Rules in organized community and other national sports programs that now exist in most areas limit the minimum age for a pitcher, the number of innings one is allowed to pitch, and the types of pitches permitted, and have most likely reduced the injury rate, although documentation is lacking.

It is apparent that osteochondritis dissecans is quite uncommon in the Little League age group of 9 to 12 years, but is more common in the older adolescents and young adults. McManama et al reported an average age of 16 years in a series of 14 patients who eventually came to surgery because of capitellar osteochondritis.[28] Studies in Little League players show a very low incidence. While this is reassuring, it may also impart a false sense of security. It may well be that the stage is set for the development of osteochondritis dissecans with repetitive throwing activities at the younger ages, but that the entity does not fully evolve or become manifest until later. With the available studies, the true incidence of this problem in baseball in the United States cannot be determined.

## Gymnastics Injuries

It has become more apparent that the tremendous forces involving the elbow in gymnastics may cause elbow damage. Priest and Weise[29] reported a series of 32 elbow injuries in female gymnasts, 30 of which were fractures or dislocations. Two individuals had osteochondrosis of the capitellum.

Subsequently, Singer and Roy[3] reported a series of seven cases of osteochondritis dissecans in young female gymnasts occurring over a relatively short period of time in a group of young women who were participating an average of 4 to 6 hours daily, which is not uncommon in serious young gymnasts. They cited Haraldsson's work on the vascular anatomy of the epiphysis of the capitellum[30] and postulated that the epiphysis underwent avascular necrosis as a result of the repetitive valgus stresses placed on a vulnerable epiphysis at a time during the development of the epiphysis when, because of its vascular supply, it was particularly susceptible.

Subsequently, Jackson and Silvino[31] have presented 10 similar cases and have indicated that this entity did not have a particularly good prognosis.

Gymnasts use their arms as weight-bearing extremities in many phases of their routines. Female gymnasts particularly have increased valgus carrying angles at the elbows, which concentrates the very large forces generated by such maneuvers as round-offs, handstands, or vaulting to the lateral side of the elbow. These large compressive forces, probably much larger than those that occur with throwing, are transmitted to the relatively small cross-sectional area of the radio-capitellar joint, resulting in very large pressures. Female gymnasts begin young, and as they excel, they spend many hours daily in their sport. It stands to reason that injuries will occur. As in baseball, the true incidence of lateral compression injuries to the elbows is unknown; but when the number of participants is taken into account, the injury rate is probably higher than in throwing sports and has been recognized only recently as a serious problem.

## Wrestling Injuries

Wrestling injuries to the elbow are usually traumatic and often quite serious, as opposed to the throwing injuries which usually occur as a result of repetitive overuse.

Published surveys indicated that 5% to 10% of all injuries occurring during wrestling were to the elbow, with forceful hyperextension being the major cause.[32, 33] Dislocations and fractures were not uncommon, and many were season-ending injuries.

## Clinical Evaluation

### History

Youngsters of any age may present with pain and tenderness in the elbow. A careful history will often suggest the diagnosis. The mode of onset of pain (whether it is acute or insidious), the location of the pain, and the presence or absence of catching or locking should be noted. Often the pain can be connected historically to a specific phase of the involved activity.

The extent of the athletic involvement of the youngster must be reviewed. It must be remembered that often these individuals are active not only in the organized team practice and game situations, but also on their own, working with a parent, coach, or teammate, and thereby subjecting their elbows to even more insult. This may be the situation with the young baseball player who practices on his own at home, or with the young gymnast who works out in a supervised setting several hours daily. Therefore, it becomes important to know not only the number of games or meets in which the athlete has participated, but also how many hours were spent in preparation and how much total time throughout the year is devoted to this activity.

## Physical Examination

Active and passive range of motion should be noted. There may be decreased extension or supination in the older, more experienced athlete, even in the absence of symptoms. The carrying angle is important, particularly in gymnasts. The sites of tenderness are characteristic for the structures involved. If it occurs on the medial side, tenderness at the epicondyle should be differentiated from soft tissue tenderness. Similarly, lateral tenderness at the radial head, joint line, or capitellum localizes the particular structures involved. The olecranon should be palpated, as well as the ulnar nerve and ulnar groove.

Swelling may be identified utilizing the normal elbow for comparison. An effusion is most accurately detected at the soft spot posterolaterally, in the interval between the lateral epicondyle and the olecranon.

The elbow should be examined for stability to varus and valgus stress, both in flexion and 20 degrees of flexion. It is important to palpate for crepitance, both medially and laterally, during active and passive movements.

An attempt should be made to reproduce the symptoms in the chronic situation. Have the young athlete reproduce the throwing motion during the examination in an attempt to reproduce the symptoms. Also, observation of the particular motion, such as the pitching delivery, can provide important information about the patient's mechanics—good or poor—which can be used in altering technique to prevent recurrence of the injury.

The entire arm, including the shoulder, cervical spine, arm, forearm, wrist, and hand should be examined carefully, and a complete neurological examination should be performed.

## Radiographic Examination

Standard anteroposterior, lateral, and oblique radiographs of the elbow will demonstrate most abnormalities.[34] In the younger child, the epiphyses may exhibit considerable variability, and comparison views of the normal side are helpful in interpretation.

In the classic Little League elbow, the medial epicondyle may be enlarged, fragmented, or slightly separated (see Fig 4). Osteochondrosis of the capitellum presents with radiolucency, such as in the 12-year-old gymnast with chronic lateral elbow pain shown in Figure 7. Figure 8 shows a loose body present in the anterior compartment which caused catching and locking in association with sports activities.

Other abnormalities may include osteochondrosis of the olecranon, as seen in Figure 11, with a comparison view of the opposite side. In adolescence, a stress fracture through the olecranon epiphysis must be differentiated from the normal unfused olecranon epiphysis.

In individuals with elbow pain in whom radiographs are normal and there is not a satisfactory response to conservative treatment, nuclear bone scans may be beneficial (Fig 12). Routine tomography is often useful in searching for loose bodies, or in better identifying osteochondritis dissecans lesions. There are occasional instances in which computerized tomography will be useful. Arthrography is rarely of benefit, and we virtually never use

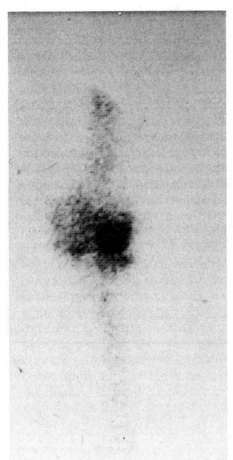

**FIG 12.**
Bone scan of the elbow of a 15-year-old pitcher with persistent lateral elbow pain and normal x-rays. Note the increased uptake in the capitellum. He eventually came to arthroscopy, where osteochondritis dissecans with a large chondral defect in the capitellum was found, with partial separation. His symptoms resolved after removal of the loose chondral fragment.

magnetic resonance imaging in the evaluation of patients with elbow problems, unless we are attempting to diagnose a complete muscle or ligament tear.

## Treatment, Rehabilitation, and Injury Prevention

Rest remains the most important initial treatment of most adolescent elbow injuries. Rarely is long-term immobilization necessary, and most problems respond to cessation of the aggravating event. Treatment of specific injuries has been discussed above in relation to each of the specific injuries.

Rehabilitation must be emphasized. As with other joints, prevention and rehabilitation of elbow injury is accomplished by strengthening the surrounding musculature. For the overhead sports, such as throwing, tennis, and javelin, this conditioning should begin with the trunk and lower extremities and proceed to shoulder, elbow, and wrist exercises. Sports like gymnastics and wrestling also require avoidance of inciting maneuvers. Modification of technique must be evaluated on an individual basis; for example, it is known that "opening" the body with throwing, i.e., bringing the arm through with the body, can reduce the valgus force at the elbow. Taking a shorter stride with the lead foot may be beneficial also.

Following any surgical procedure involving the joint, a regimen of active motion followed by active resistive exercises and progressing to light throwing at 8 weeks is an appropriate plan for rehabilitation. It is essential that the athlete be completely rehabilitated prior to returning to the sport that caused the injury. Strength, range of motion, and endurance must be normal, and rehabilitation programs should be individually prescribed depending on the particular injury and sport involved. A return to throwing may be particularly difficult, and a graduated, progressive program, such as the fungo routine, will help to prevent recurrence.

Injury prevention by proper coaching and instruction in techniques to reduce the vulnerability of the elbow, rehabilitation of previous injuries, and protective taping when necessary appear to be the most efficacious methods of minimizing the frequency and reducing the severity of elbow injuries.

## Summary

It is unarguable that the stress of repetitive throwing creates compression, shear, and distraction forces that may affect the growing epiphyses. Athletes, coaches, teachers, and parents must be made aware of these injury possibilities.

Although "macro-trauma," such as a fall from the balance beam or a severe twist during a wrestling match, is responsible for a certain percentage of elbow injuries, a large number of preventable elbow problems are due to overuse with no specific inciting event. Although few acknowledge any disability, 17% to 70% of Little League baseball pitchers clearly admit to having elbow pain at some point.

Identifying the patient at risk for development of elbow osteochondritis has proven difficult. While seen most commonly in males, it tends to be more common in certain families, in certain body types, and in those with osteochondral lesions in other parts of the body and shows approximately a 5% bilaterality. No good screening test exists to identify these children before problems develop.

Although many young athletes will complain of elbow pain at some point in their careers, most conditions follow a benign course if an early, accurate diagnosis is made. Training errors, particularly overtraining, must be identified and avoided in these enthusiastic youngsters. It is evident that the biggest contributing cause of injury is repetitive trauma to the joint. Opinions differ regarding the need to restrict the number of types of pitches thrown, innings per game, and hours of participation.

What seems evident from the injury surveys and from psychological discussion of athletic injuries is that there are a number of measures that we can take to decrease not just elbow injuries but all athletic injuries in this age group.

The emphasis of athletics in this age group should be fun and participation, not winning at all costs. This attitude must begin with the parents and coaches.

Youngsters must be encouraged to report any pain or injury when it first occurs. All organized athletic programs must have proper supervision, safe fields, and appropriate equipment. Coaching techniques must emphasize teaching strength and conditioning as well as fundamental skills.

Any child who sustains an elbow injury or complains of symptoms should be evaluated by a physician who is familiar with pediatric elbow problems.

---

## References

1. Brogdon MD, Crow NE: Little Leaguer's elbow. *AJR* 1960; 83:671–675.
2. Adams JE: Injury to the throwing arm: A study of traumatic changes in the elbow joints of boy baseball players. *Calif Med* 1965; 102:127–132.
3. Singer KM, Roy SR: Osteochondrosis of the humeral capitellum. *Am J Sports Med* 1984; 12:351–360.
4. Miller JE: Javelin thrower's elbow. *J Bone Joint Surg* 1960; 4:788.
5. Ogden JA: *Skeletal Injury in the Child,* Philadelphia, Penn, Lea & Febiger, 1982, pp 283–301.
6. Pappas AM: Elbow problems associated with baseball during childhood and adolescence. *Clin Orthop* 1982; 164:30–41.
7. Morrey BF: *The Elbow and Its Disorders.* Philadelphia, Penn, WB Saunders & Co, 1985, pp 7–42.
8. Morrey BF, Kai-nan A: Articular and ligamentous contributions to the stability of the elbow joint. *Am J Sports Med* 1983; 11:315–319.
9. Tullos HS, King JW: Throwing mechanism in sports. *Orthop Clin North Am* 1973; 4:709–720.

10. Pappas AM, Zawacki RM, Sullivan TJ: Biomechanics of baseball pitching. A preliminary report. *Am J Sports Med* 1985; 13:216–222.
11. Sisto DJ, Jobe FW, Moynes DR, et al: An electromyographic analysis of the elbow in pitching. *Am J Sports Med* 1987; 15:260–263.
12. Slocum DB: Classification of elbow injuries from baseball pitching. *Tex Med* 1968; 64:48–53.
13. Gregg JR, Torg E: Upper extremity injuries in adolescent tennis players. *Clin Sports Med* 1988; 7:359–370.
14. Tullos HS, King JW: Lesions of the pitching arm in adolescents. *JAMA* 1972; 220:264–271.
15. Grana WA, Rashkin A: Pitcher's elbow in adolescents. *Am J Sports Med* 1980; 5:333–336.
16. Woodward AH, Bianco AJ Jr: Osteochondritis dissecans of the elbow. *Clin Orthop* 1975; 110:35–41.
17. Lipscomb AB: Baseball pitching injuries in growing athletes. *J Sports Med Phys Fitness* 1975; 3:25–34.
18. Danielsson LG, Hedlund ST, Henricson AS: Apophysitis of the olecranon. *Acta Orthop Scand* 1983; 54:777–778.
19. Pavlov H: Radiology for the orthopedic surgeon. *Contemp Orthop* 1988; 17:53–56.
20. Rentrum RK, Wepfer JF, Olen DW, et al: Case report 355. *Skeletal Radiol* 1986; 15:185–187.
21. Pavlov H, Torg JS, Jacobs B, et al: Nonunion of olecranon epiphysis: Two cases in adolescent baseball pitchers. *AJR* 1981; 136:819–820.
22. Hang YS: Tardy ulnar neuritis in a Little League baseball player. *Am J Sports Med* 1981; 9:244–246.
23. Godshall RW, Hansen CA: Traumatic ulnar neuropathy in adolescent baseball pitchers. *J Bone Joint Surg* 1971; 53A:359–361.
24. Gugenheim JJ Jr, Stanley RF, Woods GW, et al: Little League survey: The Houston study. *Am J Sports Med* 1976; 4:189–200.
25. Larson RL, Singer KM, Bergstrom R, et al: Little League survey: The Eugene Study. *Am J Sports Med* 1976; 4:201–209.
26. Francis R, Bunch T, Chandler B: Little League elbow: A decade later. *Phys & Sportsmed* 1978; 6:88–94.
27. Iwase T, Ikata T: Baseball elbow of young players. *Tokushima J Exp Med* 1985; 32:57–64.
28. McManama GB, Micheli LJ, Berry MV, et al: The surgical treatment of osteochondritis of the capitellum. *Am J Sports Med* 1985; 13:11–21.
29. Priest JD, Weise DJ: Elbow injury in women's gymnastics. *Am J Sports Med* 1981; 9:288–295.
30. Haraldsson S: On osteochondrosis deformans juvenilis capituli humeri including investigation of intra-osseous vasculature in distal humerus. *Acta Orthop Scand [Suppl]* 1959; 38.
31. Jackson DW, Silvino NJ: Osteochondritis Dissecans in the female gymnast's elbow. *Arthroscopy* 1989; 5:129–136.
32. Estwanik JJ, Bergfeld JA, Collins HR, et al: Injuries in interscholastic wrestling. *Phys & Sportsmed* 1980; 8:111–121.
33. Estwanik JJ, Rovere GD: Wrestling injuries in North Carolina high schools. *Phys & Sportsmed* 1983; 11:100–108.
34. Singer KM: Radiographic evaluation of the throwing elbow, in Zarins B, Andrews JR, Carson WG (eds): *Injuries to the Throwing Arm.* Philadelphia, WB Saunders Company, 1985, pp 211–220.

# Knee Ligament Injuries in Children

## Jesse C. DeLee, M.D.,

Associate Clinical Professor, Department of Orthopaedics, University of Texas Health Science Center at San Antonio, San Antonio, Texas

## John C. Pearce, M.D.,

Venable-Stuck Fellow in Lower Extremity Reconstruction, Department of Orthopaedics, University of Texas Health Science Center at San Antonio, San Antonio, Texas

## Editor's Introduction

In the past 10 years, the recognition that knee laxity is due to multiple causes has been recognized and defined. It is not only important to distinguish physeal injury from ligamentous injury, but to develop a plan of management for both types of injury. This chapter presents a systematic approach to the evaluation and treatment of the young patient with knee laxity. Better results can be expected with prompt recognition and early appropriate treatment.

*William A. Grana, M.D.*

Recently there has been increased interest in knee ligament disruptions in the skeletally immature.* This is due to the fact that ligament injuries in children have dramatically increased with more children participating in athletic events.[16, 17, 32, 37, 53, 84, 86, 88] However, there still seems to be mystery surrounding the diagnosis and treatment of these injuries. The goal of this chapter is to present an organized approach to this problem in order to better understand the diagnosis and treatment of ligament injuries of the child's knee.

## History

In the past, injuries about the knee in children were believed to be mainly disruptions of the physis.[15, 20, 34, 53, 75, 82, 83] The physes surrounding the knee were thought to be the weak link in the stressed knee.† Rang wrote in 1974 that ligamentous injuries do not occur about the knee,[75] but he retracted this in 1983 and stated that they do occur.[76] Although boney

*See references 4, 6, 8, 10, 16, 17, 19, 22, 31, 34, 45, 49–51, 53, 58, 60, 61, 66, 78, 83.
†See references 6, 7, 10, 13, 16, 19, 20, 34, 53, 61, 78, 82–84, 87.

avulsions of ligaments were noted on radiographs, they were believed to be relatively uncommon.[75, 78]

Injured knees in children were, therefore, treated in one of two ways: (1) immobilization for non-displaced physeal plate injuries and avulsions, or (2) open reduction and internal fixation of displaced fractures and boney avulsions.[20] Little concern was given to disruption of the collateral or cruciate ligaments. In those few patients recognized to have true ligament injury, further growth was believed to alleviate their instability.[53] It has become more evident recently that children do injure their knee ligaments and that they fare no better than do adults with conservative (non-operative) treatment.*

## Epidemiology

Increased interest in children's knee injuries stems from three factors. First, there has been an increase in the participation of children in organized sports.[32, 37, 42, 53, 78, 87, 88] Goldberg[32] estimated in 1984 that 25% of girls and 50% of boys between the ages of 8 and 16 years old are engaged in competitive athletics in any 1 year. Gallagher, et al,[27] in a state-wide study, reported that 1 in 14 children presenting to emergency rooms in Massachusetts was injured in a sporting activity while only 1 in 50 was injured in a motor vehicle accident. In football alone it has been estimated that up to 81% of the children participating will suffer an injury. This represents 300,000 to 1,215,000 injured athletes in football alone over 1 year's time.[88] The knee is the area most frequently involved in these sports injuries.[64, 65] The higher incidence of knee injuries is related to the various demands and stresses applied to its supporting structures during a sporting event.[36] The knee is also exposed to direct trauma which can lead to injury.

The second factor contributing to the increased incidence of children's knee injuries is the fact that now the medical community more frequently recognizes ligament injuries in skeletally immature patients.[53] The third factor in the recent increased incidence of knee ligament injuries in children is the improved methods of diagnosis of ligamentous disruptions now being utilized in all age groups.[10, 16, 31]

## Embryology and Anatomy

Congenital anomalies of the knee occur early in the stages of fetal development.[1] The knee develops embryologically as a cleft between the mesenchymal rudiments of the femur and tibia in about the eighth week of fetal development. Vascular mesenchyme becomes isolated within the joint and is the precursor tissue of the cruciate ligaments and menisci. In the seventh to eighth weeks of development the cruciate ligaments appear as condensations of this vascular mesenchyme. These tissues become immature fibroblasts which soon develop into the cruciate ligaments. By the

*See references 10, 17, 22, 45, 46, 49, 52, 53, 58, 61, 83.

tenth week the anterior and posterior cruciate ligaments are separate structures which become independent of each other by the 18th week of development.[1]

Developmental ligament abnormalities can lead to congenitally unstable knees. The cruciate ligaments and the menisci help to shape the femoral condyles and tibial plateau of the knee, and in their absence, the intercondylar eminence of the tibia is aplastic.[29, 90] The knee is usually not solely affected, but is associated with other limb deformities such as hemimelia and leg length discrepancy.[16, 17]

Eilert[21] states that most knee problems in children younger than 12 years of age are congenital. One must be aware, therefore, of these congenital anomalies when evaluating the child with an unstable knee. In the child with clinical instability, a developmental anomaly must be considered if there is (1) no history of significant trauma; (2) an associated limb anomaly such as hemimelia, leg length discrepancy, or ball-and-socket ankle joint[14, 16, 48]; or (3) aplasia of the intercondylar eminence of the tibia on the anteroposterior radiograph graph.[29] (Fig 1). Only after a congenital malformation or anomaly has been excluded as the cause of instability, can traumatic ligament instability be considered.

## Anatomy

The anatomic relationship of the ligament origins and insertions to the physeal plates increases the stress on the physis by concentrating force to the physis which leads to its failure.[10, 13, 16, 17] All knee ligament origins and insertions, except the tibial collateral ligament insertion, are within the confines of the physeal plates of the distal femur and proximal tibia and fibula.[10, 16] (Fig 2). Therefore, when any stress is applied to the knee joint of the patient with an open physis, it is concentrated at the physeal plate of

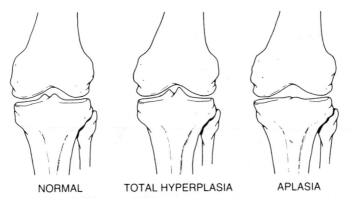

NORMAL      TOTAL HYPERPLASIA      APLASIA

**FIG 1.**
Variations in the morphologic appearance of the intercondylar eminence of the tibia. Total aphasia of the eminence suggests congenital absence of the anterior cruciate ligament.

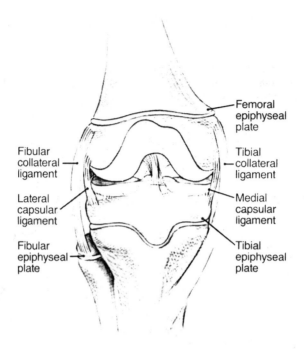

**FIG 2.**
Neither the capsular nor the cruciate ligaments cross the physeal plates except for the insertion of the tibial collateral ligament. Because of the relationship of the ligaments to the physeal plates and the relative strength of the ligaments, stress concentrates at the physeal plates, producing physeal separation rather than ligament failure.

the distal femur or proximal tibia and fibula by the collateral and/or central ligaments.[16, 17, 19, 70, 78]

## Biomechanics

### Strength of the Physeal Plate

The lower strength of the physeal plate compared to the knee ligaments, and the anatomic location of the ligament origins and insertions which concentrate forces at the physeal plate help to explain the higher incidence of physeal plate disruptions compared to pure ligament injuries.* The weakest area in the physis is the zone of hypertrophy, which is the usual zone through which physeal disruption occurs.[6, 67, 72, 82]

### Mechanics of Physeal Plate Failure

The physeal plate is protected from disruption by mamillary processes and undulations along its surface as well as by the distal attachment of the pe-

*See references 4, 6, 10, 16, 19, 50, 72, 75, 82, 89.

riosteum.[7] However, it is still the weak point when stress is applied to immature bone.[7] Bright et al[7] have demonstrated that the cartilage in the physeal plate has viscoelastic properties. Therefore, the strength of the plate depends on the total strain which is applied *and* the rate at which the strain is applied. Due to the viscoelasticity, it takes twice as much force to disrupt the physis at a rapid-loading rate than it takes when the growth plate is loaded slowly.[6] Also, Bright,[7] Harris,[38] and Tipton[89] have found reduced ductility of the cartilage with age.

In addition, physeal plate strength is affected by various hormones.[38, 39] Growth hormone produces a thicker physeal plate which is weaker in transverse loading, while estrogens cause a thinner growth plate that is stronger.

## Mechanics of Ligament Failure

The knee ligaments in the child undergo the same pathodynamic sequence of disruption as in the adult.[53] These ligaments, like the physeal plate, have viscoelastic properties and their strength is also determined by the total amount of strain and the rate at which it is applied. Cochran[11] states that under slow loading rates, ligament failures tend to occur at the ligament-bone junction, usually with a boney avulsion, while under high loading rates, ligament failures tend to occur within the body of the structures. These findings suggest that the strength of corticocancellous bone increases more rapidly than ligament strength as the loading rate increases. Rapid loading of ligaments seems to be the common denominator in injury to the adult as well as to the child.[11] Skak[86] in 1987 concluded in a series of 91 children under age 14 years that low energy was associated with ligament injuries while high energy was involved with physeal damage.[11] Therefore, with these two studies it becomes apparent that pure ligament injuries are likely to occur with low energy, rapid loading events while the physis or tendon-bone junction is injured with high energy and slow loading events.

## Diagnosis: General Principles

Careful evaluation of the history of the injury, the physical examination of the knee, and radiographs are essential for accurate diagnosis of knee ligament injuries in the skeletally immature.

## History

The history is a critical part of the knee evaluation. In the acute setting, the sport being played and the position of the limb at the time of injury are critical. Hyperextension of the knee (caused, for example, by landing on an extended knee while playing basketball) is frequently associated with anterior cruciate ligament (ACL) injury. An external rotation force applied to the knee in a valgus position can result in disruption of first the medial collateral ligament (MCL), then the ACL. An audible "pop" heard by the patient at the time of the injury strongly suggests disruption of one of the major knee ligaments, usually the ACL.[23, 31, 85] The rapid development of an effusion, usually within 12 to 24 hours, suggests a hemarthrosis. This is associated with an ACL injury, a peripheral meniscus detachment, or an osteochondral fracture, often associated with a patellar dislocation.[23, 24, 31, 42, 78, 85] The slower development of swelling suggests a reactive effusion and is usually a less sinister prognosticator of knee injury. The history of instability with weight bearing at the time of injury is often associated with significant ligament injury. Because of minimal pain during the period of time immediately following the injury, the patient may attempt to return to play, only to find that instability prevents participation. On the other hand, if severe pain is noted, a partial ligament disruption may be present. This situation demands removal of the patient from participation to prevent further damage to the incompletely torn ligament.

In the chronically unstable knee, the history provides additional information. A history of the knee giving way with a particular activity is important. The patient will often be able to relate that the knee gives way when placed in certain positions. For example, the classic description of the knee "slipping out" indicates anterior cruciate ligament insufficiency.

The symptom of giving way may also be related by the patient with a meniscal lesion. If both a ligament instability (ACL) and a meniscal lesion are present, the physical examination is essential to determine which is responsible for the patient's symptoms. The severity of instability can often be suggested by the history. The knee which gives way in normal walking is less stable than the one that gives way only with sports activity.

Locking (the inability to completely straighten the knee) will often be related by the patient. A history of locking is suggestive of a meniscal lesion, an osteochondral flap, or a loose body.

Pain may be due to ligament instability or chondral damage. By history, if pain is associated with the symptom of giving way, then either a ligamentous or meniscal pathology is the likely cause. However, if it is related to weight bearing and prolonged activity, chondral disease is the more likely problem. The importance of distinguishing pain with instability from pain with weight bearing is critical in evaluating the patient with ligament instability. Ligament reconstruction will not improve the pain of weight bearing in the patient with chondral disease. Finally, a loss of motion compared to the normal knee may be due to a structural problem (such as a loose body), a torn meniscus, an effusion, or a muscle spasm.

## Physical Examination

The examination of the injured knee is the best diagnostic tool available to evaluate the location and severity of knee injury. Examination of the child's knee is often more difficult than that of the adult.[68] Children are often frightened and unable to relax their muscles and secondary restraints about the knee, making laxity evaluation quite difficult.[25, 31] In addition, evaluation of the area of point tenderness and the use of stress x-rays are required to distinguish ligament from physeal plate injury.

The uninjured extremity is examined first. This generally helps to relax the patient by giving him an idea of how the examination of the injured knee will be performed.[31, 42, 85] It also gives the physician an idea of the natural laxity of the patient which is useful when examining the injured knee. This is extremely important when evaluating the child's knee injury. Many children have physiologic joint laxity which, in the injured knee, can produce a false-positive diagnosis of pathological ligament instability. Therefore, generalized laxity must be excluded by examination of the contralateral knee and other joints.[16, 17, 35] Hyperextension of the elbows, laxity of the shoulders, and hyperextension of the knees may be present in patients with congenital knee laxity.[35]

Following the examination of the uninjured extremity, a visual inspection of the injured knee is undertaken. The alignment of the limb in weight bearing (i.e., varus, valgus, hyperextension) is recorded. Palpation of the dorsalis pedis and posterior tibial pulses is essential with a physeal plate or knee dislocation, due to the possibility of a limb-threatening vascular injury.[42, 78] The presence of a fixed deformity usually suggests boney or physeal plate injury rather than ligament disruption. The location of ecchymosis is noted as it indicates the exact ligament and its location of injury.[69, 71] An effusion is also evident to visual inspection.

Palpation of the knee is performed after inspection. Ligament origins and insertions are palpated. If they are tender, a definite point of injury is indicated.[71] The physeal plate lines are palpated in the same manner as are the joint lines, noting specific points of tenderness which help to differentiate ligament, meniscus and physeal plate damage. If palpation suggests physeal plate injury, stress radiographs should be performed before proceeding with ligament testing.

If the growth plates are not tender, then the knee is tested for ligament laxity prior to radiographs. Passive and active range of motion are recorded as well as any associated crepitus and/or pain with motion. The order in which the laxity tests are performed is not important, but the same order of testing should be undertaken routinely. The degree of instability is recorded as recommended by the Committee on the Medical Aspects of Sports of the American Medical Association.[12] The degree of instability in any given direction is expressed as mild (1+), indicating that the joint surfaces separate less than 5 mm; moderate (2+), indicating a separation of 5 to 10 mm; or severe (3+), indicating a separation of more than 10 mm. Throughout this chapter these standards will be used to express ligament laxity. The knee is evaluated in extension and at 30 degrees of flexion for varus or valgus laxity. The central pivot ligaments are evaluated next. An anterior Lachman and flexion rotation drawer tests indicate ACL injury. A positive pivot shift, jerk, and Losee's test suggest that ACL laxity is responsible for the symptoms of instability. The anterior drawer test, positive in external or neutral rotation, indicates ACL and collateral ligament laxity.

The posterior Lachman and quadriceps active drawer tests are helpful in evaluating the PCL after acute injury. The posterior sag and posterior drawer tests are more accurate determinants of posterior cruciate ligament (PCL) injury in the chronically unstable knee. The posterior-lateral drawer and increased passive external rotation at 30 degree flexion indicates damage to the posterolateral structures.[44] The results of careful evaluation of the menisci as well as of the patellofemoral mechanism for malalignment and instability are recorded. These laxity tests are performed in the same manner as in the adult and suggest the same pathology.

## Radiographic Examination

Anteroposterior (AP), lateral, tunnel, and sunrise radiographs of the knee are viewed to identify physeal plate fractures or boney avulsions of ligaments.[91] Physeal plate widening of 8 mm or more, with or without stress, is considered to be a physeal disruption.[10, 16] Radiographs of the hip should be obtained if (1) knee films are normal, or (2) knee films are not compatible with the symptoms found in the knee examination.[13] If no deformity is noted on plain radiographs, varus/valgus and anterior/posterior stress films are obtained.[10, 13, 16, 91] Stress radiographs used to *confirm* ligament injury in the adult are essential to distinguish physeal disruptions from ligament injuries in the child. Specialized radiographic studies may be utilized to further clarify the diagnosis. These include the arthrogram, computed tomographic (CT) scan, polytomogram, and magnetic resonance imaging (MRI).[10, 13, 47] Stress radiographs and some of the specialized x-ray studies may require patient sedation either by local injection or general anesthesia.[10, 91] If general anesthesia is needed, the physician should be ready to proceed with operative treatment if indicated.

## Treatment

Once a physeal plate injury has been excluded, treatment of the specific ligament injury can be instituted. The treatment of ligament injuries about the child's knee for the most part parallels that for adults.[4, 53] The major concern in operative management of ligament injuries in the child is inadvertent damage of the physis.[16] Because of this, operative procedures are sometimes delayed or a procedure of lesser magnitude is performed in order to avoid damage of the physis.[16, 58, 61] Once the growth plate has closed, then it can be determined if further operative treatment is needed.[16]

## Medial Collateral Ligament

Medial collateral ligament injuries are usually the result of a valgus stress to the knee with the foot held stable, thus causing the medial joint line to be stressed open.[42, 52, 85] After physeal injuries have been excluded by location of point tenderness and stress radiographs,[13, 16, 17] the diagnosis and treatment plan is instituted.

## Diagnosis

The mechanism of injury is a valgus or external rotation stress to the knee. The patient presents with a painful and often swollen knee. Instability may not be present and some athletes are able to return to play immediately post-injury.

Examination of the knee may reveal an effusion which results in the knee being held in slight flexion.[85] The medial aspect of the knee is tender to palpation at either the femoral or tibial boney attachment of the MCL or in its mid-substance, depending upon the site of injury.[25, 42, 71, 85] The knee is stable to valgus stress in full extension.[25, 42, 85] The same stress, applied at 30 degrees flexion (which relaxes the posterior capsule), will cause increased discomfort and demonstrate medial joint line opening if the MCL is injured.[42, 85] The quality of the endpoint present in valgus stress is recorded as is the grade of the injury.[12]

The examination of other ligamentous structures, particularly the ACL, must reveal no laxity. The presence of a meniscal injury should be suggested by noting tenderness at the *joint line* in addition to the ligament tenderness at either its tibial or femoral attachment sites. If the ligament is injured in its mid-substance, it too will be tender on the joint line, making meniscal evaluation difficult. Routine radiographs are obtained to detect boney avulsions at the attachment of the MCL, and if these are negative, stress films are taken.

## Treatment

Once the type and severity of injury to the medial collateral ligament has been determined, and injury to the ACL, PCL, and lateral collateral ligament has been excluded, treatment can be instituted. Isolated MCL injuries (grades I to III), that is, those without associated laxity of the central pivot or lateral system, can be treated nonsurgically. Isolated boney avulsion of the MCL only requires open reduction and internal fixation if the ligaments are markedly displaced from their attachments. Otherwise, they too may be treated in a closed manner.[24, 85] Jones[49] reported on 24 high school football players ranging in age from 14 to 18 years with isolated grade III medial collateral ligament injuries which were treated nonsurgically. With his nonsurgical protocol of protected motion and strengthening exercises, these athletes returned to play in 34 days. He reported that all the patients maintained knee stability and denied any symptoms of medial collateral ligament instability at follow-up.

Treatment consists of an initial period of immobilization to diminish pain and to protect the repair response. Due to the low incidence of meniscal injuries in patients with isolated MCL injuries,[52] arthroscopy is not recommended unless the physical examination points to associated meniscal pathology. In 5 to 7 days knee motion is allowed in a hinged brace and strengthening exercises are started. Weight bearing is allowed and encouraged as soon as possible in the brace.

Straight ahead running may be started when the knee is pain-free, a full range of motion is present, and muscle strength is adequate. When the area of ligament disruption becomes non-tender to palpation and the knee has improved in its valgus stability at 30 degrees of knee flexion, running with cutting is allowed. The athlete may return to activity when the muscle tone of his injured leg equals that of the opposite leg.[46, 49] A brace may be used to provide additional varus/valgue stability.[85]

Operative repair of an *isolated* medical collateral ligament disruption is unusual.[24, 46, 49] It is indicated when there is a displaced boney avulsion of the MCL, or when there is an associated ligament injury or a reparable meniscal injury.[24, 46, 52, 85]

## Lateral Collateral Ligament

Injuries to the lateral ligaments of the knee are uncommon and usually consist of injury to the lateral collateral ligament, the arcuate ligament complex, and the popliteus tendon.[43, 53] Isolated injury of one of these three is rarely diagnosed.

## Diagnosis

The mechanism of injury is a varus stress to the knee.[43] An effusion may develop and the range of motion is usually limited by pain and/or the effusion. Palpation is helpful in determining which of the three structures is injured and where the injury is located.

In serial cutting studies of the lateral and posterior structures of the knee, Gollehon, et al,[33] Kennedy,[53] and Hsieh, et al[41] demonstrated that the lateral collateral ligament and arcuate complex function together as the principle structures resisting varus and external rotation of the tibia. The lateral collateral ligament is easily palpated with the injured leg crossed over the opposite leg in a "figure-of-four position" (Grant's test).[53] The popliteus tendon is located anterior to the fibular collateral ligament at its femoral insertion and passes posteriorly beneath the fibula to attach on the tibia. It can also be palpated in the figure-of-four position. The popliteus tendon appears to function as both a static and dynamic restraint to external rotation of the tibia.[33]

Varus stress at 30 degrees of knee flexion is used to evaluate the integrity of the lateral collateral ligament. With a varus stress applied, the amount of laxity is graded using the same system as for the medial collateral ligament injuries.[12] The posterolateral drawer test[44] and the passive external rotation at 30 degrees are used to evaluate the popliteus tendon and arcuate ligament.[43] The examiner must consider the physiological laxity present in the uninjured knee when testing these structures, especially in the patient with genu varum.

## Treatment

Treatment of these injuries is not always easy and the outcome is not predictable.[53] Isolated grade I and II injuries of the lateral collateral ligament, popliteus tendon, and/or arcuate ligament can be treated non-operatively with immobilization until comfortable and then controlled motion in a hinged brace. Strengthening and protected weight bearing begin immediately. Protection is maintained until the knee is pain-free and has a full range of motion and a strength comparable to that of the uninjured limb.

Treatment of grade III lesions of the lateral collateral ligament or popliteus tendon is undertaken in a similar fashion. Surgical repair is indicated for displaced boney avulsions of the lateral collateral ligament and/or popliteus tendon, and for combined ligament injuries to the popliteus and arcuate systems. Arthroscopy is indicated if the physical examination or MRI evaluation suggests meniscal pathology.

## Anterior Cruciate Ligament

Isolated disruptions of the anterior cruciate ligaments in children are unusual, especially in those less than 14 years old.[10, 16, 17, 19, 26, 78, 79, 90] The frequency of diagnoses of this injury has increased over recent years because of increased participation of children in sports, improved diagnostic techniques, and the knowledge that children sustain adult-type knee ligament injuries.*

Anterior cruciate insufficiency is present in two distinct groups of children.[16, 17] First, it appears in those with non-traumatic cruciate insufficiency which can be due to a generalized non-pathologic joint laxity or to congenital absence of the anterior cruciate ligament. The second group in which it is found are those patients with post-traumatic cruciate insufficiency. This is due to avulsion of either the femoral or tibial attachment of the anterior cruciate ligament or, less frequently, to a mid-substance tear.

## Non-Traumatic Cruciate Ligament Insufficiency

Many young children have inherent joint laxity in the knee, most of which resolves with growth and physical development. This physiologic laxity may give an erroneous suggestion of anterior cruciate ligament laxity in the knee. Such physiological ligament laxity involves not only the knee, but also other joints of the body such as the shoulders and elbows.[35] These children present with a positive anterior drawer test with the foot in neutral rotation and a positive Lachman's test, but with an endpoint. Associated with these findings will be a detectable pivot shift, flexion-rotation drawer, and hyperextension of the knee. These positive findings are usually bilateral, providing further evidence for the importance of examining both extremities.[13]

*See references 4, 10, 16, 21, 27, 32, 37, 53, 86.

Congenital absence of the anterior cruciate ligament is rare.[90] Developmental absence of the ACL is usually associated with other congenital abnormalities of the involved limb, such as proximal focal femoral deficiency, congenital dislocation of the knee, and leg length discrepancy.[14, 16, 48] Because of the associated limb anomalies, these patients are limited in athletic participation so the absent anterior cruciate ligament usually is not symptomatic.

Giorgi[29] reported the radiographic absence of the intercondylar eminence in knees which lack the anterior cruciate ligament. He theorized that the anterior cruciate ligament supplied traction on the tibial plateau during development that created the intercondylar eminence. In its absence, the eminence does not form, leading to the appearance of aplasia radiographically[29, 40] (see Fig 1).

## Post-Traumatic Anterior Cruciate Ligament Insufficiency

The second group of children that presents with this problem is the group with post-traumatic anterior cruciate ligament instability.[16, 17] This group can be subdivided according to the location of the ACL injury: tibial or femoral avulsion, or mid-substance tear.

Most anterior cruciate ligament injuries in children are avulsions of the ligament insertions at the tibial eminence.[16, 26, 70, 78] The ACL is attached to the tibia in a depressed area in front of and lateral to the anterior tibial spine. There is a fibrous attachment to the base of the anterior spine and a slip to the anterior horn of the lateral meniscus[30] (Fig 3). This anatomical arrangement, and the relative strength of the ligament itself compared to that of the adjacent bone and physeal plate, explains the propensity to tibial avulsions. Rinaldi and Mazzarella[77] showed that prior to fusion of the growth plates the intercondylar eminence offers less resistance to traction forces than does the ligament. Injuries that result in stretching or disruption of the anterior cruciate ligament in adults result in an avulsion of the tibial eminence in children.[4, 10, 16, 17, 55, 56, 63, 64]

Myers and McKeever[64, 65] classified tibial eminence fractures into four

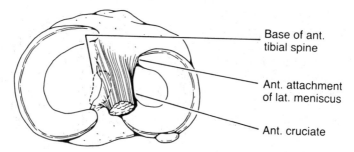

Base of ant.
tibial spine

Ant. attachment
of lat. meniscus

Ant. cruciate

**FIG 3.**
The anterior cruciate ligament inserts anterior and slightly lateral to the anterior tibial spine.

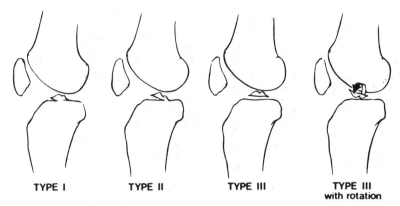

TYPE I        TYPE II        TYPE III        TYPE III
with rotation

**FIG 4.**
Meyers and McKeevers' classification of intercondylar eminence fractures based on
degree of displacement.

groups. Type I fractures are nondisplaced and type II fractures have some
elevation of the tibial eminence. Type III fractures show elevation of the
entire tibial eminence and displacement, while in type III+ injuries there is
rotation of the completely displaced eminence (Fig 4). Avulsion of the
anterior cruciate ligament at the intercondylar eminence is usually associated with severe damage to other supporting structures, such as the
collateral ligaments.[28, 45, 64, 65] It was noted initially by Garcia and Neer[28]
that tibial eminence fractures or avulsions can have associated collateral
ligament injuries. This was confirmed by Meyers and McKeever[64, 65] as
well as by Hyndman and Brown.[45] Injuries to the collateral ligaments in
conjunction with tibial spine avulsion produce a degree of ligament laxity
which is greater than that following either injury occurring as an isolated
event. For this reason, it is essential that a complete evaluation of all knee
ligaments be performed in children in whom a tibial spine avulsion is
diagnosed.[2, 28, 45, 64, 65]

Garcia and Neer[28] recommend that these tibial avulsions be treated by
closed reduction by hyperextension of the knee. Meyers and McKeever[64, 65]
treat type I and II fractures with closed reduction and immobilization, while
they treat type III and III+ fractures by open reduction and internal fixation.
In his study of 10 children less than 15 years old with tibial eminence fractures, Zariczhy[92] warns against residual displacement of the eminence following attempted closed reduction. A displaced eminence can mechan-
ically block knee extension and cause relative lengthening of the anterior
cruciate ligament. Type I tibial eminence fractures can be treated closed
with immobilization. According to most authors, type II injuries that can be
reduced are also treated closed, but those fractures in which an anatomic
reduction is not obtained should be openly reduced and fixed.[64, 65] All
type III and III+ fractures require open reduction and fixation.[64, 65, 81] The
physeal plate should not be violated when these fragments are fixed.

Avulsion of the anterior cruciate ligament from the femur is very rare. A single case was described by Eady[19] in 1982. The boney avulsion off the femur was seen on the tunnel radiograph view. This 7-year-old child underwent suture repair of the avulsed origin. The sutures were placed through drill holes in the medial femoral condyle without involvement of the physeal plate. At 15 months after surgery the patient had a stable joint.

Last, the anterior cruciate ligament may suffer a mid-substance tear. This injury, whether alone or associated with other ligament disruptions, is distinctly unusual.[4, 10, 16, 17] Primary repair of this injury has been shown to produce no better results in the child than in the adult.[4, 10, 16, 17]

## Diagnosis

The key to the diagnosis of an anterior cruciate ligament injury in the child is the history, physical exam, and specific radiographs, just as it is in the adult. The history relates a twisting or hyperextension injury followed by a loud "pop."[23, 31, 85] Isolated anterior cruciate ligament injuries are usually noncontact injuries that occur with a rapid change of position or with hyperextension. Any accompanying varus or valgus stress on the knee may result in associated medial or lateral collateral ligament injury. With an acute ACL injury, there is the rapid accumulation (within 24 hours) of a tense hemarthrosis.[16] The effusion will usually subside in a few days, leading the patient to believe that the knee is only slightly damaged. There may be associated ecchymosis at the site of injury. Range of motion may be limited by the effusion or by associated meniscal pathology.

The Lachman's, Losee's, and flexion-rotation drawer tests are present and can be elicited.[16, 42, 85] The pivot shift test is easily detected in the chronic anterior cruciate ligament deficient knee. It may be difficult to detect in the acute injury due to muscle pain and spasm. Tenderness at the medial or posterolateral joint line suggests associated meniscal pathology. Palpation of the origin and insertion of the medial and lateral collateral ligaments will detect injury of these structures. A positive anterior drawer test should suggest collateral ligament injury and anterior cruciate ligament disruption.[16, 42]

The radiographic examination is important in the skeletally immature group of patients. It is critical to obtain routine and stress radiographs in order to demonstrate avulsions and to distinguish physeal separations from ligament disruptions.[10, 13, 14, 16] An MRI may give valuable information on the location of ACL injury and the presence of associated meniscal damage.[47]

Arthroscopy should have only a limited role in the diagnosis of these injuries.[16] It is used to evaluate the menisci and to confirm the location of the ligament injury in the ACL-deficient knee.

Children with anterior cruciate ligament insufficiency fall into two groups according to the significance of their instability. First is the group that has no clinical evidence of instability. They are able to play and participate in sports with no symptoms of giving way. Second is the group in which the knee gives out in everyday activities and when the child participates in sports. Because the activity level of a child is difficult to curtail, these patients may have significant disability.

Therefore, a patient with an acute isolated mid-substance tear of the ACL should be given a period of time in which to demonstrate his instability. The fact that acute repairs of mid-substance tears of the ACL heal no better in the child than in the adult, and the fact that primary reconstruction or augmentation of a primary repair by standard methods runs a substantial risk of physeal plate damage, makes the conservative approach desirable. It is essential to inform the parents that if an episode of instability occurs, the patient's knee should be surgically stabilized to protect the menisci and articular cartilage from injury.

Children with *chronic* ACL insufficiency and "giving way" episodes are usually not functionally limited. However, these episodes of instability cause meniscal and articular cartilage damage which produce a poor long-term result. It is known that a child who has undergone meniscectomy has a poor long-term result.[16, 57, 74] Therefore, the approach taken with the child who has episodes of instability should be to stabilize the knee in order to reduce the incidence of articular cartilage and meniscal damage.

The child with an ACL-deficient knee presents a major problem in reconstruction. Any surgical procedure which is designed to restore the central pivot function of the ACL must violate the physeal plate.[16, 17, 51] Although there have been reports of good success with surgeries in which the graft crosses the growth plate, these children were older and more skeletally mature.[51, 58, 61] In this group of older patients, a physeal disruption would have less of an impact than in the younger child. If the physeal plate does have to be violated, it is not worth the risk of a physeal bar and length discrepancy in the child to do so. It may, therefore, be better to plan an extra-articular procedure (even with its tendency to stretch with time) in order to allow the growth plates to close. If the child is still active and having episodes of instability at that time, an intra-articular reconstruction may be done after the extra-articular reconstruction.

## Treatment

Operative repair of the ACL in a child follows three main principles. First, the primary reason for ACL repair is for meniscal and articular cartilage preservation. Children who lose their menisci progress to degenerative arthritis.[53, 57] Second, the surgical procedure should not violate the physeal plates. Third, the child and his family must understand that there will be limited activity until the range of motion and muscle strength have been restored. This rehabilitation period may last as long as 1 year.

Once the diagnosis of an acute anterior cruciate ligament disruption is suspected, complete evaluation of the knee is essential. An exam is done under anesthesia to confirm the ACL injury and to evaluate the secondary restraints. An arthroscopy is performed to (1) confirm the diagnosis, (2) locate the site of the ACL disruption, and (3) inspect the menisci. If a peripheral detachment of the meniscus is demonstrated, repair is indicated.[74] If the meniscus has a tear in its substance and repair is technically possible, it is recommended. If the meniscal tear produces a small, unstable meniscal fragment, excision is the treatment of choice.

If, at arthroscopy, the ACL is found to be avulsed off the tibia or femur with or without bone, a primary repair should be done.[59, 71, 79] This is performed using a Bunnell-type stitch through the ligament and then passing it through drill holes in the tibial or femoral epiphysis *without* violation of the physeal plate. These patients are immobilized with the knee bent 10 to 30 degrees for 4 to 6 weeks. This is followed by a limited range of motion in a hinged brace at 30 to 60 degrees for an additional 1 to 2 weeks. Full range of motion is then permitted. Hamstring muscle exercises are begun initially and quadriceps muscle exercises are begun at 6 months. Even with anatomic repair, residual laxity may persist. This is due to concomitant ligament injury at the time of avulsion of the tibial insertion.

The indications for a repair in an isolated mid-substance ACL tear in a child are limited to the situation in which there are grade 3(+) Lachman's and pivot shift tests in a patient with a peripheral meniscal injury that is surgically reparable. The method of mid-substance ACL repair is that of Marshall.[59] Three sutures are placed in the distal portion of the ligament and are brought out through the femoral epiphysis using two small Kirschner wires for drill holes. The proximal end of the ligament is then sutured to the distal portion using simple interrupted sutures. No sutures cross the physeal plates. The fat pad is then sutured to the cruciate ligament repair (Fig 5). An extra-articular augmentation is then performed us-

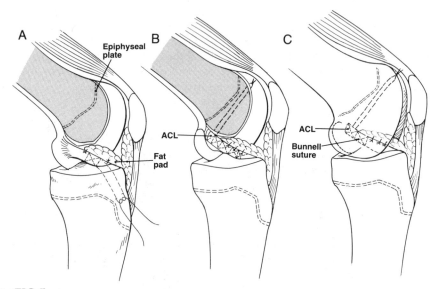

**FIG 5.**
Repair of anterior cruciate ligament. **A,** repair of tibial avulsion; **B,** repair of femoral avulsion, **C,** repair of mid-substance tear.

ing a strip of IT band 2.5 cm wide and 15 cm long. This strip is detached proximally and left attached at Gerdy's tubercle. It is then passed beneath the fibular collateral ligament and fixed to the femur, beneath an osteoperiosteal tunnel *above* the physis, with a 4.0 cancellous screw and spiked washer. The remaining IT band is brought back over the fibular collateral ligament and put back to bone below Gerdy's tubercle and fixed with a 4.0 cancellous screw and spiked washer (Fig 6). The defect in the IT band must be closed. The patient is then placed in a long leg brace with motion from 30 to 70 degrees of flexion for 4 weeks. This is followed by progressive mobilization and muscle rehabilitation.

In patients with acute ACL disruption associated with complete disruption of either collateral ligament system and/or the PCL, repair of the ACL and collateral ligaments is recommended. If the ACL injury is mid-substance, a technique similar to that of Marshall, et al[59] is utilized. Care is taken to avoid crossing the physeal plate with sutures used in the repair. Postoperative management follows that described for the ACL and collateral ligament repairs.

In a child with chronic ACL laxity, the decision to treat the patient surgically is based upon the frequency of giving way. Each episode of giving way or "slipping" produces articular cartilage shearing and potential meniscal injury. Initial treatment should consist of bracing and muscle rehabilitation. The brace is worn in sports activities. If the brace is ineffective or the patient's knee buckles in the activities of daily living, surgical reconstruction is indicated.

In most cases, an extra-articular reconstruction is performed as outlined above. If the knee is extremely unstable (grade 3+), and extra-articular reconstruction is not adequate to restore stability, then an intra-articular procedure *may* be indicated.

The "tomato stake" reconstruction described by Dr. John Bergfeld is a method of intra-articular reconstruction that does not violate the surrounding physes.[3] The chronic anterior cruciate ligament deficiency may be managed with a combined intra-articular and and extra-articular reconstruction. The remnants of the anterior cruciate ligament are exposed surgically. The proximal and distal ACL remnants are carefully teased away from the scar tissue and left intact. The remnants are augmented with either a patellar tendon or a hamstring tendon. A strip of the patellar tendon can be taken and left attached to the tibial tubercle distally. Alternatively, the semitendinosus tendon can be detached proximally and left attached distally. The patellar tendon or semitendinosus tendon is allowed to ride over the anterior border of the tibia, and is passed to the over-the-top position on the femoral condyle. The remainder of the scar tissue or fat pad is sutured around the graft (Fig 7). The extra-articular reconstruction described earlier then can be performed. There must be a careful evaluation of the secondary capsular restraints in these patients. Any posteromedial or posterolateral corner laxity should be corrected by plication of the ligament.

The patient is placed in a brace with knee motion from 30 to 70 degrees

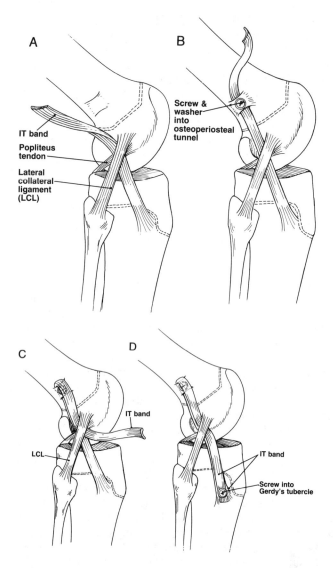

**FIG 6.**
Technique of anterolateral extra-articular reconstruction. **A,** a 2.5 cm wide by 15 cm long strip of IT band is harvested, leaving it attached to Gerdy's tubercle distally. It is then passed beneath the lateral collateral ligament. **B,** after passing beneath the lateral collateral ligament it is passed through a osteoperiosteal tunnel proximal to the physeal plate and fixed with a ligament screw and washer. **C,** the IT band is then passed distally again beneath the lateral collateral ligament. **D,** a ligament screw and washer is then used to fix the band back down to Gerdy's tubercle.

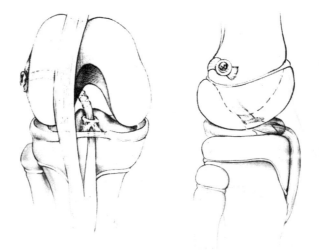

**FIG 7.**
The tomato stake procedure. The patellar tendon is left attached to the tibial tuber-cle and passed over the front of the tibia. It is fixed to the femoral origin using one suture which enters and exits through the distal femoral epiphysis and one that goes "over the top." The stump of the anterior cruciate ligament is used to agu-ment the graft.

of flexion for 4 weeks. Mobilization and rehabilitation are then instituted much the same as in an adult who has undergone a combined intra-artic-ular and extra-articular reconstruction.

One must be extremely careful in selecting patients for the "tomato stake" type repair. Although it does accomplish reconstruction of the cen-tral pivot ligament (ACL), it has two drawbacks. First, its tibial origin is too anterior and its femoral insertion often too posterior. These abnormal in-sertions result in a non-isometric reconstruction and, according to current theory, are certain to result in stretching of the reconstruction with the pas-sage of time. This may result in recurrence of the instability. Second, the use of the patellar tendon or semitendinosus tendon in this non-isometric repair leaves the surgeon with limited selections for autogenous tissue for a repeat reconstruction. For these reasons, it is best, if the clinical situation allows, to delay intra-articular reconstruction until the danger of physeal plate damage has passed and an isometric reconstruction can be per-formed.

## Posterior Cruciate Ligament

Disruption of the posterior cruciate ligament is a rare injury in the adult, and is even more uncommon in the child.[62, 73, 83] A case of posterior cru-ciate ligament injury in a 6-year-old child has been reported by Sanders, et al.[83] The posterior cruciate ligament courses from the posterior surface of the intercondylar area of the tibia in an anterior, superior, and medial direction to attach on the lateral surface of the medial femoral condyle. The tibial attachment passes distally over the posterior aspect of the tibia and blends into the periosteum, giving it a wide base.

Kennedy et al[56] demonstrated that the posterior cruciate ligament is twice as strong as the anterior cruciate ligament. This helps to explain its infrequency of injury. The posterior cruciate ligament is surrounded by the accessory ligaments of Wrisberg posteriorly and Humphrey anteriorly. These ligaments help to stabilize the knee against posterior displacement.[9] Clancy et al. noted that the posterior drawer test was significantly diminished when patients had intact ligaments of Wrisberg and/or Humphrey.[9] This decrease in posterior laxity was most apparent with the tibia internally rotated, a position which causes the ligaments of Wrisberg and Humphrey to become taut. Heller and Langeman[39] report that the ligaments of Wrisberg and Humphrey are found in equal frequency in approximately 70% of knees. They also note that the ligament of Wrisberg is at least half the diameter of the PCL, while the ligament of Humphrey is only about one third the size of the posterior cruciate ligament.[39]

## Mechanism of Injury

According to Kennedy and Grainger,[54] the posterior cruciate ligament can be injured by two separate mechanisms: first, forceful posterior displacement of the fixed tibia on the femur with the knee in 90 degrees of flexion, and second, a hyperextension injury to the knee. During hyperextension, the femoral condyles slide posteriorly on the tibia and the medial femoral condyle abuts against the posterior cruciate ligament, which is stretched. The PCL prevents further backward displacement of the femur, but if the hyperextension force continues past 30 degrees, in-substance failure or avulsion of the PCL will occur. A third mechanism of injury was reported by Donovan et al.[18] in three case reports of football players who had documented posterior cruciate ligament injuries caused by falling on the proximal tibial crest with the knee flexed at 90 degrees and the foot plantarflexed (Fig 8). Clancy[9] confirmed this mechanism of injury by reporting on ten patients with posterior cruciate ligament injuries following a fall on a flexed knee with the foot plantarflexed.

## Diagnosis

An effusion is usually not present with a PCL injury because of its intrasynovial but extra-capsular location. The posterior calf and joint line may be tender and swollen and show signs of ecchymosis due to a dissecting hematoma. Initially, the knee is painful and motion is limited. In 2 to 3 days the pain subsides and motion returns. The classic "posterior sag" or posterior drawer test may be absent initially due to the stability provided by the ligaments of Wrisberg and Humphrey.[9] If a drawer test is positive, the examiner may mistakenly believe it is an anterior drawer test if he begins the

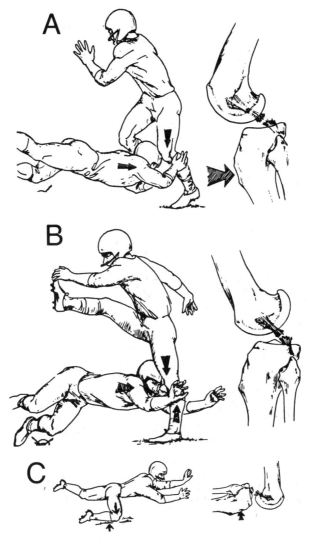

**FIG 8.**
Mechanisms of ligamentous disruption of the posterior cruciate ligament. **A,** forceful posterior displacement of fixed tibia on the femur; **B,** hyperextension of knee; **C,** blow on the proximal tibial crest with knee flexed at 90 degrees with foot fixed in plantar flexion.

examination with the tibia subluxed posteriorly rather than in its neutral position.[85]

The most accurate tests for acute PCL disruption are the "quadriceps" active drawer[15] test and the posterior Lachman test (Lachman-Trillat test). The quadriceps active drawer test is performed by placing the knee in 70

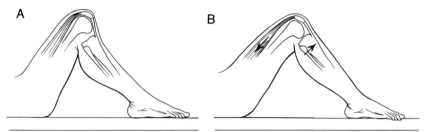

**FIG 9.**
Quadriceps active drawer test—a sensitive test for posterior cruciate injury. **A,** the knee is at 70 degrees of flexion with foot flat on examination table which allows the tibia to sublux posteriorly. **B,** the patient then contracts the quadriceps muscle while keeping the foot flat on the exam table, which will reduce the tibia to its neutral position.

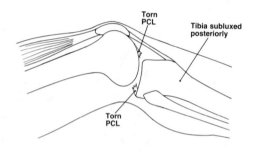

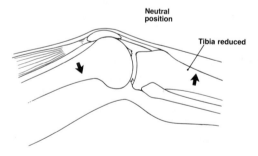

**FIG 10.**
Lachman-Trillat test (posterior Lachman). With the knee flexed 15 to 20 degrees and the distal femur stabilized, the proximal tibia is displaced posteriorly. If a definite endpoint to the posterior cruciate ligament is not felt, then the test is positive for injury to the ligament.

degrees of flexion with the foot flat on the examination table. The patient then contracts the quadriceps muscle, which is effective in pulling the tibial plateau anteriorly[15, 85] (Fig 9). The Lachman-Trillat test is accomplished by placing the knee in 15 to 20 degrees of flexion and stabilizing the distal femur in one hand and the proximal tibia in the other. The examiner must be certain that the tibia is in neutral alignment with the femur and not anteriorly or posteriorly subluxed to begin the exam. The tibia is then displaced posteriorly by the examiner against the stabilized femur. If a definite endpoint is not felt and/or there is significant displacement of the tibia posteriorly, then the test is positive for posterior cruciate ligament injury (Fig 10).

Radiographs also play an important role in the diagnosis as well. Plain radiographs may detect avulsion fractures of the femoral or tibial attachments of the posterior cruciate ligament.[5, 34, 60, 62, 63, 80] An MRI may be used to demonstrate in-substance ligament disruption, PCL avulsions with a chondral or osseous fragment, and meniscal pathology.[47] Stress films are taken to rule out a physeal plate injury.[10, 13, 16, 17]

## Treatment

Once an acute posterior cruciate ligament injury is diagnosed, treatment is directed at associated meniscal pathology and repair of the PCL if it is

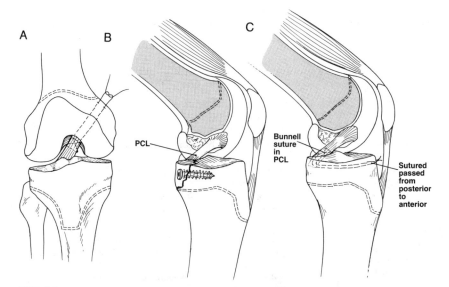

**FIG 11.**
Repair of posterior cruciate ligament. **A,** reattachment of non-boney avulsion of posterior cruciate ligament (PCL) to medial femoral condyle; **B,** screw fixation of bone fragment avulsed with PCL from tibia; **C,** reattachment of non-boney avulsion of PCL to posterior tibia.

avulsed from the femur or tibia.[5, 34, 60, 62, 63, 80] The location of the PCL injury can be determined by arthroscopy and often by MRI.[47] The MRI may show small chondral or osteochondral avulsions from the femur or tibia, which are not often seen radiographically.

The knee is first arthroscoped to confirm the location of the PCL injury, to evaluate meniscal pathology, and to visualize the chondral surfaces. Peripheral meniscal injuries are repaired and irreparable lesions excised.[74]

If the PCL is avulsed off the femur or tibia, it is repaired with intra-epiphyseal Bunnell sutures,[5, 34, 54, 60] or screw fixation of boney avulsions[5, 34, 54, 60, 80] (Fig 11). Isolated mid-substance tears are not repaired because repair of these in a child has proven to be no better than in adults[10]. Adults with chronic PCL laxity usually do not complain of instability unless there is laxity of the secondary restraints.[73] Children with chronic PCL laxity also do not usually exhibit significant functional disability. Our recommendation is to defer a formal PCL reconstruction until after physeal plate closure.

In patients with PCL disruption in conjunction with complete disruption of either collateral ligament system or the ACL, repair of the PCL, the ACL, and the collateral ligaments is recommended. If the PCL injury is mid-substance, a technique similar to that described for the ACL by Marshall et al[59] is utilized, realizing that some persistent posterior laxity is a certainty. If this is symptomatic, PCL reconstruction can be performed when physeal plate closure is complete.

# References

1. Arnoczky SP, Warren RF: Anatomy of the cruciate ligaments, in Feagin JA Jr (ed): The Cruciate Ligaments. New York, Churchill Livingstone, 1988, pp 179–195.
2. Baxter MP, Wiley JJ: Fractures of the tibial spine in children. J Bone Joint Surg 1988; 70:228–230.
3. Bergfeld J, personal communication.
4. Bradley GW, Shives TC, Samuelson KM: Ligament injuries in the knees of children. J Bone Joint Surg 1979; 61:588–591.
5. Brennan J: Avulsion injuries of the posterior cruciate ligaments. Clin Orthop 1960; 18:157–162.
6. Bright RW: Physeal injury, in Rockwood CA, Wilkins KE, King R (eds.): Fractures in Children. Philadelphia, Penn JB Lippincott Company, 1984, pp 87–172.
7. Bright RW, Burstein AH, Elmore SM: Epiphyseal-plate cartilage: A biomechanical and histological analysis of failure modes. J Bone Joint Surg 1974; 56A:688–703.
8. Chick RR, Jackson DW: Tears of the anterior cruciate ligament in young athletes. J Bone Joint Surg 1978; 60A:970–973.
9. Clancy WG, Shelbourne KD, Zoellner GB, et al: Treatment of knee joint instability secondary to rupture of the posterior cruciate ligament. J Bone Joint Surg 1983; 65A:310–322.
10. Clanton TO, DeLee JC, Sanders B, et al: Knee ligament injuries in children. J Bone Joint Surg 1979; 61A:1195–1200.

11. Cochran GV: *A Primer of Orthopaedic Biomechanics.* New York, Churchill Livingstone, 1982.
12. Committee on the Medical Aspects of Sports: Standard Nomenclature of Athletic Injuries. Chicago, American Medical Association, 1968, pp 99–101.
13. Crawford AH: Fractures about the knee in children. *Orthop Clin North Am* 1976; 7:639–656.
14. Curtis BH, Fisher RL: Congenital hyperextension with anterior subluxation of the knee. *J Bone Joint Surg* 1969; 51A:255–269.
15. Daniel DM, Stone ML, Barnett P, et al: The quadriceps active drawer. Presented at the 52nd Annual Meeting of the American Academy of Orthopaedic Surgeons, Las Vegas, Nevada, January 1985.
16. DeLee JC: ACL insufficiency in children, in Feagin JA Jr (ed): *The Crucial Ligaments.* New York, Churchill Livingstone, 1988, pp 439–447.
17. DeLee JC, Curtis R: Anterior cruciate ligament insufficiency in children. *Clin Orthop* 1983; 172:112–118.
18. Donovan TL, Benling F, Nagel DA: Posterior cruciate injury on artificial turf. *Orthop Trans* 1977; 1:20.
19. Eady JL, Cardenas CD, Sopa D: Avulsion of the femoral attachment of the anterior cruciate ligament in a seven year-old child. *J Bone Joint Surg* 1982; 64A:1376–1378.
20. Ehrlich MG, Strain RE: Epiphyseal injuries about the knee. *Orthop Clin North Am* 1979; 10:91–103.
21. Eilert RE: Arthroscopy of the knee joint in children. *Orthop Rev* 1976; 5:61–65.
22. Engebretsen S, Benum P: Poor results of anterior cruciate ligament repair in adolescence. *Acta Orthop Scand* 1988; 59:684–686.
23. Feagin JA, Curl WW: Isolated tear of the anterior cruciate ligament: Five year followup study. *Am J Sports Med* 1976; 4:95–100.
24. Fetto JF, Marshall JL: Medial collateral ligament injuries of the knee. *Clin Orthop* 1978; 132:206–218.
25. Fowler PJ: The classification and early diagnosis of knee joint instability. *Clin Orthop* 1980; 147:15–20.
26. Furman W, Marshall JL, Girgis FG: The anterior cruciate ligament. *J Bone Joint Surg* 1976; 58A:179–185.
27. Gallagher SS, Finison K, Gvyer B: The incidence of injuries among 87,000 Massachusetts children and adolescents. Results of the 1980-1981 statewide Childhood Injury Prevention Program Surveillance System. *Am J Public Health* 1984; 74:1340–1347.
28. Garcia A, Neer CS: Isolated fractures of the intercondylar eminence of the tibia. *Am J Surg* 1958; 95:593–598.
29. Giorgi B: Morphologic variations of the intercondylar eminence of the knee. *Clin Orthop* 1956; 8:209–217.
30. Girgis FG, Marshall JL, Monajem ARS: The cruciate ligaments of the knee joint. *Clin Orthop* 1975; 106:216–231.
31. Glancy GL: The injured knee in the adolescent. *J Musculo Med* 1986; 14–27.
32. Goldberg B: Pediatric sports medicine, in Scott, Nisserson, Nicholas (eds): *Principles of Sports Medicine.* Baltimore, Williams & Wilkins, 1984.
33. Gollehon DL, Torzilli PA, Warren RF: The role of the posterolateral and cruciate ligaments in the stability of the human knee. *J Bone Joint Surg* 1987; 69A:233–242.
34. Goodrich A, Ballard A: Posterior cruciate ligament avulsion associated with ipsilateral femur fracture in a 10 year-old child. *J Trauma* 1988; 28:1393–1396.

35. Grana WA, Moretz JA: Ligamentous laxity in secondary school athletes. *JAMA* 1978; 240:1975–1976.
36. Grossman RB, Nicholas J: Common disorders of the knee. *Orthop Clin North Am* 1977; 8:619.
37. Halpern B, Thompson N, Curl WW, et al: High school football injuries: Identifying the risk factors. *Am J Sports Med* 1987; 15:113–117.
38. Harris WR: The endocrine basis for slipping of the upper femoral epiphysis. An experimental study. *J Bone Joint Surg* 1950; 32B:5–11.
39. Heller L, Langeman J: The menisco-femoral ligaments of the human knee. *J Bone Joint Surg* 1964; 46B:307–313.
40. Houseworth SW, Mauro VJ, Mellon BA, et al: The intercondylar notch in acute tears of the anterior cruciate ligament: A computer graphics study. *Am J Sports Med* 1987; 15:221–224.
41. Hsieh H, Walker PS: Stabilizing mechanisms of the loaded and unloaded knee joint. *J Bone Joint Surg* 1976; 58A:87–93.
42. Hughston JC, Andrews JR, Cross MJ, et al: Classification of knee ligament instabilities, Part I. The medial compartment and cruciate ligaments. *J Bone Joint Surg* 1976; 58A:159–172.
43. Hughston JC, Andrews JR, Cross MJ, et al: Classification of knee ligament instabilities, Part II. The lateral compartment. *J Bone Joint Surg* 1976; 58A:173–179.
44. Hughston JC, Norwood LA: The posterolateral drawer test and external rotational recurvatum test for posterolateral rotatory instability of the knee. *Clin Orthop* 1980; 147:82–87.
45. Hyndman JC, Brown DG: Major ligament injuries of the knee in children. Presented at the annual meeting of the Canadian Orthopaedic Association, British Columbia, June 1978.
46. Indelicato PA: Non-operative treatment of complete tears of the medial collateral ligament of the knee. *J Bone Joint Surg* 1983; 65A:323–329.
47. Jackson DW, Jennings LD, Maywood RM, et al: Magnetic resonance imaging of the knee. *Am J Sports Med* 1988; 16:29–38.
48. Johansson E, Aparisi T: Congenital absence of the cruciate ligaments. *Clin Orthop* 1982; 162:108–111.
49. Jones RE, Henley MB, Francis P: Nonoperative management of isolated grade III collateral ligament injury in high school football players. *Clin Orthop* 1986; 213:137–140.
50. Joseph KN, Pogrund H: Traumatic rupture of the medial ligament of the knee in a four year-old boy. *J Bone Joint Surg* 1978; 60A:402–403.
51. Kannus P, Jarvinen M: Knee ligament injuries in adolescents. *J Bone Joint Surg* 1988; 70B:772–776.
52. Kannus P: Long term results of conservatively treated medial collateral ligament injuries of the knee joint. *Clin Orthop* 1988; 226:103–112.
53. Kennedy JC: *The Injured Adolescent Knee*. Baltimore, Williams & Wilkins, 1979.
54. Kennedy JC, Grainger RW: The posterior cruciate ligament. *J Trauma* 1967; 7:367–377.
55. Kennedy JC, Weinberg HW, Wilson AS: The anatomy and function of the anterior cruciate ligament. *J Bone Joint Surg* 1974; 56A:223–235.
56. Kennedy JC, Hawkins RJ, Willis RB, et al: Tension studies of human knee ligaments. *J Bone Joint Surg* 1976; 58A:350–355.
57. Krause WR, Pope MH, Johnson RJ, et al: Mechanical changes in the knee after meniscectomy. *J Bone Joint Surg* 1976; 58A:599–604.

58. Lipscomb AB, Anderson AF: Tears of the anterior cruciate ligament in adolescents. *J Bone Joint Surg* 1986; 68A:19–28.
59. Marshall JL, Warren RF, Wickiewicz TL, et al: The anterior cruciate ligament: A technique of repair and reconstruction. *Clin Orthop* 1979; 143:98–106.
60. Mayer PJ, Michell LJ: Avulsion of the femoral attachment of the posterior cruciate ligament in an eleven year-old boy. *J Bone Joint Surg* 1979; 16A:431–432.
61. McCarroll JR, Rettig AC, Shelbourne KD: Anterior cruciate ligament injuries in the young athlete with open physes. *Am J Sports Med* 1988; 16:44–47.
62. McMaster WC: Isolated posterior cruciate ligament injury: Literature review and case reports. *J Trauma* 1975; 15:1025–1029.
63. Meyers MH: Isolated avulsion of the tibial attachment of the posterior cruciate ligament of the knee. *J Bone Joint Surg* 1975; 57A:669–672.
64. Meyers HH, McKeever FM: Fracture of the intercondylar eminence of the tibia. *J Bone Joint Surg* 1970; 52A:16777–1684.
65. Meyers MH, McKeever FM: Fracture of the intercondylar eminence of the tibia. *J Bone Joint Surg* 1959; 41A:209–222.
66. Micheli LJ: Pediatric and adolescent sports injuries: Recent trends. *Exerc Sport Sci Rev* 1986; 14:359–374.
67. Mirbey J, Besancenot J, Chambers RT, et al: Avulsion fractures of the tibial tuberosity in the adolescent athlete. *Am J Sports Med* 1988; 16:336–340.
68. Morrissy RT, Eubanks RG, Park JP, et al: Arthroscopy of the knee in children. *Clin Orthop* 1982; 162:103–107.
69. Norwood LA, Hughston JC: Combined anterolateral-anteromedial rotatory instability of the knee. *Clin Orthop* 1980; 147:62–67.
70. Noyes FR, DeLucas JL, Torvik PJ: Biomechanics of anterior cruciate ligament failure: An analysis of strain-rate sensitivity and mechanisms of failure in primates. *J Bone Joint Surg* 1974; 56A:236–253.
71. O'Donoghue DH: An analysis of end results of surgical treatment of major injuries to the ligaments of the knee. *J Bone Joint Surg* 1955; 37A:1–13.
72. Ogden JA, Tross RB, Murphy MJ: Fractures of the tibial tuberosity in adolescents. *J Bone Joint Surg* 1980; 62A:205–222.
73. Parolie JM, Bergfeld JA: Long term results of nonoperative treatment of isolated posterior cruciate ligament injuries in the athlete. *Am J Sports Med* 1986; 14:35–38.
74. Price CT, Allen WC: Ligament repair in the knee with preservation of the meniscus. *J Bone Joint Surg* 1978; 60A:61–65.
75. Rang M: *Children's Fractures,* 1st ed. Philadelphia, Penn, JB Lippincott Company, 1974.
76. Rang M: *Children's Fractures,* 2nd ed. Philadelphia, Penn, JB Lippincott Company, 1983.
77. Rinaldi E, Mazzarella F: Isolated fracture avulsions of the tibial insertions of the cruciate ligaments of the knee. *Ital J Orthop Traumatol* 1980; 6:77–83.
78. Roberts JM: Fractures and dislocations of the knee, in Rockwood CA, Wilkins KE, King R (eds): *Fractures In Children.* Philadelphia, Penn, JB Lippincott Company, 1984, pp 891–945.
79. Robinson SC, Driscoll SE: Simultaneous osteochondral avulsion of the femoral and tibial insertions of the anterior cruciate ligament. *J Bone Joint Surg* 1981; 63A:1342–1343.
80. Ross AC, Chesterman PJ: Isolated avulsion of the tibial attachment of the posterior cruciate ligament in childhood. *J Bone Joint Surg* 1986; 68B:747.

81. Roth PB: Fracture of the spine of the tibia. Presented at the British Orthopaedic Association Meeting, Bristol, England, October 1927.
82. Salter RB: *Textbook of Disorders and Injuries of the Musculoskeletal System.* Baltimore, Williams & Wilkins, 1970.
83. Sanders WE, Wilkins KE, Neidre A: Acute insufficiency of the posterior cruciate ligament in children. *J Bone Joint Surg* 1980; 62A:129–130.
84. Singer IJ: Sports related knee injuries in the pediatric and adolescent athlete. *RI Med J* 1987; 70:255–263.
85. Sisk TD: Knee injuries, in Crenshaw AH (ed): *Campbell's Operative Orthopaedics,* ed 7. St. Louis, CV Mosby Company, 1987, pp 2283–2496.
86. Skak SV, Jensen TT, Poulsen TD, et al: Epidemiology of knee injuries in children. *Acta Orthop Scand* 1987; 58:78–81.
87. Steingard M, Morrison D, Schildberg W, et al: A followup study on adolescent knee injuries. *J Am Osteopath Assoc* 1987; 87:807–816.
88. Thompson N, Halpern B, Curl WW, et al: High school football injuries: Evaluation. *Am J Sports Med* 1987; 15:97–117.
89. Tipton CM, Matthes RD, Martin RK: Influence of age and sex on the strength of bone-ligament junctions in knee joints of rats. *J Bone Joint Surg* 1978; 60A:230–234.
90. Tolo VT: Congenital absence of the menisci and cruciate ligaments of the knee. *J Bone Joint Surg* 1981; 63A:1022–1023.
91. Torg JS, Pavlov H, Morris VB: Salter-Harris Type III fracture of the medial femoral condyle occurring in the adolescent athlete. *J Bone Joint Surg* 1981; 63A:586–591.
92. Zariczhy B: Avulsion fracture of the tibial eminence: Treatment by open reduction and pinning. *J Bone Joint Surg* 1977; 59A:1111–1115.

# Management of Meniscal Problems in the Young Athlete

## Kenneth E. DeHaven, M.D.

University of Rochester School of Medicine and Dentistry, Department of Orthopaedics, Section of Athletic Medicine, Rochester, New York

## Daniel C. Wascher, M.D.

University of Rochester School of Medicine and Dentistry, Department of Orthopaedics, Section of Athletic Medicine, Rochester, New York

## Editor's Introduction

Meniscal problems are far less common in the skeletally immature athlete. However, the meniscus in these younger players has a better blood supply and greater cellularity, hence greater potential for healing. The long-term results of meniscectomy in children are identical to those in adults. Therefore, better results are expected in the healing of the meniscus following repair as well as better long-term effect on the articular surface by meniscal preservation.

*William A. Grana, M.D.*

Recently there has been a marked increase in the participation of children in organized sports. In addition to increased membership in traditional sports such as football, basketball, and baseball, many children now belong to teams in soccer, hockey, and other sports. There also has been a dramatic rise in the number of girls playing interscholastic sports.

A concomitant rise in individual sports participation, such as in skiing and running, has helped fuel the growth of the number of young athletes. Although some school systems have eliminated athletics for monetary reasons, most educators feel that interscholastic athletics play an important role in the physical, social, and emotional maturation of students.

However, with the rise in athletic participation by children, physicians are seeing an increased frequency of pediatric athletic injuries. Adolescent knee injuries are often the result of contact or noncontact stresses occurring during organized competition. In particular, we have seen an increased number of meniscal tears in our pediatric population. Numerous studies have shown the poor results of clinical diagnosis in accurately predicting the pathology of children with knee injuries. Additionally, studies of

**197**

long-term results of meniscectomies in children have been uniformly disappointing. These factors have led us to undertake an aggressive approach to young athletes with meniscal injuries.

Meniscal tears are seen more frequently with increasing age in children. Tears in children under 10 years of age are exceedingly rare. The youngest patient in whom was reported a meniscal tear in an otherwise normal medial meniscus was age 4 years.[36] In younger children, meniscal injuries usually occur in congenitally abnormal menisci. In several series, all patients under 14 years with meniscal tears had lateral discoid menisci.[17, 47] Beginning in adolescence, there is a sharp increase in the frequency of traumatic meniscal tears. This is associated with increased forces being placed across the knee secondary to weight and strength gains, and with increased participation in organized athletic events which have a high risk of knee injuries.

## Anatomy

Numerous studies have documented the anatomy and vascularity of the human menisci. The meniscus is composed primarily of hypocellular fibrocartilage.[5] The majority of the collagen fibers are arranged circumferentially, which helps them to withstand the large tension loads applied in weight-bearing activities.[4] A few fibers run in a radial direction, which helps resist longitudinal splitting.

Scapinelli[37] and Arnoczky and Warren[1] described the vasculature of the human menisci. The meniscal blood flow is supplied from branches of the medial, lateral, and middle geniculate arteries. These branches form a perimeniscal capillary plexus in the surrounding capsular and synovial tissues. This plexus penetrates into the peripheral 10% to 30% of the meniscus. The portion of the lateral meniscus adjacent to the popliteal tendon was found to be void of penetrating peripheral vessels. Vascularity in the region of meniscal tears is felt to be a prerequisite for their healing.

Shim and Leung[39] performed microangiographic studies of the knee joint in child and adult cadavers. They also found a circummeniscal anastomosis which supplied the outer one third to one half of the menisci. They did not mention any differences between child and adult menisci.

In a more detailed study, Clark and Ogden[8] examined the development of menisci in prenatal and postnatal cadavers. The menisci reached their semilunar configurations early in prenatal development. Menisci in 14 week old fetuses were seen to have morphologic features of adult menisci. Histologically, there was a marked increase in cellularity and vascularity seen in the fetal specimens. After birth there was a gradual decrease in vascularity and by the age of 10 years blood vessels were located primarily in the outer one third of the menisci. However, occasional vessels could still be identified in the inner zones in contrast to adult specimens in which vessels were seen only in the peripheral one third.

The menisci also gradually undergo a decrease in cellularity with a concomitant rise in collagen fiber content. With increasing age the collagen fibers undergo organization; the majority of the fibers are oriented circumferentially and occasional fibers are arranged radially. These changes are seen between 3 and 9 years of age.

These studies suggest that meniscal injuries in the pediatric population may have greater capacity for healing, and that more centrally located tears in younger patients may be reparable. However, the majority of meniscal injuries occur in adolescents in whom the menisci have assumed the anatomic, vascular, and histologic characteristics of adult menisci.

## History

More frequently, meniscal injuries occur with noncontact stresses. A history of tibiofemoral rotational stress with the knee in a flexed position, such as occurs with cutting maneuvers in football, is common. Injuires can also occur from hyperflexion or hyperextension injuries. Varus and valgus movements can be applied to the knee by noncontact means (such as landing off-balance from a jump) or by contact from another player. The tibiofemoral compression combined with tibiofemoral rotation produce a shear force to the menisci, causing tearing to occur. The physician should inquire about previous ligament or meniscus injuries.

A thorough clinical evaluation is required prior to any treatment plan. When the patient first presents, a detailed history is taken. The examiner often must take extra time with children and adolescents to accurately pinpoint the mechanism of injury. Despite the best of efforts, the patient often will be unable to give an accurate description of the injury events. Witnesses and game films (if available) can provide additional information. There is a high incidence of collateral and cruciate ligament injury associated with meniscal tears in young athletes. It is important to inquire whether the patient felt a popping or tearing sensation as the knee gave way, and whether the patient was able to extend the knee fully and bear weight after the injury. In younger children, epiphyseal injuries about the knee must be considered in the differential diagnosis of collateral ligament injuries.

With an acute injury, the patient will most often complain of pain, swelling, locking, and giving way. Pain usually occurs immediately and is localized to either the medial or lateral compartment. Because of frequent collateral ligament injuries, the pain is not always confined to the joint line but often extends along the course of the fibers of the involved ligament.

The occurrence of hemarthrosis after a knee injury suggests an anterior cruciate ligament injury. Treatment is directed towards the cruciate ligament injury, but the physician should remember the frequent association of meniscal tears with anterior cruciate ligament (ACL) disruptions. The typical effusion seen in isolated meniscal injuries develops gradually over a 2 to 3 day period.

Locking often occurs after acute meniscal injuries, especially displaced bucket-handle lesions. Typically the knee lacks 15 to 45 degree of full extension. Sometimes the patient or a bystander is able to manipulate the knee to reduce the meniscus and achieve full extension. The physician must carefully ascertain whether the patient had the ability to extend the knee fully immediately after injury, because developing hemarthrosis from other injuries can cause the inability to extend the knee joint fully a few hours after the injury.

At the time of injury the patient also often states that the knee "gave way." In isolated meniscal injuries, the immediate pain can cause a reflex inhibition of the quadriceps musculature and a collapse of the limb. In acute or chronic cruciate ligament injuries, the instability usually occurs prior to any painful sensation.

In the chronic meniscal tear, the patient will often recall an acute episode followed by gradual improvement. However, the patient remains limited by joint line pain on the side of the meniscal tear. Intermittent locking episodes may occur and the patient may refer to a "trick knee." Giving way may occur secondary to pain, similar to acute injuries. The degree of functional limitation that results from chronic meniscal injuries depends on the severity of the tear and the extent of functional demands on the meniscus.

## Physical Examination

The physical examination must include a complete examination of the knee. Particular attention should be directed to the patellofemoral joint, acute or chronic ligamentous instability, and the possibility of epiphyseal injuries. The following are areas of particular interest in an examination for suspected meniscal pathology. The physician should carefully examine for the presence of an effusion, especially in acute injuries. Range of motion should be recorded and compared to the uninjured extremity; a lack of full extension should be searched for carefully. Subtle differences in knee extension can be detected by having the patient lie prone with his legs from mid-thigh down hanging off the end of the table. The cause of any lack of full extension (pain, effusion, mechanical block) should be ascertained. The medial and lateral joint lines should be palpated in their entirety for specific points of tenderness. The McMurry test (circumduction maneuvers with the knee flexed, eliciting pain or a click) can demonstrate otherwise occult posterior horn tears. Quadriceps muscle atrophy usually accompanies chronic meniscus injury and thigh circumference should be measured from a standard reference point.

## Diagnostic Tests

Plain radiographs should be used to evaluate all acute and chronic knee injuries. Although no abnormalities will be seen in isolated meniscal injuries, associated boney lesions must be excluded. X-rays should include standard anteroposterior (AP) lateral, Merchant patellofemoral, and tunnel views (to best demonstrate osteochondritis dessicans). Stress x-rays should always be obtained in acute injuries with varus or valgus laxity and open epiphyses.

In chronic or subacute suspected meniscal injuries, further diagnostic studies can assist in establishing the correct diagnosis and planning appropriate treatment. Double contrast arthrography can accurately detect many meniscal tears. The reported accuracy of this study has ranged from 60% to 97%.[12, 18, 25, 34] Medial meniscal tears are usually well visualized. The region of the posterior horn of the lateral meniscus can be difficult to evaluate because of shadows caused by the popliteus tendon hiatus. In young athletes, however, arthrography has been reported to be less effective. Obviously, the cooperation of the patient and the skill of the arthrographer play a great role in the effectiveness of this technique.

More recently, newer imaging techniques have been utilized to detect meniscal injuries. Manco et al[29] reported that computerized tomography (CT) of the knee without contrast had an overall diagnostic accuracy of 91%. Some of the advantages of CT scanning listed by these investigators are: (1) it is an easily performed, noninvasive procedure; (2) it allows better visualization of the posterior horn of the lateral meniscus; and (3) it provides a clearer anatomic picture compared to arthrography.

Magnetic resonance imaging (MRI) has also been advocated for the diagnosis of meniscal tears. Polly et al[35] reported a 98% diagnostic accuracy for tears of the medial meniscus and a 90% diagnostic accuracy for tears of the lateral meniscus using this technique. The advantages of MRI were those of a noninvasive procedure, the elimination of exposure to ionizing radiation, and good delineation of the posterior horns. However, Silva and Silver[40] found only a 45% diagnostic accuracy of MRI in evaluating meniscal tears. They advised against the use of MRI as a routine diagnostic test for meniscal lesions.

All special imaging techniques for meniscal tears can be expected to have great variability in results depending on the sophistication of the scanning equipment and the skill and experience of the radiologist. Noninvasive techniques may have an advantage for younger children, but they still require the patient to remain motionless for 20 to 30 minutes. CT or MRI may have an advantage in suspected posterior horn tears of the lateral meniscus. The orthopaedist must choose any diagnostic work-up based upon clinical examination, index of suspicion, and the experience level of available local radiographers.

These diagnostic tests should be pursued to help direct treatment. A negative study can be reassuring to both the patient and the physician that a trial of conservative therapy is indicated. Likewise, a positive study can provide impetus for timely operative treatment. Diagnostic studies can also help identify reparable tears, which can help the physician and the patient to plan for a more extensive operative procedure and a longer rehabilitation period.

## Arthroscopy

The orthopaedist should use arthroscopy as both a diagnostic and a therapeutic modality in both acute and chronic knee injuries in adolescents. Examination of acute injuries in children is often difficult, especially if other major knee pathology has occurred. Diagnostic arthroscopy yields an accurate assessment of meniscal injuries in acute hemarthrosis of the knee. Eiskjaer and Larsen[14] reported only a 32% accuracy of clinical diagnosis in acute hemarthrosis of the knee in 25 children. Several recent articles have documented the usefulness of arthroscopy in diagnosing chronic knee complaints in children. In the above series, only 34 of 76 clinically suspected chronic meniscal tears were confirmed by arthroscopic examination. Suman et al[43] showed the accuracy of clinical diagnosis of meniscal injuries to be 42% in patients under 13 years old and 56% in patients 14 to 17 years old. The most common "incorrect" clinical diagnoses were meniscal tears and discoid menisci. Morrissy et al[33] found similar results and stated that arthroscopy was useful in children with doubtful clinical diagnoses who remained symptomatic despite conservative treatment. Bergstrom et al[3] performed arthroscopy on 15 children, each with a clinical diagnosis of a torn meniscus. Only 3 of the 15 children were found to have a meniscal injury at arthroscopy.

Other diagnostic tests were rarely utilized in the above series, which may explain the high number of clinical diagnostic errors. Some authors feel that arthrography is unreliable in children. However, utilization of some of the newer imaging modalities may help to increase the diagnostic accuracy for meniscal injuries.

Arthroscopic examination is best performed under spinal or general anesthesia. Complete anesthesia allows for a thorough ligament examination. Adequate visualization can be obtained in knees with acute hemarthrosis by first completely draining the knee and then utilizing a constant irrigation flow. Knees with severe capsular injuries are considered unsuitable for arthroscopy, as large amounts of fluid can extravasate into the soft tissue. Neurovascular compression syndromes have been reported. A tourniquet may be used, but inflation should be avoided, if possible, if an open procedure is anticipated.

Most authors utilize a 5 mm arthroscope in children, and we have found this to be adequate. Usually, no technical difficulties are encountered, and the larger arthroscope affords better visualization of the joint. The entire knee must be systematically searched for other pathology. The menisci should be thoroughly probed and any tears that are encountered should be assessed for their stability. Creating additional posteromedial or posterolateral portals, or passing the 70 degree arthroscope back through the intercondylar notch, will allow more complete visualization of the posterior horns of the menisci.

## Conservative Management

Patients with both acute and chronic knee injuries may be managed best initially by a conservative management program. In acute grade I and II collateral ligament injuries with associated joint line tenderness, it may be difficult to accurately assess the menisci in children. There should be no hemarthrosis or anterior cruciate ligament instability detected. The joint line tenderness could be secondary to rupture of the collateral ligament fibers, or rupture of the underlying meniscus. In this situation, it is appropriate to treat the collateral ligament injury. Our management consists of a hinged splint with motion allowed in the comfort range. Full motion should be reached as soon as possible. Progressive resistance exercises of the quadriceps, hamstrings, and hip abductors, and a graduated running program should then be instituted. If the patient recovers fully with no meniscal symptoms, then either there was no meniscal pathology, or else a minor tear healed spontaneously. If, after adequate rehabilitation, the athlete continues to have symptoms of meniscal pathology but shows improvement in the collateral ligament findings, the physician should proceed with a diagnostic work-up and arthroscopy, as with any suspected meniscal tear.

Children with chronic knee symptoms often present with vague knee complaints. Examination frequently shows mild effusion, abnormal patellofemoral signs, and joint line tenderness, but no block to extension. There are usually associated quadriceps atrophy and muscular weakness, and an initial program of rehabilitation is indicated. Progressive resistance exercises should be instituted, using the isometric quadriceps technique. Athletic participation should be avoided initially and non-steroidal anti-inflammatory medication is usually helpful. When the muscle strength of the injured limb reaches 90% of that of the uninvolved extremity, the patient may gradually resume athletic training as tolerated. If the symptoms resolve, it usually indicates that no meniscal pathology existed in spite of the joint line tenderness and that inadequate or no rehabilitation following a minor injury accounted for the symptoms. Patients who fail to improve warrant further diagnostic evaluation.

## Surgical Treatment

The primary goals in the treatment of meniscal injuries in young athletes are relieving the symptoms caused by the tear, preserving maximal function, and preventing long-term degenerative changes. A secondary goal should be a return to full activity as soon as possible. The specific therapeutic approach will be dictated by the location of the tear, any associated ligament injury, the age of the patient, and whether the tear is acute or chronic. The menisci play an important role in the transmission of forces across the knee joint. Numerous studies have shown poor long-term results following the meniscectomy in adults[23, 27, 44] and children.[16, 30, 32, 44, 45, 47] Therefore, particular emphasis should be placed upon retaining as much functional meniscus as possible when treating children.

Most grade school and high school athletes will participate in sports only on a recreational level when they reach adulthood; the majority have not decided on career choices. Upon reaching adulthood, many adolescents will place greater demands on their knees in the workplace than on the playing field. The physician constantly needs to remind himself, the patient, and the patient's parents that the primary goal in rehabilitation is maximal long-term knee function rather than simply a quick return to interscholastic athletics. Thus, for tears in which a meniscal repair (and the minimum 6-months' absence from sports) offers the best chance of unimpaired long-term knee function, partial meniscectomy should not be performed merely to return the child to athletics in a shorter time frame.

There are four major options for the treatment of meniscal injuries: (1) not treatment at all; (2) meniscal repair; (3) partial meniscectomy; and (4) total meniscectomy. The exact method chosen in the pediatric population depends on the nature of the meniscal pathology and the status of the remainder of the knee joint. This underscores the need for thorough clinical evaluation and diagnostic testing prior to making decisions regarding surgical treatment.

## Untreated Meniscal Tears

Not all meniscal tears require treatment, as some tears will heal with conservative treatment and others will not be symptomatic. Even partially damaged menisci continue to have biomechanical function if the meniscus is stable and the peripheral circumferential fibers are intact. Casscells[7] has stated "when in doubt, leave it in." Questionable tears can be left alone and, if they prove to be problematic, they can be treated later with partial excision. However, once removed, the torn meniscus can never to replaced. The meniscus does not have the ability to reliably regenerate following excision. The majority of tears which we have left untreated have been partial thickness, longitudinally oriented, vertical tears. These occur primarily on the femoral surface of the lateral meniscus and on the tibial surface of the medial meniscus. They usually are located in the vascular outer one third of the posterior zones of the menisci. These tears are often incidental findings in a knee with other more significant pathology. In our experience, anterior cruciate ligament tears have been present in over 80% of knees in which meniscus tears have been left untreated. Full thickness tears can also be left alone if they are short (approximately 5 mm) and if they are stable to probing. The physician should not be able to displace the portion of the meniscus central to the tear more than 3 mm from the intact outer rim. Small radial tears that involve less than the inner one third of a meniscus can also be left alone, as they are rarely symptomatic. In general, every effort should be made to retain stable meniscal tissue, especially in an unstable knee.

In our experience, approximately 5% of all meniscal tears have been categorized as stable and treated conservatively. In conjunction with the sports trauma group from Linkoping University in Sweden, we have followed 75 patients with 80 "stable" meniscal tears that have been left alone.[46] At arthrosocpy, no effort was made to freshen up the torn edges of the meniscus other than probing with a nerve hook to assess for stability. Patients with isolated stable meniscal lesions were treated with partial weight bearing for approximately 1 week. The remaining patients had associated acute and chronic anterior cruciate ligament injuries and required postoperative immobilization and appropriate anterior cruciate ligament rehabilitation. Seventy of these injuries were vertical longitudinal tears (25% of which were full thickness) and 10 were radial tears. Thirty-two tears were reevaluated by arthroscopy at an average of 26 months after injury. Seventeen of the 26 longitudinal tears had completely healed, but none of the 6 radial tears had healed. Six patients have required further treatment of their meniscal tears: 4 had extension of their tears during athletic activities and underwent partial meniscectomy; and 2 had persistent symptoms from their original tear and had meniscus repair. In patients less than 20 years of age, 3 of 5 vertical longitudinal tears had healed on reexamination, 1 tear was unchanged but asymptomatic, and 1 tear was unchanged but was associated with persistent symptoms and required partial meniscectomy.

We have not found any statistical difference in healing between tears in stable versus unstable knees. In the majority of cases, these tears have occurred in knees with associated major knee injuries. In these cases, it is prudent to leave the stable meniscal injuries alone. Healing will occur in the majority of the injuries and most of the remaining tears will remain asymptomatic. In knees with isolated stable meniscal tears, treatment becomes a matter of judgement. In young athletes without mechanical symptoms (i.e., locking, giving way), a period of conservative treatment and rehabilitation is warranted before exposing the child to the risk of even partial meniscectomy at an early age.

## Meniscal Repairs

Although in the mid-1800s Annandale in Edinburgh reported the first meniscal repair, and in the 1930s King[28] demonstrated in dogs the ability of peripheral tears to heal, the concept of repair of isolated meniscal tears became popular only in the last 10 years. Work on the vascular anatomy of the meniscus demonstrated that the outer 10% to 33% of the meniscus had an adequate blood supply for healing.[1, 28, 37] Some studies have indicated that the extent of vascular penetration into the body of the meniscus is even greater in skeletally immature children.[1, 8, 39] Numerous authors have documented the ability of peripheral tears to heal.[13, 20, 38] Others have reported successful repairs of anterior central detachments.[19, 42]

Peripheral tears are by far the most common reparable tears encountered in the young athlete. Peripheral tears occur most commonly in the posterior horns and more frequently in the medial meniscus than in the lateral meniscus. Meniscal tears that are considered for repair should be complete vertical tears longer than 1 cm located in the periphery of the meniscus.[11] Both acute and chronic tears can be repaired, but acute tears tend to have more favorable healing rates. Preoperative arthrography or other imaging often identifies tears suitable for repair, particularly for the medial meniscus. With acute tears, our current philosophy is to repair all reparable tears if other surgical procedures are to be performed (i.e., ACL repair or reconstruction); if no other surgery is planned, a trial of 4 to 6 weeks of immobilization followed by protected rehabilitation can be entertained, since spontaneous healing of acute peripheral tears has been documented to occur. The predictability of spontaneous healing has not been delineated, however.

All meniscal tears that are going to be repaired should have arthroscopic examination prior to suturing. The extent of the tears should be ascertained with certainty and precision. The menisci should be thoroughly probed and subjected to varus and valgus stress during the arthroscopic exam; posterior visualization through the intercondylar notch is almost always required to define the extent of posterior tears of the medial meniscus. Meniscal tears that are definitely suitable for repair are vertical, longitudinal tears within the vascular zone that are greater than 1 cm in length and have a meniscus body of good quality. Repeat tears that meet these criteria can be successfully repaired also. Meniscal tears with the aforementioned characteristics but with questionable vascularity can also be considered for repair.

An in vivo assessment of vascularity can be performed arthroscopically. By avoiding tourniquet inflation, bleeding at the tear can be assessed. The presence of bleeding from the torn meniscal tissue ensures adequate vascularity for repair. Lack of observable bleeding does not exclude vascularity; the pressure of the irrigating fluid can shut down the meniscal capillary circulation. When no bleeding is observed, a decision regarding vascularity must be made based upon the location of the tear. Tears less than 3 mm from the menisco-synovial junction can be considered vascular; tears over 5 mm from this point are considered to be in the avascular portion of the meniscus. Tears 3 to 5 mm from the menisco-synovial junction have questionable vascularity. In skeletally immature patients, tears in this region are more likely to be within the vascular zone. If the surgeon elects to repair a tear in an area of questionable vascularity, healing enhancement techniques should be utilized. We routinely perform synovial and meniscal rim abrasions to stimulate a vascular healing response. Arnoczky et al[2] have recently reported that fibrin clot helps enhance healing of meniscal lesions in the avascular zone in dogs. However, the human applications of fibrin clot enhancement are not currently known. Radial tears near the anterior or posterior osseous attachments, and acute, complete radial tears in the middle one third also can be considered for repair, but these are of questionable suitability. Scott et al[38] documented poor healing rates in double longitudinal tears.

Reparable meniscal tears within 2 mm of the menisco-synovial junction can be repaired by either arthroscopic or open techniques. Although some physicians prefer arthrosocpic repair of these menisci,[38] we favor an open procedure. This provides direct exposure of the torn meniscal edges and allows careful freshening of the torn surfaces. Freshening of these surfaces enhances the vascularity of the tear and, we believe, promotes healing. Vertically oriented mattress sutures are then carefully placed to achieve an accurate and anatomic repair without perforating the intact body of the meniscus. The details of the procedure are well described elsewhere.[11, 13] In addition, the risk of neurovascular injury is diminished by utilizing the open technique.

We use arthroscopic techniques in tears more than 2 mm central to the menisco-synovial junction because open repair is either technically more difficult or impossible at this site. Our personal preference is to repair posterior horn tears using an inside-out technique, but we find an outside-in technique to be easier to carry out in anterior horn tears. Middle third horn tears can be repaired using either technique. When repairing posterior horn tears, the surgeon should always use a posterior incision and retract and protect the neurovascular structures to avoid injury. In younger children with greater likelihood of vascularity in more central tears, arthroscopic repair techniques have greater applicability. Arthroscopic repair is also required in oblique tears and in radial tears that are judged to be suitable for repair.

Both Stone[42] and Goletz and Clancy[19] have reported on tears of the anterior horn of the medial meniscus from its osseous attachment repaired by an open technique. In our experience these have been rare lesions. The clinical presentation is different from other meniscal tears; pain occurs with full extension at the anterior medial joint line. Examination elicits joint line tenderness along the medial aspect of the patellar tendon. Arthroscopy demonstrates increased mobility of the anterior horn with probing, with full extension, or with valgus stress. These tears are repaired via a standard anterior medial arthrotomy; sutures are placed through the perimeniscal tissues or through drill holes in the tibia (as described by Stone).

Our rehabilitation protocol following meniscal repair is based upon two fundamental principles. First, a period of early protection is required to maximize the healing response. Second, maturation of the healing response is necessary before subjecting the repair to significant stresses. Postoperatively, the patient's knee is immobilized at 45 degrees for 2 weeks, followed by gradual protected motion and weight bearing over the next 4 weeks. More vigorous motion and progressive resistance exercises are then initiated 6 weeks following surgery. Crutches are discarded when the patient can lift 15 pounds with the quadriceps muscles, which usually occurs at around the seventh postoperative week. A controlled running program (jogging to half speed) and cycling is then allowed during the 3 to 6 months postoperative period. Hard running and agility activities are delayed until after 6 months. The athlete can usually return to competition by

6 to 8 months after operation. If a ligament repair or reconstruction has been carried out, we follow our standard protocol for those procedures, which satisfactorily protects the meniscus repair also.

The results of meniscal repairs have been quite gratifying, especially when compared to the long-term results of meniscectomies. Some authors have noted greater success of healing in lateral meniscal repairs. Acute tears also tend to heal more frequently than chronic tears. Hamberg et al[20] reported a 16% repeat tear rate using an open repair, but half of the repeat tears occurred in sites distant to the repair. All of the patients with clinically good results who consented to second-look arthroscopies demonstrated healing tears. However, most of these patients were adults with an average age of 27 years. Scott et al[38] reported on 178 arthroscopic repairs followed for an average of 2 years. Sixty-two percent had healed completely by arthrographic or arthroscopic criteria, 16% had healed incompletely, and 21% had failed to heal. Sixty-eight meniscal repairs were performed on patients under 19 years of age. The investigators saw no statistically increased healing rate in their pediatric population.

We have studied a group of 80 meniscal repairs for 2 to 9 years (average 5 years) in patients with an average age at repair of 21 years.[13] Our youngest patient was 12 years old. We have seen 9 repeat tears; only three were at the repair site. Six of the 9 repeat tears were in 16 ACL-deficient knees that were not stabilized. Only 2 of 38 tears in ACL reconstructed knees have had repeat tears, which matches the re-tear rate in patients with normal anterior cruciate ligaments. Most patients were asymptomatic; there were occasional complaints of giving way and swelling in patients with chronic ACL-deficient knees, and of mild pain and stiffness in patients with ACL reconstructions. Forty-two of 44 patients with isolated meniscal repairs had no athletic limitations. No symptoms directly referable to meniscal pathology were found. Although re-tears occur more frequently in ACL-deficient knees, we still repair menisci in highly selected cases (modest functional demands, mild to moderate laxity) without ligament reconstruction (62% of relatively unselected patients were doing well at the time of their last follow-up). In summary, we have found meniscal repair to give excellent clinical and functional results in properly selected tears in properly selected patients.

## Partial Meniscectomy

Although we favor an aggressive approach to repairing meniscal tears in young athletes, the majority of meniscal injuries do not meet the criteria for meniscal repair. Approximately 75% of the meniscal injuries we see require partial meniscectomy. Arthroscopic partial meniscectomy yields gratifying relief of symptoms and affords a much shorter rehabilitation time compared with traditional total meniscectomy.[6, 26, 31] However, arthroscopic partial meniscectomy sometimes requires great technical skill, as not all tears present the same degree of difficulty. If the surgeon is unable to perform an adequate arthroscopic partial meniscectomy, he should abandon this procedure re prep and re drape, and proceed with an open arthrotomy without hesitation. Arthroscopic instruments employed through an arthrotomy can often yield a very satisfactory partial meniscectomy. Even if partial meniscectomy is not possible, a well-done traditional meniscectomy is better than a poorly performed arthroscopic partial meniscectomy that is left that way.

The techniques of arthroscopic partial meniscectomy are well described elsewhere. Generally, a 25 or 30 degree arthroscope is employed with a video camera and monitor. A variety of instruments placed through different portals allow for cutting large portions of menisci or trimming smaller fragments. The exact technique used depends upon individual preference and experience as well as the location and extent of the tear. All unstable meniscal tissue should be excised while retaining as much peripheral rim as possible. This allows relief of symptoms, yet preserves maximal function of the meniscus. Smooth contouring of the remaining rim is recommended to help prevent re-tearing of the meniscus.

Rehabilitation after arthroscopic meniscectomy is similar to that after open meniscectomy, except that the time required is much shorter. Isometric quadriceps-setting exercises and active range of motion exercises are begun immediately. Unsupported ambulation can begin in 1 to 3 days as tolerated. Strenuous training can usually begin at 7 to 14 days and most young athletes can return to competition in 3 to 4 weeks post-surgery.

Arthroscopic meniscectomy generally produces little short-term morbidity. The theoretical advantages of partial meniscectomy have been supported by studies comparing partial to total meniscectomy with a 5- to 10-year follow-up. Tapper and Hoover[44] noted that bucket-handle tears with the peripheral rim left intact had the highest percentage of excellent results in their series. McGinty et al[31] showed much improved functional results after partial meniscectomy compared with total meniscectomy. The partial meniscectomy group also had 50% fewer post-meniscectomy radiographic changes as described by Fairbanks.[15] Cargill and Jackson,[6] and Jackson and Dandy[26] also noted less discomfort and fewer radiographic abnormalities in their patients with partial meniscectomies.

None of these studies specifically analyzed partial meniscectomies in children. Tapper and Hoover[44] did note an overall less favorable result in children in their series. Manzione et al[30] had 5 partial meniscectomies in their group of 20 children and their results were identical to their patients with total meniscectomy.

Although no firm clinical evidence supports an advantage for partial meniscectomy over complete meniscectomy in young athletes, there are theoretical advantages. Any remaining stable meniscus should provide some stability and assist with load transmission across the knee joint. Hargreaves and Seedhom[22] found that load transmission across the menisci dropped from 85% to 35% after partial medial meniscectomy and from 75% to 50% after partial lateral meniscectomy. Stress on the areas of articular contact doubled or quadrupled if the entire medial or lateral meniscus was excised. Similar findings were seen with in vivo animal experiments.[9] More biomechanical analyses and clinical studies with longer follow-up periods need to be performed, but our current approach is to perform partial meniscectomies on young athletes with unstable tears that do not meet the criteria for repair.

## Discoid Lateral Meniscus

The discoid lateral meniscus is a congenital abnormality. The incidence varies from 2% to 16% but appears to be much higher in Japanese populations.[17, 24, 41] Discoid menisci are more prone to injury. However, some can cause pain and mechanical symptoms in the absence of a tear, while others remain intact and symptom-free. Discoid lateral menisci frequently present initially during childhood. Common symptoms are pain with ordinary activities, giving way, locking, and snapping. Discoid menisci are probably the most frequent cause of meniscal symptoms in children under 10 years old.

Depending upon the location and extent of a tear in a discoid lateral meniscus, a total or subtotal meniscectomy may be required. Excellent functional results are generally obtained following complete excision,[17, 24] but early degenerative changes have been seen. Symptomatic discoid menisci that are intact or have central tears are best treated by partial meniscectomy. Techniques have been developed for arthroscopic partial meniscectomy. Hayashi et al[21] recommend leaving a 6 to 8 mm rim of meniscus to minimize the chance for subsequent tears while providing adequate tissue for meniscus function. Early results of partial excision of discoid menisci have also been excellent,[17, 21] but no long-term studies are available to compare them to total meniscectomies.

## Total Meniscectomy

We rarely perform total meniscectomy in our current practice; however, a few indications remain. The first indication is a major tear in association with a large parameniscal cyst. Open en bloc resection of the entire meniscus and the cyst is our procedure of choice. Another indication for total meniscectomy is a major disruption of all the circumferential fibers, such that the meniscus is torn into two separate pieces. A final indication may result from consideration of the particular surgeon's skill with arthroscopic techniques. It is worth emphasizing again that a well-done traditional meniscectomy is better than a poorly performed arthroscopic meniscectomy.

When performing an open traditional meniscectomy, the plane of resection should be just on the meniscus side of the menisco-synovial junction. This avoids weakening the deep capsular fibers of the collateral ligament complex. A second incision is utilized to ensure complete removal of the posterior horn of the medial meniscus without damaging the articular surfaces.[10] Postoperatively, patients are kept on crutches until they can walk without a limp. Isometric quadriceps muscle exercises are begun immediately, followed by a progressive resistance program. Usually patients return to strenuous training in 4 to 6 weeks after surgery.

Numerous studies have documented disappointing clinical and radiographic results after traditional total meniscectomy. Tapper and Hoover[44] noted that 50% of their patients had troublesome symptoms and 80% had degenerative changes on radiographs. Medlar et al[32] followed 26 children with isolated meniscectomies for 8 years and noted 46% fair and 11% poor results. They found ligament laxity, early degenerative arthritis, and symptomatic knee pain in the majority of patients. Manzione et al[30] also found unsatisfactory results in 60% of their pediatric patients with isolated meniscectomy followed for 5.5 years. Children followed after meniscectomy in Finland[45] showed 30% with intermittent pain with activity, although only 10% had degenerative changes on roentgenograms. Zaman and Leonard[47] in New Zealand had only 42% of children symptom-free 7.5 years following meniscectomy. Clearly, total meniscectomy in children is not a benign procedure. One can only anticipate further degenerative changes in younger patients as they are followed for longer periods of time.

## Conclusion

Meniscal injuries in young athletes are seen with increasing frequency during adolescence. Discoid lateral menisci frequently present in younger children. Diagnosis of meniscal tears can be difficult in children; radiographic studies and diagnostic arthroscopy should be used to obtain a precise diagnosis. In young athletes with meniscal tears we favor a selective treatment approach: stable tears are best managed conservatively; unstable tears should be repaired if possible or else treated with partial meniscectomy; and rare indications still exist for total meniscectomy by arthroscopic or open methods. By preserving as much functional meniscal tissue as possible, this selective approach should yield relief of symptoms and hopefully minimize the long-term problems seen after meniscectomy.

## References

1. Arnoczky SP, Warren RF: Microvasculature of the human meniscus. *Am J Sports Med* 1982; 10:90–95.
2. Arnoczky SP, Warren RF, Spivak JM: Meniscal repair using an exogenous fibrin clot. *J Bone Joint Surg* 1988; 70A:1209–1217.
3. Bergstron R, Gillquist J, Lysholm J, et al: Arthroscopy of the knee in children. *J Pediatr Orthop* 1984; 4:542–545.
4. Bullough PG, Munuera L, Murphy J, et al: The strength of the menisci of the knee as it relates to their fine structure. *J Bone Joint Surg* 1970; 52B:564–570.
5. Cameron HU, MacNab I: The structure of the meniscus of the human knee joint. *Clin Orthop* 1972; 89:215–219.
6. Cargill A O, Jackson JP: Bucket-handle tear of the medial meniscus. *J Bone Joint Surg* 1976; 58A:248–251.

7. Casscells SW: The place of arthroscopy in the diagnosis and treatment of internal derangements of the knee. *Clin Orthop* 1980; 151:135–142.
8. Clark CR, Ogden JA: Development of the menisci of the human knee joint. *J Bone Joint Surg* 1983; 65A:538–547.
9. Cox JS, Nye CE, Schaefer WW, et al: The degenerative effects of partial and total resection of the medial meniscus in dogs' knees. *Clin Orthop* 1975; 109:179–183.
10. DeHaven KE: The knee, in Goldstein LA, Dickerson RC (eds): *Atlas of Orthopaedic Surgery,* ed 2. St. Louis, CV Mosby, 1981, pp 405–477.
11. DeHaven KE: Injuries to the menisci of the knee, in Nicholas JA, Hershman EB (eds): *The Lower Extremity and Spine in Sports Medicine.* St. Louis, CV Mosby, 1986, pp 1119–1157.
12. DeHaven KE, Collins HR: Diagnosis of internal derangements of the knee. *J Bone Joint Surg* 1975; 57A:802–810.
13. DeHaven KE, Black KP, Griffiths JH: Open meniscus repair: Technique and two to nine year results. *Am J Sports Med,* in press.
14. Eiskjaer S, Larsen ST: Arthroscopy of the knee in children. *Acta Orthop Scand* 1987; 58:273–276.
15. Fairbanks TJ: Knee joint changes after meniscectomy. *J Bone Joint Surg* 1948; 30B:664–670.
16. Fowler PJ: Meniscal lesions in the adolescent: The role of arthroscopy in the management of adolescent knee problems, in Kennedy JC (ed): *The Injured Adolescent Knee.* Baltimore, Williams & Wilkins, 1979, 43–76.
17. Fujikawa K, Iseki F, Mikura Y: Partial resection of the discoid meniscus in the child's knee. *J Bone Joint Surg* 1981; 63B:391–395.
18. Gillies H, Seligson D: Precision in the diagnosis of meniscal lesions: A comparison of clinical evaluation, arthrography, and arthroscopy. *J Bone Joint Surg* 1979; 61A:343–346.
19. Goletz T, Clancy WG: Symptomatic dislocation of the anterior horn of the medial meniscus. Presented at the annual meeting of the American Orthopaedic Society for Sports Medicine, Big Sky, Montana, 1980.
20. Hamberg P, Gillquist J, Lysholm J: Suture of new and old peripheral meniscus tears. *J Bone Joint Surg* 1983; 65A:193–197.
21. Hayashi LK, Yamaga H, Ida K, et al: Arthroscopic meniscectomy for discoid lateral meniscus in children. *J Bone Joint Surg* 1988; 70A:1495–1499.
22. Hargreaves DJ, Seedhom BB: On the "bucket handle" tear: Partial or total meniscectomy? A quantitative study. *J Bone Joint Surg* 1979; 61B:381.
23. Huckell JR: Is meniscectomy a benign procedure? *Can J Surg* 1965; 8:254–260.
24. Ikeuchi H: Arthroscopic treatment of the discoid lateral meniscus. *Clin Orthop* 1982; 167:19–28.
25. Ireland J, Trickey EL, Stoker DJ: Arthroscopy and arthrography of the knee. *J Bond Joint Surg* 1980; 62B:3–6.
26. Jackson RW, Dandy DJ: Partial meniscectomy. *J Bone Joint Surg* 1976; 58B:142.
27. Johnson RJ, Kettelkamp DB, Clark W, et al: Factors affecting late results after meniscectomy. *J Bone Joint Surg* 1974; 56A:719–729.
28. King D: The healing of semilunar cartilages. *J Bone Joint Surg* 1936; 28:333–342.
29. Manco LG, Kavanaugh JH, Lozman J, et al: Diagnosis of meniscal tears using high-resolution computed tomography. *J Bone Joint Surg* 1987; 69A:498–502.

30. Manzione M, Pizzutillo PD, Peoples AB, et al: Meniscectomy in children: A long term follow-up study. *Am J Sports Med* 1983; 11:111–115.
31. McGinty JB, Geuss LF, Marvin RA: Partial or total meniscectomy. *J Bone Joint Surg* 1977; 59A:763–766.
32. Medlar RC, Mandiberg JJ, Lyne ED: Meniscectomies in children. *Am J Sports Med* 1980; 8:87–92.
33. Morrissy RT, Eubanks RG, Park JP, et al: Arthroscopy of the knee in children. *Clin Orthop* 1982; 162:103–107.
34. Nicholas JA, Freiberger RH, Killoran PJ: Double-contrast arthrography of the knee. *J Bone Joint Surg* 1970; 52A:203–220.
35. Polly DW, Callaghan JJ, Sikes RA, et al: The accuracy of selective magnetic resonance imaging compared with the findings of arthroscopy of the knee. *J Bone Joint Surg* 1988; 70A:192–198.
36. Saddawi ND, Hoffman BK: Tear of the attachment of a normal medial meniscus of the knee in a four-year-old child. *J Bone Joint Surg* 1970; 52A:809–811.
37. Scapinelli R: Studies on the vasculature of the human knee joint. *Acta Anat* 1968; 70:305–331.
38. Scott GA, Jolly BL, Henning CE: Combined posterior incision and arthroscopic intra-articular repair of the meniscus. *J Bone Joint Surg* 1986; 68A:847–861.
39. Shim S, Leung G: Blood supply of the knee joint. *Clin Orthop* 1986; 208:119–125.
40. Silva Jr, I, Silver DM: Tears of the meniscus as revealed by magnetic resonance imaging. *J Bone Joint Surg* 1988; 70A:199–202.
41. Smilie IS: *Injuries of the Knee Joint,* ed 4. Edinburgh, Churchill Livingstone, 1970.
42. Stone RG: Anterior central meniscus tears. Presented at the Second Congress of the International Arthroscopy Association, Kyoto, Japan, 1978.
43. Suman RK, Stother IG, Illingworth G: Diagnostic arthroscopy of the knee in children. *J Bone Joint Surg* 1984; 66B:535–537.
44. Tapper EM, Hoover NW: Late results after meniscectomy. *J Bone Joint Surg* 1969; 51A:517–526.
45. Vahvanen V, Aalto K: Meniscectomy in children. *Acta Orthop Scand* 1979; 50:791–795.
46. Weiss CB, Lundberg M, Hamberg P, et al: Non-operative treatment of meniscal tears. *J Bone Joint Surg* 1989; 71A:811-822.
47. Zaman M, Leonard MA: Meniscectomy in children: A study of fifty-nine knees. *J Bone Joint Surg* 1978; 60B:436–437.

**Part IV**

# *Rehabilitation*

Edited by
JENNIFER A. STONE, M.S., A.T.C.

# Health Care Delivery Systems for the Adolescent Athlete

## Teresa A. Hazucha, M.A., A.T.C.

Director, St. Ann's HEALTHletics, St. Ann's Hospital, Westerville, Ohio

## Donna L. Hull, M.S., A.T.C.

Head Athletic Trainer, Dublin City Schools, Dublin, Ohio

In the past 2 decades there has been a steady growth in the number of adolescents participating in interscholastic athletic programs and organized community recreational sports programs. It is now estimated that approximately one half of all male and one fourth of all female adolescents participate in some kind of organized athletic program, either at school or in community programs.[1] Nearly 6 million males and females have been estimated to participate in interscholastic athletics alone each year.[2]

Where there are athletes inevitably there will be injuries. Projections from the National Athletic Trainers' Association (NATA) Injury Surveillance Studies reveal that 23% of the nation's male and female basketball players were sidelined by injury at least once during the 1987–1988 season.[2] Thirty percent of the nation's 273,000 high school wrestlers sustained time-loss injuries which precluded their athletic participation. In football the statistics are even more dramatic. A 3-year study conducted by the NATA revealed that 36% of interscholastic football players sustained a time-loss injury during this period. Eleven percent of high school football injuries were classified as major, resulting in the player being sidelined for more than 3 weeks.[3]

These statistics lead to questions regarding what health care delivery systems are available to the adolescent and whether there are unique challenges in treating the adolescent athlete. Identifying the adolescent's pattern of health care usage, his age-appropriate needs, and the variety of health care delivery systems currently available to him will be the primary focus of the material presented in this chapter.

## Pattern of Health Care Usage

The adolescent athlete presents special challenges to the health care practitioner. The practitioner is challenged not only by the determination of age-appropriate needs and activity-appropriate care, but also by the adolescent's episodic pattern of health care. Adolescents tend to use health care services differently than do younger, school-age children who are brought in by their parents. There is little obligatory contact with health care professionals among the adolescent population, and these individuals are rarely threatened by life-endangering physical illness.[4] Adolescents rarely make time for routine preventive or health maintenance visits but seek episodic care instead.[5] Direct parental coordination in health care often is relinquished during adolescence for the young person's pursuit of independent interaction with the health care provider. The general physical wellness of this population discourages routine health interactions with a professional. Injury and illness prevention, anticipatory guidance, wellness education, and situational injury rehabilitation are services not often pursued by the adolescent as a routine aspect of health care. Blum and associates' 1988 report raises concern in its finding that adolescents have been the only population in the United States which has not experienced an improvement in health status in the past 30 years.[6]

Part of the strategy for improving health care for these young people involves individualizing approaches to particular communities or populations of adolescents, such as adolescent athletes. Athletics frequently forms the basis of the adolescent's episodic visits to health care practitioners. Interscholastic sports physicals, sports camp examinations, and sports injury care provide opportunities for medical professionals to have impact on adolescent health. Because adolescents seek health care only intermittently, health care providers must maximize their efforts during each visit to meet age-appropriate concerns and needs. Of note, encouraging the expression of adolescent concerns is a part of adolescent health care equally as important as addressing the physical needs associated with injury or illness.

## Age-Appropriate Care

Age-appropriate care can contribute significantly to the adolescent's healthy transition into adulthood. The health care needs of this age demand more than prompt physical diagnosis and systematic injury treatment. Specifically, there are three important areas of emphasis which are essential in meeting the particular needs of the adolescent athlete: injury prevention,[7-9] anticipatory guidance,[9] and rehabilitation[4, 7, 10] of injury or illness. The goal of age-appropriate care is to permit adolescents to enter adulthood free of the residual effects of childhood and adolescent trauma, and to arm them with the practical information and support necessary to make lifelong health choices as adolescents and adults.

## Prevention

The injury statistics provided by the NATA indicate that an opportunity exists to improve adolescent health by targeting the adolescent athlete population in injury prevention and risk reduction programming. Risk reduction programming instituted on the interscholastic level incorporates the evaluation of athletic facilities, instructional equipment, protective equipment, conditioning programs, coaching techniques, and school-based sports injury policies and practices. Identifying areas of high risk and working actively to eliminate or minimize them will contribute to the prevention of injury and re-injury associated with athletics.

Overuse and overtraining injury is a genre of injury entirely new to organized adolescent sports.[10] The causes of many common overuse and overtraining injuries such as tendonitis, stress fractures, and patellofemoral tracking problems must be recognized in order to intervene effectively in the injury cycle and prevent recurrence.[8] Knowledge of age-appropriate, scientifically based, and safe training techniques is invaluable to the health care provider actively involved with the treatment of adolescent sports injuries.

## Anticipatory Guidance

Through anticipatory guidance health care practitioners can be influential in fostering independence in the adolescent, educating the adolescent in responsible personal health care, and educating and guiding the adolescent in the selection of positive, health-promoting behaviors.

Part of the enthusiasm of those who work with teenagers derives from the fact that it is during adolescence that independence is established and many lifelong health behaviors are integrated. Adolescents are enthusiastic and receptive to positive educational information which will assist them in pursuing their independence. Athletics provides an ideal opportunity to guide and instruct adolescents in lifelong health behaviors related to nutrition, weight loss and gain, conditioning, stress management, substance abuse, and responsible personal health care.[4] Failing to provide adolescent athletes with professional resources in response to their enthusiastic inquiries is to forgo a "teachable moment" which could contribute to positive lifelong health choices. Health care professionals must be knowledgeable regarding both the depth and breadth of athletic health care. Referral to allied health care professionals such as exercise physiologists, athletic trainers, nutritionists, psychologists, and others can provide the breadth of information that adolescent athletes require to integrate positive lifelong health choices.

The health care professional is looked to for guidance and support by both the adolescent and his parents. Parents and adolescents require repeated reassurance and support regarding both normal adolescent developmental issues and normal injury symptomatology associated with trauma. It is during adolescence that biological, psychological, and social factors focus the young person's attention on inner states.[9] This increased self-concern leads to an increased frequency in reporting physical symptoms[11] and emotional distress.[12] Reports indicate that nearly 40% of students think about their health often, and almost 20% worry about it all the time.[9] Younger teenagers report more concerns and symptoms than do older teenagers.[9] However, between the ages of 12 and 17 years, satisfaction with body weight and physique decreases.[9] The health care provider must be careful not to allow excessive concerns to develop over innocent symptoms and normal physical development. Caring reassurance combined with the education of young people about common symptoms, symptom progression, and the normal sequence of injury resolution is an important part of adolescent health maintenance. Parental worry about the physical and mental development of the adolescent is common also.[9] The health care provider's task is to address the parent's concerns, the adolescent's concerns, and the injury situation. In many cases the adolescent patient and/or his parents are seeking education and calming reassurance rather than solely diagnosis and injury management. In injury situations, the adolescent must be assured that treatment is available and relief possible. Because of their focus on inner body states, their inexperience with injury and illness, and their inexperience with the health care system, adolescents seek reassurance and reinforcement that the injury or illness can be resolved and that they can be returned to a state of wellness. Information on the progression of symptoms and treatment and timely reevaluation both assist in diminishing patient anxiety and parental concern.

## Rehabilitation

Perhaps one of the greatest contributions the health care practitioner can make to adolescent medicine is to assist the adolescent in making a healthy transition to adulthood free of the residual effects of childhood and adolescent trauma. Health care practitioners must view themselves as adolescent advocates responding not only to the immediate injury and activity needs but also to the long-term, lifelong activity goals of the adolescent as emerging adult. Traumatic injuries and overuse/overtraining injuries to the musculoskeletal system incurred in adolescence can predispose the patient to a chronic injury cycle or a lifelong limitation in full function if rehabilitation is not pursued to resolve the injury. Rehabilitation usually receives little emphasis after a childhood injury except in severe cases.[10] However, there is a need for intervention at the time of initial musculoskeletal injury onset to avoid injury recurrence.[4] Children are at risk not only for re-injury, but also for new injuries resulting from compensatory behavior.[4] Short-term adolescent goals such as continued association with a positive peer group may be denied by failure to rehabilitate the patient to the previous state of wellness. The chronic injury recurrence cycle is disruptive to the adolescent and denies him the opportunity to achieve competence in and a positive experience from his physical endeavors.[4] At this time when health-forming behaviors are being established, the denial of a positive experience and continuous athletic participation may in fact influence the rejection of physical activity as a lifelong wellness choice. The exercise habits learned in childhood and adolescence have a major impact on subsequent adult lifestyles.[13] A full return to the state of health which was present prior to injury or trauma is an essential standard of care where possible if we are to expect adolescents to emerge as healthy, active adults. Rehabilitation is an important element in the healthy transition from adolescence to adulthood.

## Health Care Delivery Systems

There are a variety of health care delivery systems available to the adolescent athlete. However, statistical information tracking the utilization rates of medical services by the adolescent athlete is insufficient. Therefore, the information presented here will focus on identifying the variety of health care delivery systems which are available and the major characteristics of each. Information will be included on physician services and the diversity of interscholastic athlete health care services. An overview of current medical trends (including information on emergency centers, sports medicine clinics, and health maintenance organizations) which are having an effect on the delivery of health care to adolescent athletes will be presented also.

## Physician Services

Consulting with a physician is the traditional first step into the health care system. Surveys indicate that a variety of physicians and medical specialists are caring for the adolescent athlete. Physicians actively involved in adolescent sports medicine include primary care and family physicians, pediatricians, and orthopedic surgeons, to name a few.

Primary care physicians make up a significant portion of all physicians practicing sports medicine. Within the American College of Sports Medicine (ACSM), primary care physicians form the largest group within the "Medicine" section. However, it should be noted that few of these physicians practice sports medicine on a full-time basis.[15]

Historically, nonsurgical physicians have been involved in sports medicine from the beginning by virtue of their administering physical examinations and giving medical clearance for young people to participate in organized sports. Once the athlete is cleared for participation, the physician caring for the injured athlete on the athletic field or in his private office becomes of interest. An injured adolescent athlete may be seen first by his primary care or family physician. In addition, a number of injured athletes may be seen by the team physician; statistics indicate that many times the team physician is a primary care specialist.

What medical specialists are involved as team physicians for athletic programs? In a 1987 analysis of 29,000 team physicians, 23% of the physicians responding classified themselves as family practitioners.[14] In addition, 17% classified themselves as orthopaedic specialists and 13% as general practitioners.[14] General surgeons, internal medicine specialists, obstetrician/gynecologists, osteopaths, and pediatricians were other specialists responding with 4% or greater participation.

With a significant number of musculoskeletal injuries occurring in adolescent athletics it seems appropriate that a number of orthopaedic surgeons are working as team physicians. However, it appears that an even greater number are available as team consultants. The pattern appears to be one in which the primary care team physicians will refer to the orthopaedic surgeons when their specialized services are required.

It also seems appropriate for a great number of pediatricians to be involved as team physicians, for adolescent athletes and there are pediatricians serving as interscholastic team physicians. However, as noted by Luckstead, comparatively few pediatricians are actively involved in youth sports[16] despite the fact that, based on their medical expertise and anticipatory guidance, they are well suited to provide health care to adolescent athletes.

Perhaps the reason that such a significant percentage of primary care physicians are involved as team physicians is proximity. Culpepper and Niemann analyzed the health care personnel in 131 public and private secondary school athletic programs in Alabama.[17] The results of their study indicate that of the class 1A public schools (those schools with the samllest student enrollment), 60% were located more than 10 miles away from the nearest medical facility. Among the class 4A public schools (those schools with the largest student enrollment), 90% were located less than 10 miles from the nearest medical facility. In addition, only 30% of the 1A schools reported having a physician who lives in the community, compared to 90% of the 4A schools. Perhaps of greater significance though, was the fact that only 55% of all schools reported having a team physician. The primary care or family physician represented 65.8% of all team physicians and 100% of the team physicians for 1A and 2A schools.

## Characteristics and Medical Education of Team Physicians

A significant amount of material has been written about the characteristics and medical training of team physicians. However, this information becomes even more relevant when matching health care services with the age-appropriate needs of the adolescent athlete is considered.

As discussed earlier, the interscholastic team physician typically is a primary care physician interested in the community and athletics.[14] This individual works as a part-time volunteer whose training as a team physician tends to be informal. Many physicians gain experience by volunteering to assist other team physicians.[14] The time committed to an interscholastic sports program varies among physicians. Traditionally, the team physician is a "game" physician who is present at varsity football games and perhaps at select high-risk events such as wrestling, gymnastics, or ice hockey. One also may find the team physician present at high-visibility sports, such as basketball.

There appears to be variability in the team physician's level of training and expertise in adolescent medicine. In addition, at the present time sports medicine is not viewed as a medical specialty. Therefore, until recently, future team physicians did not have access to formalized sports medicine training in medical school or through their residency programs. However, primary care physicians today have the opportunity to apply to a limited number of primary care sports medicine fellowships located throughout the country.[14–18] Generally, enrollment is limited and the number of interested applicants is high. To be eligible for such a fellowship, the candidate must be board-eligible in family practice, pediatrics, or another primary care specialty. Emphasis in these programs is placed on sport-specific musculoskeletal injuries, select illnesses and their effects on athletic performance, the prevention of athletic injuries, exercise science, and nutrition. Physicians currently working with adolescent athletes frequently find themselves answering questions posed by the athlete or the athlete's parent on injury prevention, limitations and safeguards, physical conditioning, and nutrition.[1]

## Interscholastic-Based Athlete Health Care

It has been estimated that less than 10% of the nation's secondary schools provide an adequate athletic health care program.[17, 19] One factor contributing to this health care inadequacy is the lack of qualified on-site personnel.[7, 17, 19] The inadequacy becomes a significant concern when viewed in light of injury statistics which reveal that 55% to 60% of all injuries to athletes occur on site in practice sessions.[20] The qualifications of the on-site personnel providing athletic health care currently is highly variable. Personnel assuming these responsibilities range from team physicians, to certified athletic trainers, school nurses, emergency medical technicians, coaches, and adolescent student trainers.

The certified athletic trainer (ATC) is trained specifically to provide clinical athlete health care services, injury prevention and risk reduction programming, and supervision of age-appropriate, scientifically-based, safe athletics. The athletic trainer's educational background and formal training in athlete health care, exercise sciences, and health and safety supervision specifically prepares him to act as a knowledgeable health care professional in the delivery of these services. Even though these specifically trained allied health care professional exist, utilization of them by secondary schools remains low. According to statistical information provided by the NATA, there are more than 20,000 high schools in the United States, 15,000 of which sponsor football programs. At the present time, only 16% of those high schools have ATCs or other professionals with equivalent credentials on staff.[3, 21]

Statistics are not available as to the percentages of schools using non-athletic trainer health care professionals to meet athletic health care needs. Physician involvement with school sports programs was discussed earlier. Other health care professionals who are providing elements of on-site health care to the interscholastic athlete include school nurses and emergency medical technicians. The services of emergency medical technicians appear to be limited primarily to on-site medical coverage of high-risk sports contests.

Coaches are often thrust into the role of health care provider by default due to the lack of on-site, trained health care professionals. The qualifications of coaches to assume health care responsibilities are quite limited. According to the National High School Athletic Coaches Association (NHSACA), no full-scale, standardized certification system exists for coaches.[22] High school coaches by and large are not required to be formally educated in exercise science, athletics, coaching, or athlete health care. Fifteen states do require limited workshops for coaches which may include such topics as chemical and substance abuse, the psychology of coaching adolescents, and the recognition and management of athletic injuries.[22] This lack of training places coaches in the precarious position of being required to assume the comprehensive responsibilities of athlete health care without formal training.

A corollary concern to the lack of on-site qualified personnel is the lack of a systemic approach to high school athlete health care.[7, 23, 24] A systematic health care program for athletes consists of injury prevention and risk reduction programming, and age-appropriate, scientifically-based supervision of athletes. Injury recognition and management, rehabilitation, and education and counseling programming also should be included. A systematic athlete health care program is built upon a team comprised of multiple health care professionals.

## Current Medical Trends—Emergency Rooms/Centers and Urgent Care Centers

Hospital emergency rooms (ERs), free-standing emergency centers (FECs), and urgent care centers (UCCs) are all medical facilities which may be utilized by the adolescent athlete. Life-threatening illnesses and injuries sustained by an athlete generally are referred to the ER. In addition, non–life-threatening illnesses and injuries such as sprains, strains, and contusions also may be treated initially in the ER.

There is a certain degree of reassurance and convenience in the fact that ER services are available 7 days a week for 24 hours a day. The accessibility to trained medical personnel in the ER is particularly helpful for those community and school programs that lack qualified, trained medical personnel on site at athletic events. The injured athlete may find himself being transported to the ER as the first step of medical intervention.

Free-standing emergency centers (FECs) are defined as medical facilities which provide episodic emergency care 24 hours a day, 7 days a week.[25] FECs offer services similar to a hospital emergency room, but are physically separated from the hospital. UCCs are defined as medical facilities that provide episodic care for minor medical emergencies during certain hours.[25]

Accessibility and convenience are two reasons patients utilize FECs and urgent care centers. The average waiting time to be seen in such a facility is generally shorter than that of a hospital emergency room.[25] Unlike most physician's offices, appointments are not necessary; this encourages walk-in patients who perceive they need some form of medical attention. It may be the convenience factor which is most attractive to the athletic patient who is looking for immediate medical intervention. For the adolescent athlete however, concern may arise regarding the type of medical specialist treating the athlete, the continuity of care, and the establishment of rehabilitation and follow-up program which minimizes the length of time the athlete is removed from activity.

## Current Medical Trends—Sports Medicine Centers

There has been a rapid growth in the number of sports medicine centers (SMCs) throughout the country.[26] Serving as the catalyst for this growth has been the increased participation of the public in organized and informal fitness and recreational sports programs, as well as the growth of interscholastic athletics.[26, 27] With this growth in participation has come the demand for comprehensive and specialized treatment of sport-related injuries.[27, 28] Sports medicine centers have become an alternative health care delivery service for the adolescent athlete.

The exact number of adolescent athletes seen in SMCs for sport-related injuries is not known. However, in a study conducted by Esterson, 56% of 48 SMCs stated that high school athletes comprise the majority of their patients.[27] In a study by Kegerreis and colleagues,[28] high school athletes were ranked as the second largest client population to utilize the surveyed SMCs. A similar finding was noted in a study by Weidner.[26] These studies imply that a significant number of adolescent athletes are receiving health care services in SMCs. Services commonly offered by these facilities include the diagnosis, treatment evaluation, and rehabilitation of injuries.[27] Additional services such as fitness evaluations, exercise prescriptions, and lifestyle counseling also may be available.[26]

A variety of physicians and allied health care professionals provide these services at the SMCs. Physicians commonly affiliated with SMCs include orthopedists, cardiologists, family physicians, osteopaths, and podiatrists.[14, 26, 28] Allied health care professionals such physical therapists, physical therapists who are also NATA-certified athletic trainers, NATA-certified athletic trainers, and exercise physiologists are employed commonly by SMCs.[26, 28] Other health care professionals who may be found working in SMCs include nurses, health educators, athletic trainers (non-certified), psychologists, and nutritionists. While this is not a comprehensive professional listing, it demonstrates the variety of medical specialists an injured athlete may come into contact with when seeking care at a SMC. The variety of medical services and personnel involved with SMCs may be explained by the fact that sports medicine is multidisciplinary and is not regarded as its own medical specialty.[26] At the present time there are no guidelines for the staffing of personnel at SMCs or for the services they provide.[29]

## Current Medical Trends—Health Maintenance Organizations and Preferred Providers

Health maintenance organizations (HMOs) and preferred provider organizations (PPOs) have become significant health care provider forces. Current estimates indicate that nearly 1 out of every 10 Americans subscribe to an HMO or PPO as their primary payor of medical services, and projections indicate that this number may rise to 33% of the population by 1995.[30]

Although there are individual differences between each HMO and PPO policy, all are designed to restrain the rising cost of health care. These organizations attempt to control health care costs by negotiating fees for service with providers, by structuring financial incentives to discourage inefficient use of hospital ancillary services, and by consolidating administrative costs. Another method of cost restriction frequently used by HMOs is to require subscribers to enter the health care system by first consulting a primary care physician. Under this system, the primray care physician has become identified as the "gatekeeper" to the entrance and referral system of health care.[31]

The potential impact of these alternative health care delivery systems on the adolescent athlete is significant. It would be advisable for team physicians and health care professionals working with adolescent athletes to note the rising number of athletes who are insured by an HMO or PPO. All medical personnel need to be concerned with the timeliness of appropriate medical intervention and continuity of care for the adolescent athlete. In order to provide continuity of care, it is important for the team physician to develop a positive working relationship with the primary care physicians in the community.[1, 7] It appears it also will be important for team physicians to develop a positive working relationship with the primary care physicians who are actively practicing in the community's HMOs and PPOs. However, the impact of HMOs and PPOs will be felt not only by the team physician, but by all medical personnel providing health care for the adolescent athlete. They all will need to understand the timing of referral systems and the avenues of access to medical specialists such as orthopaedic surgeons and physical therapists.

One potential area of concern, however, centers around the experience of HMO and PPO practitioners in treating sports medicine–related injuries. Another area of concern centers around establishing communication channels and continuity of care between the athlete's team medical personnel and the HMO or PPO medical personnel.

## Conclusion

The injured adolescent athlete presents unique challenges to the health care provider. An understanding of these challenges may be obtained by identifying the adolescent's pattern of health care usage and age-appropriate needs. The potential exists to improve the level of care of the injured athlete by recognizing this pattern of usage and matching age-appropriate needs with available health care delivery systems.

A variety of health care delivery systems are available to the adolescent athlete. However, statistical information as to the specific patterns of utilization of these systems by adolescents does not exist, and only an overview can be presented. A systematic athletic health care program for the adolescent may be enhanced by maximizing the available health care delivery systems and striving to build a multidisciplinary health care team.

## References

1. Shaffer TE: The physician's role in sports medicine. *J Adolesc Health Care* 1983; 3:227–230.
2. National Athletic Trainers' Association (NATA): Study shows 23 percent of high school basketball players injured this year (press release). Dallas, Texas 1988.
3. National Athletic Trainers' Association (NATA): 3-year study finds "major injuries" up to 20 percent in high school football (press release). Dallas, Texas, 1989.
4. Smith NJ: Some health care needs of young athletes. *Adv Pediatr* 1981; 28:187–228.
5. Schicher A, Beck A: School-based follow-up care for sports physicians. *J Sch Health* 1988; 58:200–202.
6. Blum RW: Preparticipation evaluation of the adolescent athlete. *Adolesc Athlete* 1985; 78:52–69.
7. Zlotsky NA: Secondary school sportsmedicine. *Conn Med* 1981; 45:625–627.
8. Micheli LJ: Overuse injuries in children's sports: The growth factor. *Orthop Clin North Am* 1983; 14:337–360.
9. Orr D: Adolescence, stress, and psychomotor issues. *J Adolesc Health Care* 1986; 7:97S–108S.
10. Micheli LJ: Pediatric and adolescent sports injuries: Recent trends. *Exerc Sport Sci Rev* 1986; 14:359–374.
11. Pennebaker JW: *The Psychology of Physical Symptoms.* New York, Springer–Verlag, 1982.
12. Carver C: A cybernetic model of self attention process. *J Prev Soc Psychol* 1978; 37:1251–1281.
13. McKeag DB: Adolescents and exercise. *J Adolesc Health Care* 1986; 7:1215–1295.
14. Samples P: The team physician: No official job description. *Phys Sportsmed* 1988; 16:169–175.
15. Howe WB, McKeag DB: Primary care sports medicine: A part-timer's perspective. *Phys Sportsmed* 1988; 16:103–114.
16. Luckstead EF: Pediatric team physicians. *Pediatrics* 1986; 78:941–942.
17. Culpepper ML, Neimann KM: Professional personnel in health care among secondary school athletes in Alabama. *South Med J* 1987; 80:336–338.
18. Strauss RH: Sports medicine training heads in the right direction. *Phys Sportsmed* 1987; 15:47.
19. Stopica C, Kaiser D: Certified athletic trainers in our secondary schools: The need and the solution. *Athletic Training* 1988; 23:322–324.

20. National Athletic Trainers' Association (NATA): Facts on sports-related injuries in boys and girls high school basketball (press release). Dallas, Texas 1988.
21. National Athletic Trainers' Association (NATA): NATA News. 1989; 1:10.
22. Zakariya SD: Before the new season kicks off, get a game plan to cut sports injuries. Am Sch Board J 1988; 7:23–26.
23. Rice SG, Schlotfeldt JD, Foley WE: The athletic health care and training program. West J Med 1985; 142:352–357.
24. National Athletic Trainers' Association (NATA): NATA News. 1989; 1:10.
25. Gilman TA, Bucco CK: Alternative delivery systems: An overview. Top Health Care Financ 1987; 13:1–7.
26. Weidner TG: Sports medicine centers: Aspects of their operations and approaches to sports medicine care. Athletic Training 1988; 23:22–26.
27. Esterson PS: Sports medicine centers in the United States: The personnel, patients, and services. J Orthop Sports Phys Ther 1980; 1:222–225.
28. Kegerreis S, Malone T, Greenwald L, et al: Survey of scholastic athletic health care and sports medicine clinics. J Orthop Sports Phys Ther 1983; 5:78–81.
29. Hage P: Sports medicine clinics: Are guidelines necessary? Phys Sportsmed 1982; 10:165–177.
30. Lee KE, Lee KJ: HMOs and PPOs: Pointers and pitfalls Conn Med 1985; 50:753–757.
31. Taggart MP, Wartman SA, Wessen AF: Communication influences on the choice of primary care. Med Care 1987; 25:671–674.

# Unique Factors in Rehabilitating the Young Athlete

## Julie Ann Moyer, Ed.D.

Adjunct Professor, University of Delaware, Newark, Delaware; Adjunct Professor and Athletic Trainer, Delaware Technical and Community College, Wilmington, Delaware; Clinical Assistant Professor, Thomas Jefferson University, Philadelphia, Pennsylvania; Director, Pike Creek Sports Medicine, Physical Therapy, Wilmington, Delaware

Children are not just little adults. Young athletes have many biological and psychosocial differences as compared to older athletes, and consequently they require specific rehabilitation modifications when injured. Because of physical skill and psychological immaturity, young athletes (1) are prone to injuries; (2) require special goal-setting considerations; (3) need specific equipment and protective padding modifications; and (4) require exercise and modalitic treatment modifications, as compared to the athletic adult (Table 1).

---

**TABLE 1.**
**Factors Which May Contribute to Increased Injuries in Children**

1. Children are becoming taller, heavier, and less fit.
2. Children are less emotionally and structurally mature and stable as compared to adults.
3. Improper coaching skills.
4. Inappropriate equipment, playing facility, and officiating.
5. Some children are overtrained; their training program is often structured in the same manner as an adult's program.
6. Children have decreased muscle strength, decreased cardiac output, and decreased skeletal maturity as compared to an adult.
7. Children often compete against other children of the same age regardless of the opposing child's size.
8. Children are physiologically more stressed by excessively hot and cold temperatures.

---

# General Rehabilitation Considerations

## Rehabilitation Goals in Sports Medicine

Goal setting is an essential component of all rehabilitation programs. Goals, established after a comprehensive initial evaluation and subsequent re-evaluations, help direct the youth's treatment management program. The two primary rehabilitation goals in prepubescent sports medicine are the prevention of injuries and the return of an injured athlete to his previous level of competition as safely and quickly as possible.

The number one goal in youth sports medicine is the prevention of injuries. This is best achieved by (1) proper in-season and off-season conditioning; (2) a pre-participation physical examination; (3) good nutrition and diet; (4) education of the athlete, parents, and coaches to the various aspects associated with the prevention, treatment, and rehabilitation of sports injuries (including proper coaching techniques); and (5) the assurance of a safe playing environment and equipment.

The second goal of youth sports rehabilitation, the quick and safe return of an athlete to play, can be achieved by adhering to four rehabilitation principles: (1) rehabilitation must be adapted to the individualized needs of the athlete; (2) rehabilitation should not aggravate the disorder; (3) the therapy program should be performed in orderly, progressive steps; and (4) rehabilitation should be well-rounded. Also, the exercise program should be changed periodically to avoid boredom. The uninjured parts of the body should continue to be exercised in order to reduce further injury when the athlete returns to his sport. The children should be actively involved in a home program with their parents or coach. And, realistic goals should be set with the youth, allowing for constant re-evaluation and respective goal modification.

Another factor that must be considered in goal setting is the mental and emotional maturity of the child. Injury may produce a wide variety of psychosocial reactions. Both child and adult athletes will vary in terms of injury denial, depression, cooperation, pain tolerance, motivation, anger, guilt, fear, and the ability to adjust to injury. The final rehabilitative goal that must be achieved before the youth is able to return to the sports environment is the passing of a functional test. It is therefore essential that the health care practitioner work closely with the parents and coach when rehabilitating an injured youth.

## Musculoskeletal Differences

An apparent biological difference between prepubescent and postpubescent children involves the musculoskeletal system. Prepubescent children are less structurally mature and stable as compared to adults.[47] Prepubescent children have decreased muscular strength, and are becoming taller, heavier, and less fit.[20] Because of this growth, children must make mechanical adjustments to compensate for increased moments of inertia.[16a]

Because a child's ligamentous structure is up to three times stronger than the skeletal and cartilagenous structures, there are fewer ligamentous and more boney injuries in prepubescent children.[25] A boney injury of major concern in youth is injury to the epiphysis. Approximately 10% of all skeletal injuries in children occur at the epiphysis, but only about 5% of epiphyseal injuries inhibit proper skeletal growth.[30] Approximately 50% of all injuries to long bones in childhood are at the epiphyseal plate.[18] Besides direct trauma, boney damage can also be caused by recurrent overloading of the growth plate by high-intensity, repetitive overtraining.[36, 47]

## Equipment and Protective Padding

Equipment and protective padding must be modified to the anatomical size, skill level, strength capacity, emotional maturity, and psychological understanding of the young athlete. On strengthening equipment, the lever arm length, seat depth, and starting resistance must be adapted for the child. In order to prevent injury, regular sports equipment such as baseball bats, mouth protectors, shoulder pads, shoes, and field hockey sticks must also be adapted to the individual size and needs of the child.

## Summary of General Rehabilitation Considerations

1. Goal setting is an essential component of all rehabilitation programs.
2. The two primary goals in youth sports medicine are the prevention of injuries and the safe return of the athlete to play as quickly as possible.
3. A functional test must be passed before an athlete can return to play.
4. There are many factors which contribute to increased injuries in children including decreased fitness; decreased emotional and structural maturity; inappropriate equipment, playing facilities, and officiating; and improper coaching techniques.
5. Because a child's ligamentous structure is up to three times stronger than the skeletal and cartilagenous structures, there are fewer ligamentous and more boney injuries in prepubescent children.
6. Ten percent of all skeletal injuries in children occur at the epiphysis, but only 5% of these injuries inhibit proper skeletal growth.
7. Fifty percent of all injuries to long bones in childhood occur at the epiphyseal plate.

## Rehabilitative Exercises and the Prepubescent Athlete

Exercise is an essential component of all rehabilitation programs, especially those for young athletes. Exercise must, however, be performed with good judgment in youth because it can increase the stress to epiphyseal plates and lead to growth disruptions. By increasing blood flow, exercise may influence epiphyseal plate closure and thus modify growth. However, if exercise is performed bilaterally and equally, any growth change associated with increased blood flow should be bilateral and should not cause a skeletal imbalance.

There are many different forms of exercise that are helpful in a youth's rehabilitation program. These exercises include isotonics, isokinetics, endurance activities, range of motion exercises, proprioceptive/balance and agility activities, and sport-specific exercises.

## Isotonics: Weight Lifting and Weight Training in Preadolescence

The American Academy of Pediatrics distinguishes weight training from weight lifting by definition. Weight training is defined as repetitive submaximal conditioning, while weight lifting involves the lifting of maximal weight for sport.[1, 22] Because weight training uses submaximal resistance and creates the positive effects of sports conditioning, the American Academy of Pediatrics, along with many other researchers, recommends properly supervised weight training for youths.[8] However, due to its high potential for causing injury, weight lifting is not advised for preadolescent youths.[1, 8]

The components of a good prepubescent weight training program should include general exercises for all major body parts and specific exercises geared toward strengthening the muscles used by the youth in his particular sport.[1] Weight training and other strengthening exercises should be only one aspect of a comprehensive youth fitness or rehabilitation program. Other aspects are (1) warm-up, (2) range of motion exercises, (3) endurance exercises, (4) proprioceptive and general balance activities, (5) coordination and agility skills, (6) sport-specific activities, and (7) warm-down. Preadolescent isotonic weight training should be performed only by emotionally responsible youths who are properly supervised by knowledgeable coaches, and who have first undergone a pre-participation physical examination.[8]

Early research suggested that prepubertal males could not produce significant strength gains during weight training due to low levels of circulating androgens.[1] However, more recent findings indicate that prepubescent males produce significantly greater strength gains in specific muscle groups as compared to pubescent and postpubescent males after participating in a structured resistive exercise program.[33] An increase in strength as high as 52% was noted in prepubertal males who received proper supervision and training performed in a slow, gradual, nonballistic manner.[40]

The following weight training program guidelines should be adhered to as part of a youth's conditioning program: (1) emphasis should be placed upon concentric, submaximal lifting throughout the full range of motion; (2) 1 to 3 sets of 6 to 15 repetitions should be performed 2 to 3 times per week; (3) lifting should be performed weight-free until proper technique is verified; and (4) after 15 repetitions are properly performed, weight may be added in 1- to 3-pound increments.[8]

## Isokinetics

Isokinetics is a form of resistive exercise in which maximal power is applied throughout the entire range of motion by accommodating resistance against a lever moving at a fixed speed. Isokinetics can be performed both eccentrically (lengthening contraction) and concentrically (shortening contraction). Although most research involving isokinetics utilizes adult subjects, concentric isokinetic human output patterns are similar between prepubertal males and adults.[46]

When exercising concentrically, isokinetic training at 180 degrees/sec until the point of 50% muscular fatigue produces an overflow of strength gains when re-tested at speeds from 60 degrees/sec to 300 degrees/sec.[42] When exercising concentrically in a traditional repetition/set format instead of a 50% muscular fatigue format, decreased torque values are found with increased speeds.[14] Fast speed isokinetic rehabilitation produces significantly greater strength increases at high, more functional speeds and causes increased cross-sectional areas of fast twitch – A fibers.[41] In contrast, no significant decreased torque values are found with increased speeds when performed eccentrically.[14]

Although it would be optimal to exercise a limb to a velocity similar to actual sports performance speeds, this is often impossible. For example, actual human maximal limb velocity during knee extension averages 900 degrees/sec to 1,105 degrees/sec, but most isokinetic rehabilitation equipment does not exceed 300 degrees/sec.[31] It is therefore suggested that when rehabilitating the prepubertal athlete isokinetically, full velocity spectrum speeds should be used when exercising concentrically, whereas only one mid-spectrum speed should be used when exercising eccentrically (except for specific modifications for specific disorders).[14, 31, 41, 46] Instead of traditional sets and repetitions, exercise should be performed to 50% muscular fatigue.[42]

## Range of Motion Exercises

Stretching is an important part of a rehabilitation program for athletes of all ages. However, special considerations must be taken during the ranging of children due to the increased stress it may produce at the skeletal attachment sites of the muscles, tendons, and ligaments. Because of this potential epiphyseal damage, injuries that occur near growth plates need to be stretched conservatively. Aggressive range of motion exercises may aggravate this area and disrupt normal growth.

## Endurance Exercises

In terms of cardiovascular fitness, children are unfit.[22] During the normal activities of daily living, children seldom achieve a heart rate of greater than 160 beats/minute.[11] After an injury, children are even less active. Therefore, it is important to have an endurance aspect of exercise at an intensity capable of producing a heart rate greater than 160 beats/minute (approximately 60% of the maximum heart rate) for 25 to 30 minutes.[11] Aerobics will also assist in decreasing the percentage of body fat. Approximately 20% of adolescent individuals are obese.[29] It is necessary to maintain or improve the youth's aerobic capabilities, maintain good body weight, and strengthen the uninvolved areas of the body while rehabilitating an injured area.

## Other Forms of Therapeutic Exercise

Other forms of therapy which are beneficial in a prepubertal rehabilitation program include, but are not limited to, postural exercises, balance exercises, mobilization, proprioceptive neuromuscular stimulation (PNF) techniques, and hydrotherapy. When an injury occurs, a secondary characteristic that often develops is abnormal postural change. All exercises should reinforce good postural tone and skeletal alignment in children. The development of proper posture in childhood may retard the development of many different disorders in adulthood. Postural changes can lead to muscular imbalances and future thoracic outlet, temporomandibular joint, and low back disorders, to name a few.

Wobble (balance) boards are essential rehabilitation equipment. Wobble boards stimulate the mechanoreceptor feedback mechanisms, thus enhancing proprioception and improving function.[4] Wobble boards are especially helpful in lower extremity and low back disorders.

Joint mobilization is a therapeutic technique in which the practitioner oscillates skeletal components of a patient's joint in an attempt to achieve normal joint space. In comparison to the adult, the young athlete may be affected more positively by mobilization or mainpulative techniques used on joints which are prone to marked degenerative changes with age, such as the sacroiliac joint.[44] However, caution again must be used due to the skeletal immaturity of a child.

Proprioceptive neuromuscular facilitation is a therapeutic technique that is primarily based upon neurophysiologic mechanisms involving the stretch reflex, and that facilitates or inhibits motor output and improves range of motion.[35] When combined with cryotherapy, PNF provides significant improvements in flexibility.[5] Because of its neuromuscular mass movement approach, PNF may be superior to a traditional weight training program at enhancing athletic performance.

Hydrotherapy, also known as swim or aqua therapy, primarily consists of exercise performed in the water. This environment is safe and unique in promoting range of motion, muscle strengthening, relaxation, and endurance. Due to the fact that the body weight is reduced by approximately 90% in shoulder-deep water, the young athlete is able to perform the exercises easier than on the traditional land environment. Except for children who fear the water, this form of physical therapy is extremely pleasing to most youths. Hydrotherapy is a fun and productive adjunct to a traditional sports rehabilitation program.

## Summary of Rehabilitation Exercises for Young Athletes

1. Exercises must be performed bilaterally and equally; they must include both the involved and uninvolved extremities.

2. The injured prepubertal athlete must maintain normal cardiovascular status through aerobic conditioning. A heart rate of at least 60% of the maximum heart rate must be sustained for 25 to 30 minutes 3 to 5 times per week during the rehabilitation or conditioning session.

3. Special consideration should be used when performing range of motion exercises and mobilization. Excessive stress may cause further damage at the boney attachment of the ligaments. Mobilization may be more effective in children than in adults, but it must be performed with caution.

4. Isokinetic concentric training should use full velocity spectrum speeds; isokinetic eccentric training requires only a single mid-spectrum speed. Exercise should be performed to 50% muscular fatigue.

5. A rehabilitation program must be comprehensive and must include a warm-up, range of motion exercises, strength and power exercises, endurance training, proprioception/balance activities, coordination and agility skills, sport-specific training, and a warm-down.

6. Isotonics should be performed submaximally, concentrically, and throughout the full available range of motion. One to 3 sets of 6 to 15 repetitions should be performed 2 to 3 times per week, with weight increases in 1- to 3-pound increments after 15 repetitions are properly performed. Intensity, range of motion, repetitions/sets, and frequency may be modified for specific disorders.

7. Proprioceptive neuromuscular facilitation (PNF) is an effective alternative to isotonics in improving strength and range of motion.

8. The stimulation of mechanoreceptor feedback mechanisms, and thus the enhancement of proprioception and function, may be activated with the use of a wobble board.

9. All youth rehabilitation programs should encourage normal postural alignment.

10. Hydrotherapy is a fun and productive adjunct to a traditional rehabilitation program.

## Therapeutic Modalities and the Prepubescent Athlete

Heat, cold, light, sound, massage, electricity, wrapping, traction, and compression devices have been used for many years to treat and rehabilitate injuries. As early as the Panhellenic games of the ancient Greek civilization, athletic trainers utilized some of these rehabilitation techniques to treat sports-related injuries.[9, 15]

Many of the modalitic approaches to the treatment and rehabilitation of sports injuries utilize energy from the electromagnetic spectrum. The primary responses of this energy are heat production and the stimulation of excitable tissue. Therapeutic modalities which utilize electric energy include ultraviolet radiation, infrared radiation, microwave diathermy, shortwave diathermy, and alternating current/direct current electrical nerve/muscle stimulators.

## Principles and Methods of Temperature Exchange

The body emits heat into the environment via conduction, convection, conversion, radiation, and evaporation.

Conduction is the exchange of heat from a warmer object to a cooler object through direct contact. An example of conductive heating is a hot pack application. Convective heating is the exchange of heat between a surface and water on air moving past that surface. For example, placing an extremity into a whirlpool with still water produces conductive heating; whereas turning on the agitator and causing the water to move constitutes convective heating.

The process by which electromagnetic energy passes into the skin and, after meeting a specific type of tissue resistance, converts the energy into heat, is known as conversion heating. This type of heating includes short-wave diathermy and microwave diathermy.

Radiation is the propagation of energy in the form of electromagnetic waves. Infrared and ultraviolet modalities emit forms of radiation in order to produce a therapeutic, photochemical response.

Heat is also emitted from the body via evaporation. Evaporation of water occurs on the skin (with and without sweating) and through the lining of the respiratory tract. Evaporation is a critical form of excess heat emission necessary during increased workloads. When the environmental temperature exceeds the skin temperature, the body activates sweat glands. Sweating is used in an attempt to cool the skin. As an individual becomes acclimatized to a hot environment, the amount of sweat produced is increased; however, children acclimatize at a much slower rate than adults and have a lower sweating capacity as compared to adults.[6]

## Temperature and Hot/Cold Application

**Cold Application.**—It is easier for a young athlete to protect himself from excessively cold temperatures than from very hot temperatures; therefore, the body's thermoregulatory system is more geared to protect overheating.[2]

When a child is exposed to cold, peripheral circulation is reduced along with decreased skin temperatures. This reduction lowers the temperature difference between the skin and the environment, thus minimizing the amount of heat lost by the body. Cold causes the skin's blood vessels to constrict. The blood is thereby displaced from the skin's superficial veins to deep veins, thus increasing the blood volume from the skin to the central circulatory system.[2, 24] Cooling of the central core is minimized by an exchange of heat between the deep veins and their neighboring arteries.[2, 24, 38]

Two other ways that a child's body protects itself from excessive cold is through natural insulation and an increased metabolic rate. Children with increased body fat are more insulated and thus are better protected against cold injury. An increased metabolic rate causes an increase in heat production, and also helps to protect the child from cold injury.

Exercising in cold water does not keep an individual warm—it actually has the opposite effect. Cold also causes decreased tissue conductance. A 15 m/sec drop in nerve conduction velocity occurs for every 10°C fall in temperature.[43]

Since a child's surface area to mass ratio is higher than an adult's, there is a greater speed of transfer and relative quantity of heat and cold exchange between the body and the environment. That is, whether hot or cold, the greater the temperature difference between the environment and the body, the greater the effect on the child.[6]

**Heat Application.**—Exposure to heat causes vasodilation in the skin, venous return from the extremities via superficial veins, increased tissue conductance, decreased splanchnic blood flow, and increased cardiac output. Under normal conditions, approximately 5% of the blood pumped by the heart travels to the skin.[2] As the temperature of the skin increases, this percentage may increase to more than 20%.[2]

Exercise, both alone and especially when combined with heat application, produces an increase in metabolic rate and an increase in bodily heat production. Children produce more metabolic heat per unit of mass than do adults. Therefore, children receiving exercise and/or heat application are more susceptible to overheating.[6]

A decrease in deep muscle blood flow also occurs, which may account for decreased strength output after heat application; however, some research suggests otherwise.[26, 28, 37] Due to conflicting data on heat/cold application and strength output, psychological factors must be considered. Research has shown that self-predicted performance has a significant influence on a subject's ability to generate isometric strength after therapeutic heat and cold applications.[26]

## Methods of Therapeutic Hot/Cold Applications

Various forms of therapeutic heating include hot packs, hot whirlpools, infrared radiation, ultraviolet radiation, shortwave diathermy, microwave diathermy, and ultrasound. Hot packs are generally stored in a hydroculator at a pre-established temperature for adult treatment ranging from 140°F to 160°F.[21] Since excessive temperatures affect children to a greater degree than adults, and because hydroculator temperatures can be regulated only slightly, hot packs should be applied with extra towels between the skin and the pack when used with children. Treatment duration should not exceed 20 minutes.

**Hot Whirlpools.**—Unlike most hydroculators, the temperature of the hot whirlpool is adjustable and can be lowered significantly for children. Hot whirlpools for an adult should never exceed 115°F for therapy for an extremity, but are usually set at 104°F. The maximum safe adult exposure to heat is 113°F for 30 minutes.[21]

For children, the whirlpool temperature for therapy of an extremity should not exceed 104°F, and should usually average 100°F, for 15 to 20 minutes. If a contrast whirlpool bath is used, the temperature of the hot whirlpool should not exceed 100°F and the temperature of the cold whirlpool should not be lower than 62°F. As with all treatment modalities, these temperature ranges may be modified for more sensitive youths. Also, all indications, contraindications, and precautions should be reviewed before using any treatment modality.

**Cold Application.**—A layer of toweling should be placed between the young athlete and the cold pack. This towel may be moistened with warm water in order to increase the rate of cold absorption and improve the initial comfort level. If a cold whirlpool or ice bath is preferred, the temperature should not be lower than 55°F, and should average 62°F. If lower body cooling is performed, the young athlete may tolerate treatment better if he "hugs" a hot pack during treatment. Cold duration and frequency should not exceed 20-minute intervals.

Chemical cold packs should be used only in emergencies when ice or cold gel packs are not available. Chemical cold packs may leak and cause chemical burns, and they do not sufficiently decrease the temperature of the area being treated.[19] Also, vapocoolant sprays should be used with extreme caution; the young athlete should never be allowed to self-apply these cold sprays. Cold compression units and other devices that circulate cold water or fluorocarbons (Freon) over the injured site may be used if the temperature does not fall below 55°F.

**Radiation.**—Two types of radiation are ultraviolet and infrared. Ultraviolet and infrared radiation are superficial forms of heating that are not used frequently in sports medicine.

Ninety-five percent of infrared energy is absorbed by human skin, with the maximum depth of penetration being 3 millimeters.[21] The intensity of the dosage is based upon the child's tolerance; that is, the temperature should be comfortable and easily tolerated by the youth. Treatment duration for an adult is usually 30 to 45 minutes, but should average 25 to 30 minutes for a child.

Ultraviolet radiation can be a very dangerous treatment modality and produces both photochemical and biological effects. Ultraviolet radiation has been found to produce good healing effects with skin conditions such as psoriasis and acne vulgaris (pubescent), but it may also produce serious negative effects such as eye damage or skin cancer. Hypersensitivity to this treatment is common with children taking photosensitizing drugs.

The intensity and duration of ultraviolet radiation is extremely variable. Any young athlete requiring such treatment must first undergo minimal erythema dose testing (the minimum ultraviolet radiation dosage required to produce, within a few hours, a slight reddening of the average white skin) in order to determine a safe initial dosage and progression plan.[21]

**Diathermy.**—Therapeutic deep heating, also known as diathermy, primarily involves shortwave diathermy, microwave diathermy, and ultrasound.[21] Shortwave diathermy and microwave diathermy utilize electrical energy in the electromagnetic spectrum, while ultrasound utilizes acoustic energy. The goal of this type of heating is to produce a sufficient rise in deep tissue temperature without heating the overlying tissues to such a degree that damage will result. Since the temperature receptors that tell the brain when too hot a temperature intensity exists are superficial, and since diathermy tries to minimize the superficial tissue temperature while heating the deeper tissues, a patient's heat tolerance cannot be used as a determinant of treatment intensity. Diathermy must therefore be used with extreme caution because it may destroy tissues even if the child does not feel a burning sensation.

Shortwave diathermy transfers its energy to deep tissues via high-frequency currents, and penetrates to a maximum depth of 3 cm. Since the skin, acting as a capacitor, experiences decreased impedances with increased frequencies, most of the energy supplied by shortwave diathermy will be dissipated to the majority of the tissue.[39] Microwave diathermy is a form of electromagnetic energy which penetrates maximally to a 5-cm depth. Microwave diathermy is rarely used in the United States. Both shortwave diathermy and microwave diathermy have a treatment time of approximately 20 minutes.

The intensity of shortwave diathermy treatment is based upon feedback from the patient; the treatment should be warm and comfortable. There is no current method to measure the quantity of high-frequency current that the treated area has received. Likewise, microwave diathermy allows the practitioner to record the intensity output of the machine, but information as to the exact distribution of energy and tissue temperature is not given by the equipment.

Ultrasound, utilizing the transmission of acoustic energy, involves more localized heating and a shorter treatment time as compared to the other diathermies. It is therefore more easily tolerated by children. Ultrasound can be combined with drugs (phonophoresis) in order to non-painfully drive medication to an injured site. Ultrasound produces both thermal and nonthermal effects, has a more reliable dosimetry system, and can include selective heating.[21, 23]

Ultrasound produces only a minimal rise in superficial tissue temperature, while penetrating to depths up to 5 centimeters.[21] The average dosage intensity ranges from 0.1 to 1.5 watts/cm$^2$. However, if the youth experiences any sensation greater than a very mild warmth, the intensity should be lowered. Time of application is generally 3 to 10 minutes per treatment field.

## Diathermy, Blood Flow, and Limb Discrepancy

Diathermies, because of their deep heating effects, can adversely affect the epiphyses of young athletes. If deep heating modalities that exhibit a superficial tissue tolerance to heat lower than boney/epiphyseal tolerance must be used, there are certain parameters the practitioner must observe. As long as the dosage is low enough not to cause superficial and soft tissue injuries such as swelling, burns, and muscle spasms,[50] and as long as the frequency of treatment is kept to a minimum,[7] then diathermy may be used with caution over the epiphyses of growing children. However, diathermy application to the epiphyseal plates of growing children is not recommended. The practitioner should attempt to avoid the application of any modality which may promote epiphyseal arrest.

Boney growth changes may actually be due to blood flow changes to the epiphysis. High, nontherapeutic doses of thermal electromagnetic radiation produce local hyperthermia and have been shown to cause a decrease in bone growth, whereas moderate doses have produced small amounts of growth.[7, 50] Some research found no boney growth changes with microwave diathermy application.[13] If thermal modalities such as hot or cold packs, whirlpools, and shortwave diathermy are utilized within the therapeutic doses over the boney growth plate of the injured extremity, it may be appropriate to apply the same treatment to the contralateral limb in order to maintain equal limb lengths.

Although research has suggested that if therapeutic doses of ultrasound are applied over the bone, no detrimental effects of growth will occur,[21] ultrasound to the epiphysis must still be used with extreme caution.

Even though ultrasound causes a high degree of reflection on the bone's surface, there still exists a high coefficient of bone tissue absorption.[23] Overdoses of ultrasound may produce pathological fractures.[21] Individuals with less than 8 centimeters of soft tissue covering the bone require a lower wattage of ultrasound energy in order to avoid pain and possible damage.[21] Since children have less soft tissue covering bones as compared to adults, and a high coefficient of ultrasound absorption, lower superficial temperatures as compared to boney temperatures (and therefore a lack of superficial tissue cueing), and a chance of pathological fractures with overdoses, ultrasound should be used with extreme discretion over the growth plates of the prepubertal athlete.

## Electrical Stimulation and Other Therapeutic Techniques

There are various alternating current and direct current electrical muscle and nerve stimulators which are used therapeutically in sports medicine. The effects of electrical stimulation include decreased pain, substitution of muscle work, decreased spasticity and muscle spasm, introduction of medication into the body (iontophoresis), retardation of atrophy, decreased adhesion formation, improved amino acid transport, increased skin adenosine triphosphate (ATP) concentrations, decreased edema, increased circulation of blood and lymph fluids, improved osteogenesis in cases of nonunion or congenital pseudoarthrosis, and accelerated wound healing.

**Iontophoresis.**—Iontophoresis is a very useful means by which to transfer therapeutic ions into the body. Both steroidal and nonsteroidal drugs may be utilized. Some beneficial ions and radical include acetate for calcium deposits, copper for sinusitis, calcium for spasmodic conditions, magnesium for muscle relaxation, and iodine for decreased scar formation.[17] Many of the documented concentrations and quantities of the medications used with iontophoresis are based upon the average adult body weight; therefore, modifications should be used when introducing these ions and radicals to children.

**Stimulation and Strength.**—Electrogalvanic stimulation, especially when combined with exercise, is capable of improving the strength of both uninjured and, particularly, injured muscles.[3, 12, 16, 45, 48] Electrogalvanic stimulation has been found to be valuable in improving the thigh circumference and quadriceps muscle strength of post-meniscectomy patients,[48] in improving the strength of uninjured abductor digiti quanti muscles,[12] and in improving the strength of uninjured quadriceps muscles.[16] However, electrical stimulation may increase isometric strength only; significant gains in isokinetic power are rare.[3]

Based upon the current literature, it is suggested that electrical stimulation to muscles can be combined with exercise to produce strength gains. Electrical stimulation should be used only when dealing with injured or weakened muscles. And, because of possible changes in bone growth with electrical stimulation, electrodes should rarely be placed over boney growth plates.

**Microcurrent Electrotherapy.**—Microcurrent electrotherapy neuromuscular stimulation (MENS) is a fairly new and controversial treatment modality different from other forms of electrotherapy in that it utilizes a low microamperage current versus a higher milliamperage current. Because of this low-level current, the athlete seldom feels any sensation. Proponents of this modality believe that MENS is more comfortable, gentle, pain relieving, and has more significant tissue healing properties as compared to other forms of electrotherapy.[34] Skeptics believe that there has not yet been enough independent research performed with MENS in order to truly determine its effectiveness. Until further research is undertaken, especially with microcurrents and boney growth plates, the use of MENS therapy with prepubescent children is not recommended.

**Interferential Therapy.**—Interferential therapy strategically crosses two medium-frequency alternating currents in order to produce a therapeutic low-frequency current of inconsistent waveform amplitude.[39] Since excitable tissue can only be stimulated at low frequencies (generally below 150 Hz), and since the low-frequency current produced by interferential stimulation usually ranges from 10 to 150 Hz, interferential therapy appears to be a very successful means of therapeutic tissue stimulation and pain relief. As with all forms of electrical stimulation, the current should be applied over boney growth plates only in medically essential situations.

**Laser Biostimulation.**—Laser biostimulation irradiates local skin areas with a low-powered laser in order to produce a variety of therapeutic effects, including wound healing.[10, 17] Although laser biostimulation was first used more than a decade ago in eastern Europe, it has been used only in limited areas in the United States since 1982. And, as of January 1989, it has been approved by the Food and Drug Administration only as an investigational device. Due to the lack of approval by the Food and Drug Administration and the lack of research on the use of this treatment in children, laser biostimulation is not recommended for use on the prepubescent athlete.

**Traction.**—There are many different types and methods of spinal traction. Traction may be performed manually, posturally, or with mechanical devices. One device that is gaining popularity is gravity lumbar traction. When dealing with youths, gravity traction involving inversion therapy (hanging upside-down) should be used prudently due to the diverse physiological effects it may produce including increased heart rate, blood pressure, and growth plate changes.

**Massage.**—Massage is the manipulation of body tissue to cause a variety of physiological responses such as muscle relaxation and sedation, improved return of blood and lymph fluids, and retardation of adhesion formation.[21] There are various massage techniques that may be employed in sports medicine, and there are several guidelines that should be followed when massaging youths: (1) minimize pain, (2) loosen tight clothing but provide proper draping, and (3) when able, combine massage with stretching. Shiatsu, a Japanese method of massage, usually combines massage and exercise in such a way as to apply gradual therapeutic pressure to the body's surface followed by gentle stretching.[27] This blending of massage and stretching is recommended for the young athlete when increased flexibility and decreased muscle fatigue are desired rehabilitation goals.

## Summary of Therapeutic Modalities

Therapeutic modalities produce a variety of physiological responses primarily involving changes in blood flow. General recommendations for the use of therapeutic modalities on prepubescent athletes include:

1. Lower intensities due to slightly increased cold temperature limits and decreased hot temperature limits.
2. Shorter treatment durations which lower the overall dosage and allow the impatient child to tolerate the length of the treatment time better.
3. More frequent checks on the child to assure a proper treatment.
4. Increased use of psychological aids such as noises and sounds from a machine.
5. The use of extreme caution when applying any treatment modality over the epiphyses of children.

## References

1. American Academy of Pediatrics: Weight training and weight lifting: Information for the pediatrician. *Phys Sportsmed* 1983; 11:157–161.
2. Astrand PO, Rodahl K: *Textbook of Work Physiology.* New York, McGraw-Hill Book Company, 1977.
3. Boutelle D, Smith B, Malone T: A strength study utilizing the electrostim 180. *J Orthop Sports Phys Ther* 1985; 7:50–53.
4. Burton AK: Trunk muscle activity induced by three sizes of wobble boards. *J Orthop Sports Phys Ther* 1986; 8:27–29.
5. Cornelius W, Jackson A: The effects of cryotherapy and pNF on hip extensor flexibiltiy. *Ath Train* 1984; 19:183–199.
6. Davidson M: Heat illness in athletes. *Ath Train* 1985; 20:96–101.

7. Doyle JR, Smart BW: Stimulation of bone growth by shortwave diathermy. *J Bone Joint Surg* 1963; 45A:15–24.
8. Duda M: Prepubescent strength training gains support. *Phys Sportsmed* 1986; 14:157–161.
9. Durant W: *The Life of Greece*. New York, Simon & Schuster, Inc, 1939.
10. Enwemeka CS: Laser biostimulation of healing wounds: Specific effects and mechanisms of action. *J Orthop Sports Phys Ther* 1988; 9:333–337.
11. Gilliam TB, MacConnie SE, Geenen DL, et al: Exercise programs for children: A way to prevent. *Phys Sportsmed* 1982; 10:96–108.
12. Goonan MR, Guerrieo GP, Weisberg J: The effects of electrical stimulation of normal abductor digiti quinti on strength. *J Orthop Sports Phys Ther* 1985; 6:343–346.
13. Granberry WM, Janes JM: The lack of effect microwave diathermy on rate of growth of bone of the growing dog. *J Bone Joint Surg* 1963; 45A:773–777.
14. Hageman PA, Gillaspie DM, Hill LD: Effects of speed and limb dominance on eccentric and concentric isokinetic testing of the knee. *J Orthop Sports Phys Ther* 1988; 10:59–65.
15. Harris HA: *Greek Athletes and Athletics*. London, Hutchinson Co, 1964.
16. Hartsell HD: Electrical muscle stimulation and isometric exercise effects on selected quadriceps parameters. *J Orthop Sports Phys Ther* 1986; 8:203–209.
16a. Jensen RK: Effect of a 12-month growth period on the body moments of inertia of children. *Med Sci Sports Exerc* 1981; 13:235–242.
17. Kahn J: Nonsteroidal iontophoresis. *Clin Manag* 1987; 7:14–15.
18. Kennedy JC: *The Injured Adolescent Knee*. Baltimore, Williams & Wilkins Co, 1979.
19. Knight KL: *Cryotherapy Theory, Technique, and Physiology*. Chattanooga, Tenn, Chattanooga Corp, 1985.
20. Kozar B, Lord RM: Overuse injury in the young athlete: Reasons for concern. *Phys Sportsmed* 1983; 11:116–122.
21. Krusen FH, Kottke FJ, Ellwood PM (eds): *Handbook of Physical Medicine and Rehabilitation*. Philadelphia, WB Saunders Co, 1971.
22. Legwole G: New verse same chorus: Children aren't fit. *Phys Sportsmed* 1983; 11:153–155.
23. Lehmann JF: Diathermy, in Krusen FH, Kottke FJ, Ellwood PM (eds): *Handbook of Physical Medicine and Rehabilitation*. Philadelphia, WB Saunders Co, 1971.
24. Luciano DS, Vander AJ, Sherman JH: *Human Function and Structure*. New York, McGraw-Hill Book Co, 1978.
25. Michel LJ: Epiphyseal fractures of the elbow in children. *Am Fam Physician* 1980; 22:107–116.
26. Moyer JA: *The Effects of Predicted Versus Actual Performance Responses on Motor Tasks With Implications to Vocational Education and Rehabilitation* (dissertation). Temple University, Philadelphia, 1986.
27. Namikoshi T: *Shiatsu and Stretching*. New York, Japan Publications Inc, 1985.
28. Grose JE: Depression of muscular fatigue curves by heat and cold. *Res Quart* 1958; 29:20.
29. Pate RR: A new definition of youth fitness. *Phys Sportsmed* 1983; 11:77–83.
30. Pappas AM: Epiphyseal injuries in sports. *Phys Sportsmed* 1983; 11;140–148.
31. Parker MG: Characteristics of skeletal muscle during rehabilitation: Quadriceps femoris. *Ath Train* 1981; 4:122–124.

32. Pediatric aspects of physical fitness, recreation, and sports: Competitive athletics for children of elementary school age. *Pediatrics* 1981; 67:927–928.
33. Pfeiffer RD, Francis RS: Effects of strength training on muscle development in prepubescent, pubescent, and postpubescent males. *Phys Sportsmed* 1986; 14:134–143.
34. Picker RI: Microcurrent therapy—harnessing the healing power of bioelectricity. Unpublished data, 1988.
35. Prentice WE, Kooima EF: The use of proprioceptive neuromuscular facilitation techniques in the rehabilitation of sports-related injury. *Ath Train* 1986; 21:26–31.
36. Rarick GL, Steefeldt V: Characteristics of the young athlete, in Thomas JR (ed): *Youth Sports Guide for Coaches and Parents.* Washington DC, AAHPER, 1976.
37. Robins AC: The effect of hot and cold shower baths upon adolescents participating in physical education classes. *Res Quart* 1942; 13:373–380.
38. Rowell LB: Human cardiovascular adjustments to exercise and thermal stress. *Physiol Rev* 1974; 54:75–78.
39. Savage B: *Interferential Therapy.* Boston, Faber & Faber, 1984.
40. Shankman GA: Strength training injuries in young athletes. *The First Aider* 1988; 57:1, 12.
41. Thomee R, Renström P, Grimby G, et al: Slow or fast isokinetic training after knee ligament surgery. *J Orthop Sports Phys Ther* 1987; 8:475–479.
42. Timm KE: Investigation of the physiologic overflow effect from speed-specific isokinetic activity. *J Orthop Sports Phys Ther* 1987; 9:106–110.
43. Vangaard L: Physiological reactions to wet-cold. *Aviat Space Environ Med* 1975; 46:33.
44. Walker JM: Age-related differences in the human sacroiliac joint: A histological study; implications for therapy. *J Orthop Sports Phys Ther* 1986; 7:325–334.
45. Walmsley RP, Letts G, Vooys J: A comparison of torque generated by knee extension with a maximal voluntary muscle contraction vis-a-vis electrical stimulation. *J Orthop Sports Phys Ther* 1984; 6:10–17.
46. Weltman A, Tippett S, Janney C, et al: Measurement of isokinetic strength in prepubertal males. *J Orthop Sports Phys Ther* 1988; 9:345–351.
47. Wilkerson J: Strength and endurance training of the youthful performer, in Strong CH, Ludwig DD (eds): *The Olympic Ideal, 776 BC to the 21st Century.* Bloomington, Proceedings of the National Olympic Academy IV, 1980.
48. Williams RA, Morrissey MC, Brewster CE: The effect of electrical stimulation on quadriceps strength and thigh circumference in meniscectomy patients. *J Orthop Sports Phys Ther* 1986; 8:143–146.
49. Winton FR, Bayliss LE: *Human Physiology.* Boston, Little, Brown & Co, 1955.
50. Wise CS, Castleman B, Watkins AC: Effect of diathermy on bone growth in the albino rat. *J Bone Joint Surg* 1949; 31A:487–500.

# USA Hockey: A Vision for the 1990s

## Keith Blase

Assistant Executive Director, Amateur Hockey Association of the United States,
Colorado Springs, Colorado

Ice hockey has experienced tremendous growth throughout the world, and in particular in the United States, during the last 15 to 20 years. Once considered a rough winter sport for men, limited primarily to those parts of the country which provided natural ice surfaces, ice hockey is now played by both men and women of all ages from coast to coast. The number of American players is estimated to be approximately 300,000 and, although participation in the United States is still concentrated in New England, Michigan, and Minnesota, few areas have been left untouched by the sport's growth.

Since the United States' Olympic gold medal victory in 1980 at Lake Placid, New York, team registration as recorded by the Amateur Hockey Association of the United States (AHAUS/USA Hockey) has grown steadily from 10,490 teams in 1980 to a record high of 14,347 teams during the 1987–1988 season. This upward trend is expected to continue.

Nearly 75% of the more than 14,000 teams registered with AHAUS are for children under the age of 17 years old. It is important to note, however, that tremendous growth is also being experienced at the adult level (age 20 years old and over).

One key factor in the growth of hockey at the amateur level has been the expansion of professional hockey. From the early 1940s until 1967, the National Hockey League (NHL) was composed of only 6 teams. In 1967–1968 the league underwent its first expansion and doubled its size to 12 teams and 2 divisions. Since then, the league has added 6 more teams through a second expansion and 3 more teams through a merger with the World Hockey Association to bring the total number of teams to 21.

Increased opportunities to play beyond the AHAUS and college programs are now providing incentive to more young athletes. The number of Americans playing professional hockey at all levels in both North America and Europe has grown to approximately 300 during the 1987–1988 season.

Another important factor influencing growth in the United States has been the increased exposure to and awareness of international and Olympic hockey. More and more of our young athletes are aspiring to represent

245

their country in world or Olympic competition in lieu of or prior to moving on to professional competition. This Olympic dream has helped to attract participants to the sport.

## Overview

Although AHAUS is the national governing body for amateur ice hockey in the United States and has jurisdiction over the club system that conducts programs for its over 14,000 registered teams, it must work cooperatively with the two other major amateur components of the sport in the United States, high schools and college/university programs.

Most of the players participating in the USA Hockey programs are between the ages of 8 and 17 years old. A high school player is typically between the ages of 14 and 17 years old. High school hockey programs are often coordinated with AHAUS activities (as registered members) while they are also governed by the National Federation of State High School Associations. The college/university programs then take over where most club and high school activities terminate.

The difficulties presented by this organizational structure are evidenced in conflicting policies, regulations, and playing rules, although a great deal of effort has been made in recent years to standardize these factors in the spirit of cooperation and for the betterment of the game.

## High School Hockey

While AHAUS has approximately 900 high school teams among its members, there is a substantial number of additional high schools that conduct varsity and/or club programs in ice hockey and do not belong to AHAUS. These non-member varsity high school programs usually come under the jurisdiction of the National Federation of State High School Associations. They are generally independent of AHAUS and have their own rules, regulations, and schedules. In places where the independent high school program co-exists with AHAUS programs, there is usually some degree of overlap.

In areas where both varsity high school and AHAUS programs exist, athletes are often forced to choose between them. This is partly because of scheduling conflicts, but also because many state high school associations have regulations prohibiting a high school athlete from playing on an outside team (i.e., Minnesota, Massachusetts, and Colorado).

Private schools with varsity and/or intramural teams also conduct significant hockey programs and sometimes exist outside both the National Federation of State High School Associations and AHAUS structures. These teams compete against each other within their own private school leagues as well as engage in supplemental competition against public schools, college junior varsity teams, or AHAUS teams.

The private schools generally have well-supported, well-run programs from the standpoint of both development and competition. Some conduct ice hockey programs for their female students as well. These schools seem to be able to integrate their competitive athletic programs into those of the proximate high school and club teams with minimal conflict. However, players from private schools are generally precluded by their educational institutions' athletic regulations from playing on an outside team during the regular hockey season.

## Colleges/Universities

U.S. colleges also conduct major programs in ice hockey. Approximately 53 National Collegiate Athletic Association (NCAA) member colleges have division I varsity ice hockey programs, in 4 major conferences: the Western Collegiate Athletic Conference (WCHA); the Central Collegiate Hockey Association (CCHA); the Hockey East (HE); and the Eastern Collegiate Athletic Conference (ECAC). Additionally, there are 72 NCAA division II–III schools with men's varsity programs and 16 National Junior College Athletic Association (NJCAA) member programs. Both the NCAA and the NJCAA conduct their own programs and are not directly affiliated with AHAUS other than in a cooperative manner, although some schools are members. Both the NCAA and the NJCAA conduct national ice hockey championships.

The U.S. college hockey program has become an increasingly important source of players for United States national teams competing in international competitions at the world tournament and Olympic levels. In 1960 there were only a few college players on the U.S. National/Olympic team that won the gold medal in Squaw Valley. However, by 1976, 19 of the 20 athletes on the American team had spent some time in the college hockey system.

Although some college programs find it difficult to loan their players periodically to United States national teams for international competition, it is becoming increasingly more common and acceptable. The importance of their participation at this level of competition to their overall development is being recognized by both coaches and administrators alike.

## The Role of the National Governing Body

### AHAUS

These letters are seen across patches, pins, and instructional manuals. They represent the Amateur Hockey Association of the United States, Inc. (now doing business as USA Hockey) which is the governing body for all amateur ice hockey in this country. As such, the stated objectives of this association are as follows:

1. To foster, develop, advance, encourage, and regulate the game of ice hockey as an amateur sport in the United States.
2. To educate and train players, coaches, officials, parents, and administrators.
3. To promote, encourage, and assist in the formation of regional, dis-

trict, affiliate, and, where appropriate, special jurisdictional amateur ice hockey associations as local governing bodies of amateur ice hockey through their affiliation with this association.

4. To affiliate with and cooperate with other national or international amateur ice hockey organizations.
5. To establish and maintain uniform tests of amateur standing and uniform playing rules for amateur ice hockey within its jurisdiction.
6. To conduct, promote, and assist in the conduct and promotion of local, district, regional, national, and international amateur hockey contests and tournaments through constituent, sanctioned, or affiliated organizations.
7. To register and sanction active amateur hockey leagues, clubs, and players in the United States.

However, these objectives represent just a small part of the AHAUS. The purpose of the association is to administrate a well-organized youth sports program for those interested in playing amateur ice hockey in this country. Its goals include educating participants, administrators, parents, coaches, officials, fans, and others in the game of ice hockey while encouraging more people to become involved in the program.

The AHAUS is divided into 11 registration districts throughout the United States. Each district has a registrar to register teams, a referee-in-chief to register officials and organize clinics, and a coaching program director to administrate an educational program for coaches.

For players, the AHAUS conducts annual regional and national championships in various age classifications, sponsors regional and national summer development camps at the United States Olympic Training Center, studies and makes recommendations for protective equipment, distributes awards, and provides an excellent insurance plan.

For coaches and officials, the AHAUS conducts clinics and produces training manuals and films through the Coaching Achievement Program and the Officiating Program. These programs can enrich the knowledge of either a coach or an official through careful study, training, and examination. The AHAUS also promotes uniformity in playing rules and their interpretations.

The AHAUS has not forgotten parents either, supplying these vital members of amateur hockey with a "Parent's Guide To Youth Hockey," which includes tips on buying equipment, the rules of the game, the role parents should play, and much more.

Another publication which keeps players, coaches, officials, and parents in touch with the AHAUS is "American Hockey," published ten times a year. As the main communication vehicle for the AHAUS, the magazine is read by over 130,000 subscribers a year.

Finally, the AHAUS acts as a clearinghouse for information to assist local organizations in finding solutions to problems at the grass roots level, and annually publishes the "Official Guide" of the AHAUS by-laws, constitution, rules and regulations, board of directors, officers, affiliate associations, and staff.

Along with these stated objectives, the board of directors also has established a "philosophy of youth hockey" which hopefully will help to guide the direction its member clubs will take in the promotion and development of the game at the grass roots level. Since more than 75% of the nearly 14,000 registered teams play in the age classifications of "7 years or under", "9 years or under", "11 years or under", "13 years or under", "15 years or under", and "17 years or under", AHAUS is attempting to emphasize the educational and recreational values of ice hockey.

The AHAUS *recommended* guidelines for youth hockey encourage a noncompetitive environment in which children and youths can learn basic hockey skills without distractions that are often associated when too great an emphasis is placed on winning. Mastering the fundamental skills and learning the fun of playing this sport are essential to the development of a lifelong interest in hockey. Programs must be conducted in a manner which accommodates the number of new players who wish to play hockey and reduces the number who become disenchanted and drop out.

These voluntary guidelines are directed toward children's programs, but they must be implemented by adults if they are to influence youths. Coaches, parents, administrators, and rink operators must all do their part to ensure that the AHAUS philosophy and its guidelines are upheld as follows:

1. For players in the age classification of "through 17 years or under", team schedules should include at least two practices for every game.

2. The recommended maximum number of games per season by age classification is (a) 15 games for "9 years or under"; (b) 20 games for "11 years or under"; (c) 30 games for "13 years or under"; (d) 35 games for "15 years or under"; and (e) 45 games for "17 years or under".

3. Youngsters through the "11 years or under" age classification should play their games at or near their program site. Travel of greater than ten miles from the program site should be limited to no more than three games per season.

4. Starting times for games by age classification should be no later than (a) 7 pm for "9 years or under" and "11 years or under"; (b) 8 pm for "13 years or under"; (c) 9 pm for "15 years or under"; and (d) 10 pm for "17 years or under".

5. Any practice session scheduled before 3 pm should be set up so that the earliest times are reserved for the older age classifications.

6. Scoring records should be de-emphasized at the age classifications of "9 years or under", "11 years or under", and "13 years or under".

7. Awards should be inexpensive and based on significant achievements. The most gratifying reward that any player can receive is the joy that comes from the skill development that contributes to team success.

8. An opportunity to practice and play under the direction of a good coach is the primary prerequisite to skill development. Players should be given ample opportunities to develop to the limit of their potential, regardless of their abilities.

9. The recruitment of players, on a widespread geographic basis, for the

establishment of youth division "elite teams," whose purpose is to win games and championships and to satisfy the self-interests of adults and organizations, is discouraged.

10. It is recommended that adult volunteers emphasize the formal education of players and deemphasize excessive competition and professionalism in the youth age classifications.

## Evolution of Ice Hockey

For purposes of discussion, the evolution of ice hockey in the United States may be broken down into four eras representing separate decades: era I (the sixties); era II (the seventies); era III (the eighties); and era IV (the nineties).

## Era I—The Sixties

This period represented one of increasing public awareness of ice hockey. More people become aware of its existence and were drawn to participation. Much of this interest and growth can surely be associated with the 1960 gold medal victory by the United States at the Olympic Games in Squaw Valley, California.

As mentioned earlier, during the latter part of this decade the National Hockey League underwent its first expansion, growing from 6 to 12 teams, and thereby exposed the game to more people.

Also during this period of time, ice rinks began to appear all over the country. They were built by private entrepreneurs as well as by municipalities. This, of course, created more opportunities for individuals to participate in the sport.

## Era II—The Seventies

The seventies were characterized by an increasing awareness of European hockey. This awareness evolved for several reasons. First, U.S. participation in world and international events increased during this decade. Second, the 1972 Super Series (Team Canada vs. Soviets) took place. Third, there was increased participation in the NHL by European players. And fourth, summer hockey programs began to become popular for all ages toward the latter part of the decade.

This era was also characterized by the beginning of an awareness that ice hockey's volunteer coaches and officials needed to be educated.

## Era III—The Eighties

The eighties have been characterized by a greater growth of support materials for the education of coaches, officials, parents, and administrators than during any other period of the game. Printed materials and videos are readily available. Coaches and players have access to a wealth of information giving them the potential to be the most knowledgeable coaches and players in the history of the game.

Available support tools currently include technical support people in each district; manuals; videos; seminars for coaches at all levels; manuals translated from materials from Czechoslovakia, Sweden, and Canada; and nutritional, fitness, and safety information.

Additionally, there has been an explosion in the effort to develop our athletes into elite level performers through development camps and programs.

The improvements resulting from this growth have been substantial. The education of our coaches has led to better practices with multiple coaches participating (team coaching concept). In turn, this has led to an improvement in the skill instruction aspect of coaching. Our coaches are doing a better job of teaching skills than ever before. At the national level, our efforts to provide opportunities for training and competition to the potential elite athlete have tripled during this decade. AHAUS currently conducts 14 programs for players between the ages of 15 and 23 years each summer.

Although there has been tremendous progress during this decade, the eighties have not been free of problems. We have identified several areas of concern which must be addressed if we are to continue to experience growth and prosperity. These are discussed as follows:

**Facilities.**—Ice rinks and facilities have closed nationwide as a result of increasing operating and insurance costs. There are very few privately owned facilities anymore; most facilities are currently owned and operated by municipal governments. This is a limiting factor in future growth.

**Cost of Participation.**—The cost of individual participation in this sport has risen as a result of upwardly spiraling costs for ice time, equipment, and insurance.

**Overemphasis on Competition.**—Competition is being stressed at too early an age, thus driving some youngsters from the game. At the beginning of the season, the children try out and then are split up into different levels. This sytem is well organized but the categories are perhaps too well defined for the youngsters who are just starting out. They are judged too quickly at a time when athletic skills vary widely amongst children who are close in age. This means of classifying is sometimes too strict, giving the children a false sense of their talents. This classification scale also separates youngsters from their friends who might be far off on some other team.

For those who practice recreational hockey, getting on the ice can be a bit of a problem. The practice times that are available are often the least desirable ones. The best times are reserved for the best teams.

The injustices get worse during the games. The stronger and better players get to play first and are almost always on the ice. The less talented players, of course, learn nothing by sitting on the bench. Participation by all team members exists in name only.

Some coaches show favoritism toward certain players because they are related or are friends of the family.

Finally, the emphasis on competition becomes truly excessive when organizers schedule tournaments during the week, thus forcing the players to miss school.

So the spirit of competition, which can be a great self-motivator, has become misunderstood, ruining what should be an experience that sharpens skills and self-confidence for each player.

**Coaches Identifying with Winning.**—Coaches at many levels have lost sight of their true objective and identify too much with winning.

For all the people who coach conscientiously, there are just as many who forget that the real reason for coaching is to be there for the players, not to flatter their own egos. When this happens, they favor the biggest, the strongest, and the most talented players. Their goal becomes winning at all costs, much to the detriment of the players.

If the coaches act this way, it is probably because they lack a more long-term vision. Winning is their only goal because other goals escape them (i.e., education, strategies, team spirit). They are criticized for not being current in hockey itself.

As for the parents, they are difficult to please. Coaches who work at the recreational level are accused of being too demanding. Those who are in charge of the elite teams are often told that they are not good enough. Unfortunately, under these circumstances, some coaches put undue emphasis on winning in order to gain a little bit of consideration.

**Overaggressiveness.**—Overaggressiveness has become a common problem which has resulted in the loss of much of the skill aspect of the game. Players are subjected to this type of pressure as early as 14 years of age.

The coaches that stress winning show quite a bit of aggressiveness themselves. This can be exhibited toward the players whom the coaches call every name in the book when they miss a pass or a goal, or fail to show enough aggressiveness in their play. As for the opponents, some coaches do not miss any chance to verbally insult them, preferably when the referee's back is turned, to give the spectators an extra treat. This humiliation of the referee gives the coach his own bit of pleasure, too.

As for the referees themselves, they are constantly being yelled at for not knowing the rules or for not enforcing them. The officials are not infallible, but what the coaches fail to realize is the disastrous effect their behavior has on the players. The coaches contribute to the development of aggressive behavior by their questionable conduct.

**Injuries.**—Injuries as a result of overaggressive behavior are on the rise. There are several contributing factors which experts often point to.

1. Increased protective equipment is being worn. Players are now wearing "a suit of armor" and they often have no fear of injury. Thus, they take stupid chances and expose themselves to possible injury.

2. Too often it is incorrectly believed that the rules of youth hockey are the same as those of professional hockey. In truth, rules are adapted to the age of the players. For example, checking is prohibited at the "11 years or under" age level. However, rules in general are insufficiently enforced, due

to ignorance or to just letting things pass in the heat of the game. For whatever reason, a serious effort must be made to correct this situation.

**Pressure.**—Ambitious parents who apply excessive pressure on their children have become increasingly prevalent.

Psychologists believe that before a child reaches puberty, his conduct already conforms to the conduct of his parents, or at least to what they have planned for him. Parents who want to make their child into "the next great hockey player" can be fairly sure of success, especially if they are an unfailing presence in the stands at every game. But in the heat of the match these ambitions too often degenerate. Parents sometimes will yell insults and hassle their child, and may also call the coach or the referee incompetent. These parents, who are not in the majority, poison the atmosphere and ruin the game for their child and for everyone.

Parents, coaches, and referees may forget that the players are too young to share their adult objectives. Winning interests the players less than the game itself, at least up to a certain age. Their desire to play is hampered by this adult behavior and they become upset. In certain areas, the competitive spirit is reduced to the domination of one player over another.

Those of us involved in the sport believe it is healthy to openly examine these issues in an effort to bring about a solution. The solutions to these problems and issues, of course, will assist us in our efforts to propel the sport of ice hockey into the 1990s.

## Into the 1990s—Challenges for the Next Decade

With the growth of ice hockey during the 1980s has come the realization that problems do exist which must be addressed. Our ability to identify these problems and successfully deal with them is the key to the future growth and development of ice hockey in the United States.

**Facilities.**—Difficulties associated with facilities range from their nonexistence to their unavailability. Most natural ice surfaces are found in the northern regions of the country for limited periods of 2 to 6 months a year. The present costs of building and maintaining an ice rink are considerable, and other activities often compete with hockey for the use of the facility, especially if it is designed as a multipurpose structure. Furthermore, preferential treatment for publicly owned facilities in terms of lower insurance rates, lower taxes, and lower utility rates makes it less desirable for private concerns to underwrite the construction and maintenance of rinks. These factors often curtail the number of ice surfaces being built and the number of months the facilities are open for use. A final critical point is the fact that there are currently only nine international-size ($100 \times 200$ feet) rinks in this country. AHAUS must encourage the building of new rink facilities around the United States, particularly those that meet the international standards. Most international-size rinks must be built in order to give the U.S. players more experience on the larger surface.

**Participation Cost.**—AHAUS must make an effort to find low-cost methods of providing opportunities for new participants to play the game. It is fast becoming known as a "rich man's sport." Obviously, many of the needs in program implementation and support are closely connected to funding. National Hockey League and United States Olympic Committee grants to AHAUS have been of great assistance. However, additional sources of funding need to be secured, possibly through expanding the number of corporate sponsorships, public sector donations, and contributions from equipment manufacturers and suppliers.

The rising cost of insurance is a major contributing factor to the rising cost of participation. With assistance from the federal government, an attempt must be made to place limits on the legal liability of amateur sports bodies. This is a problem facing all sports, not just ice hockey.

**Overemphasis on Winning.**—As the national governing body for ice hockey, AHAUS must help amateur hockey regain the perspective of serving the well-being and education of the child as a whole. It must place a new emphasis on the philosophical guidelines which have already been established by the AHAUS youth council and spread it throughout all levels of the sport.

This philosophical basis includes developing and establishing a truly recreational philosophy for those participants under the age of 13 years old, promoting excellence in those players aged 14 to 20 years old, and helping our adult volunteers to exercise responsible behavior.

Youth hockey should emphasize the needs of the participants. Children participate in sports for simple reasons. They want to have fun, make friends, and develop physical skills. Youth hockey must serve the players. Emphasis must be placed on sportsmanship, the desire to win according to the rules, and an appropriate acceptance of defeat by the loser.

Amateur hockey must become a sport which is accessible to all: children, adolescents and adults; boys and girls; good players and not-so-good players, according to each individual's abilities and desire to play.

**Player Development.**—We must convince more and more of our players to train year-round for hockey. Specifically, we must convince them to train to improve strength, quickness, flexibility, power, agility, balance, and endurance. Participation in other sports such as tennis, baseball, basketball, and soccer may also help to enhance these same qualities.

We must convince more of our coaches to better prepare their players through the use of off-ice training. Both individual and team skills and tactics may be practiced off of the ice.

During the eighties we noted an increased emphasis on and improvement in the area of skill development. Building on this improvement, we must concentrate on teaching tactics and concepts. We must teach our players to "read and react". We must emphasize the concept of "support". The importance of the four players without the puck is essential to create options. Movement should be made with a purpose, either to support or to create pressure. We must teach players to deceive opponents by doing the unexpected rather than the obvious. We need to teach players to "save their ice" so they can take passes from the proper angle while moving.

Players should utilize the triangle approach in the attacking zone. And players should regroup in the neutral zone.

Increased support for a full-time national team in the 1990s should be considered, as it would provide motivation to remain in the sport, elite competition opportunities, an ongoing training mechanism for our Olympic program, and visibility for AHAUS. To this end, funds for team preparation and international competition are particularly necessary.

**Ethical Responsibilities.**—Many amateur hockey administrators, coaches, and officials at all levels of the game have become concerned about the trends that have been creeping into the game today. Stick work and overaggressive play are on the increase and so is the number of serious injuries, specifically spinal injuries. The National Hockey League has become a dangerous role model often used by ambitious coaches and parents pushing their players to excel. Coaches seem to have lost a certain degree of respect for the game. Administrators at both the amateur and professional level of the sport must be willing to accept some of the responsibility and to work along with coaches and referees to put things back in perspective. This calls for leadership!

It is very easy to blame the referees for not calling enough infractions. Yet, the same individuals who complain about this are too often the first to complain when the referees call too many infractions and do not allow the players to "play the game."

We must work to bring integrity back into the game. Coaches, administrators, and referees together must insist on some basic limits. There are certain values that are important to the future well-being of the game, and it is up to all parties involved to play a major role in turning things around.

## Summary and Conclusion

Effective grass roots programs, coupled with the influence of professional hockey and the Olympic movement have tripled the number of Americans playing ice hockey since 1971. This rapid growth has also resulted in numerous problems which have been identified and must be addressed by the leadership of our sport if the sport is to continue to prosper and grow. We are on the threshold; we have the knowledge; we are encouraging the development of facilities; and we are increasing the number of highly skilled players.

The 1990s may become known as the "Golden Years of USA Hockey" if we all make a commitment to place a higher priority on the following concepts:

1. A total approach to player development both on and off the ice and from the young to the old.
2. A greater emphasis on performance within specifically defined values.
3. A continued commitment to educational and training programs for coaches, referees, and administrators.

4. Additional research and development in the area of injury prevention and treatment and adherence to safety measures, including rule changes, designed to keep the game safe for the participant.
5. Continued cooperation and coordination among the several organizations administering amateur hockey programs.
6. The development of more ice rinks, particularly those of international size.
7. Aggressive, dynamic, and visionary leadership.
8. And finally, a de-emphasis on winning and a re-emphasis on participation and fun.

# Index

Fatigue (cont.)
   overtraining as cause of,
     108–110
   pathogenic weight-control
     behavior as cause of, 109
   postviral fatigue syndrome as
     cause of, 105
   psychological problems as
     symptoms of, 107–108
   respiratory disorders as cause of,
     111
   sleeplessness as cause of, 110
   smokeless tobacco as cause of,
     110
   viral hepatitis as cause of, 104
   in young athletes, 101–114
   definition of, 102
   heart disorders as cause of, 112
   hyperventilation as cause of, 111
   ozone inhalation as cause of, 111
   pregnancy as cause of, 112
   seasonal allergic rhinitis as cause of,
     111
   tachyarrhythmias as cause of, 112
Federation de International de Ski,
   15
Fitness level, initial, as potential
   determinant in young athletes,
   47
Fractures
   intercondylar eminence, types of,
     181
   intra-articular, 131–132
   stress
     as chronic injury, 138
     of olecranon, 160, 161

**G**

Gender as potential determinant of
   trainability in young athletes,
   47
Grant's test, 178
Growth
   acute and chronic injury effects on,
     127–146
   as cause of chronic injury,
     137–138
   of musculoskeletal system,
     128–130
   soft tissue, 130

Growth plates
   anatomy of, 128, 129
   injury of, 131, 133
     acute, 130
     chronic, 138
Gymnastics
   elbow injury due to, 162–163
   osteochondritis dissecans due to,
     163
   osteochondrosis due to, 162
   predicting performance in, 19–20

**H**

HE (see Hockey East)
Health, psychosocial and sports, 116
Health care
   age-appropriate, 218–221
   anticipatory guidance in, 219–220
   interscholastic-based athletic,
     223–224
   rehabilitation as part of, 220–221
   usage patterns of, 217–218
Health care delivery systems for
   adolescent athletes, 217–228
   physician services in, 221–222
   pediatricians as part of, 222
   team physicians in, 222–223
Health Maintenance Organizations,
   current medical trends in, 226
Heart disease, congenital, 89, 92–94
   as cause of exercise-related sudden
     death, 112
   postoperative, 89, 94–95
Heart disorders as cause of fatigue,
   112
Heart murmurs, types of, 91
Heat in rehabilitation, 236, 237
   methods of, 237–239
Hepatitis, viral, as cause of chronic
   fatigue, 104
Heritability
   effect on elite performances,
     22–24, 26
   estimates of variables, 23
HMOs (see Health Maintenance
   Organizations)
Hockey
   ice (see Ice hockey)
   USA (see USA Hockey)
Hockey East, 247

Whirlpools, hot, in rehabilitation, 237–238
Wolff-Parkinson-White syndrome, 96, 97–98
Wrestling
 elbow injury due to, 163

predicting performance in, 18–19

**Y**

Youth (*see* Athletes, prepubescent; Athletes, young; Children; specific entries)